PLANT BREEDING FROM LABORATORIES TO FIELDS

Edited by **Sven Bode Andersen**

Plant Breeding from Laboratories to Fields
http://dx.doi.org/10.5772/3362
Edited by Sven Bode Andersen

Contributors

Maira Milani, Márcia Barreto De Medeiros Nóbrega, Halagappa Shashidhar, George Tryphone, Deogracious Protas, Luseko Chilagane, Paul Kusolwa, Susan Nchimbi-Msolla, Guo-Liang Jiang, Vladimir Zhukov, Alexey Y. Borisov, Igor Tikhonovich, Oksana Yurievna Shtark, Sudhir Shukla, Maria Carlota Vaz Patto, Pedro Mendes-Moreira, Carla Brites, Maria Bronze, Silas Pego, Mara Lisa Alves, Elsa Mecha, Genyi Li, Santelmo Vasconcelos, Sandra Brammer, Ana Christina Brasileiro-Vidal, Ana Rafaela Oliveira, Liane Balvedi Poersch, Sandra Patussi Brammer, Harsh Raman, Rosy Raman, Nicholas Larkan

Published by InTech

Janeza Trdine 9, 51000 Rijeka, Croatia

Copyright © 2013 InTech

Notice

Publishing Process Manager Ana Pantar
Technical Editor InTech DTP team
Cover InTech Design team

Additional hard copies can be obtained from orders@intechopen.com

Plant Breeding from Laboratories to Fields, Edited by Sven Bode Andersen
p. cm.
ISBN 978-953-51-1090-3

For EU product safety concerns:
IN TECH d.o.o., Prolaz Marije Krucifikse Kozulić 3, 51000 Rijeka, Croatia,
info@intechopen.com or visit our website at intechopen.com.

Meet the editor

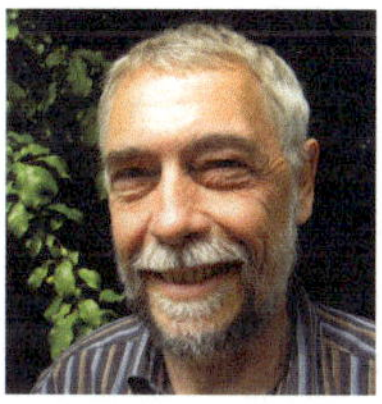

Sven Bode Andersen is a Professor of Plant Breeding at the Department of Plant and Environmental Sciences, Faculty of Science, University of Copenhagen, Denmark. He received a M.Sc. in Agronomy (Horticulture) in March 1980. In June 1983, he obtained a Ph.D. in Agronomy (Plant Breeding) with the thesis on Haploid production in plant breeding. He became the professor of Plant Breeding in May 2003. His research focuses on the following: Biotechnology for Plant Breeding, Doubled haploid systems, protoplasts, Molecular markers for Diversity analysis and genetic dissection of important traits, Quantitative trait analysis of resistance, quality and yield.

Contents

Preface

Breeding of crop plants to make them more adapted to human agricultural systems has been on-going during domestication the last 10 000 years. However, only recently with the invention of the Mendelian principles of genetics and the subsequent development of quantitative genetics during the twentieth century has such genetic crop improvement become based on a general theory. During the last 50 years plant breeding has entered a molecular era based on molecular tools to analyse DNA, RNA and proteins and associate such molecular results with plant phenotype. These marker trait associations develop fast to enable more efficient breeding. However, they still leave a major part of breeding to be performed through selection of phenotypes using quantitative genetic tools. The ten chapters of the book illustrate this development.

Genomics and Marker Assisted Breeding

Future plant breeding will move much beyond the conventional genetic barriers consisting of the species limits. Different crops derived from different species are the result of evolution, during the past thousands of years to a certain extent driven by humans. Only recently have we come to understand that our crop plants have arisen through genetic bottle necks since only a minor part of globally existing genetic diversity has been searched for agriculturally useful genes. Since crops are the result of evolution they are genetically related and well-functioning genes from one crop may be useful also in other related crops exchanged through species hybridisation, or in the case of distantly related or different types of organisms through genetic engineering.

Much understanding of relations between crop plants has been obtained through in situ hybridization techniques described in detail by Brammer et al. (Chapter 1) for the triticae family, which beautifully pictures the principles of synteny; the fact that chromosomal arrangements of genes are partially maintained over millions of years of evolution. Combined with the rapid development of new techniques of molecular genetic markers (Li et al. Chapter 2), which will efficiently detect desired alleles of a gene during breeding operations, our window of breeding, still mainly within species, may open widely during the next future to more frequently exploit new genes across traditional species barriers. It may also open up for general use of the still existing widely diversified wild crop relatives.

Such use of molecular markers for marker assisted breeding described by Jiang (Chapter 3) is based on the principles of genetic linkage, so that markers surrounding or inside a gene affecting a breeding trait, tend to be inherited together with the trait and therefore completely or partially can reveal the phenotype of the plant. With further development in the number of such molecular markers, which can be analysed for a lower prize, the use of marker assisted breeding can be expected to move from breeding of mainly simply inherited to more complex traits, comprising large numbers of quantitative trait loci (QTL) affecting different important breeding traits (genomic selection).

Until now the development of marker assisted breeding for semi-quantitative traits have developed most for the breeding of more horizontal types of disease resistance, like resistance to blackleg of rapeseed (Raman et al, Chapter 4) and horizontal resistance to several common bean diseases (Tryphone et al, Chapter 5). These chapters demonstrate well the process of dissection of conventionally quantitative traits of disease resistance into chromosomal sections (QTL) covered with genetic markers. The result is a limited number of genes or QTL with known chromosomal locations, different alleles with different effects as well names for each gene. This makes possible the planning of breeding operations to backcross or stack (pyramide) such resistance to an extent previously not possible with conventional breeding. In particular these developments in the breeding of more complex types of disease resistance may find great use to breed cultivars with more durable disease resistance than when more simply inherited sources of resistance are used.

Crop Breeding for Complex Phenotypes

Limitation in water supply is a major constraint to food production world-wide and it is expected to intensify with future climate change. Better genetic tolerance to such drought conditions, which should result in improved exploitation of available water, however, is a highly complex trait controlled by different genes for different plant development stages and with severe interactions between genes of the crop and its growing environment (Shashidhar et al, Chapter 6). This results in rather long term breeding programs the success of which highly depends on good choice of breeding material, target region of cultivation and multisite selection environment.

Most land plants have developed various types of symbiosis with microorganisms, which may have major impacts on the plant's nutrient supply. These central biological phenomena are mostly known fromlegume-rhizobium interactions (Zhukov et al, Chapter 7), but they are still used only to a limited extend to breed e.g. legume crops with higher nitrogen fixation rates. Recent molecular developments and improved understanding of the complex plant microbe interactions in such symbiosis may enable future systematic breeding for legume crops with higher nitrogen fixation to reduce the need of nitrogen fertilizer in future agriculture. Furthermore, better understanding of the principles of beneficial plant microbe interactions in the legume system may enable the breeding of other crops for improved beneficial symbiosis with microorganisms.

The chapter by Mishra et al (Chapter 8) on opium poppy is a good example of the complex breeding of an important medicinal plant. Desire of high contents of alkaloids combined with good adaptation to cultivation methods turns improvement of the crop into highly complex breeding programs, which may be simplified in the future through better understanding of the regulation of synthetic pathways.

Another example of improvement of an industrially important crop to a large extent produced by small growers on marginal land is the breeding of Castor (Ricinus communis) (Milani et al, Chapter 9). The castor oil produced from the plants feeds several different types of chemical industry, and breeding for high oil content combined with adaptation to cultivation system leads to complex breeding programs, where choice of plant material, targeted growers and type of cultivar is essential for success.

Finally the use of participatory plant breeding, where farmers growing a crop in an area are involved in breeding and maintenance of their plant material (Vaz Patto et al, Chapter 10) illustrates the potential of shared ownership among farmers for a high quality local type of maize. Particularly in times with strong concentration of breeding activities into relatively few breeding companies enforcing intellectual property rights on cultivated material this example from Portugal stands out as a means to preserve a special local production.

Sven Bode Andersen, Professor Phd
Faculty of Science,
University of Copenhagen, Danmark

Section 1

Genomics and Marker Assisted Breeding

Chapter 1

Genomic *in situ* Hybridization in Triticeae: A Methodological Approach

Sandra Patussi Brammer, Santelmo Vasconcelos,
Liane Balvedi Poersch, Ana Rafaela Oliveira and
Ana Christina Brasileiro-Vidal

Additional information is available at the end of the chapter

http://dx.doi.org/10.5772/52928

1. Introduction

In several plant groups, especially those with polyploid complexes as *Triticum* (the wheat genus, Poaceae), related species can be used as important sources of genes. In the tribe Triticeae as a whole, which comprises other important cereals as barley (*Hordeum vulgare*) and rye (*Secale cereale*), there are high rates of successful interspecific hybridization [1-2]. Due to the ease in obtaining these hybrids, plus the high amount of available information on the genomes of the species, the interspecific hybrids are potentially useful for the genetic improvement of these crops [3-4]. Thus, the hybrids and their derivatives from breeding programs can be analyzed by means of different approaches, aiming the full knowledge on the phenotypic constitution of the plant material for its subsequent utilization.

Many cytogenetic methods can be applied during the process of crop improvement, mainly regarding the characterization of chromosome types among accessions of a germplasm collection [5-6]. Since the discovery of the nucleic acid hybridization reaction by Hall & Spiegelmann [7], and later by using fluorescent detection rather than radioactive isotopes [8], the fluorescent *in situ* hybridization (FISH) and its variations have been largely employed in karyotype characterization of plants [9]. The technique basically consists on the pairing of a given probe (a DNA or RNA fragment) with a specific sequence on the target genome, aiming to indicate its exact location in a chromosome.

When the objective is to distinguish parental chromosomes (or chromosome segments) in an interspecific hybridization or the distinct genomes of an allopolyploid, the entire genome of one parent should be labeled and used as probe [10]. In this case, the technique is called genomic *in situ* hybridization (GISH). On the other hand, the genome of the second parent (unlabeled) is used as blocking DNA, aiming to avoid non-specific hybridizations due to the similarity of the two parental genomes. Thus, both parental genomes (the probe and the blocking DNA) must be used together in the same hybridization mixture. The proportion probe:blocking DNA should be adequate to avoid the detection of the second parent (see Fig. 1).

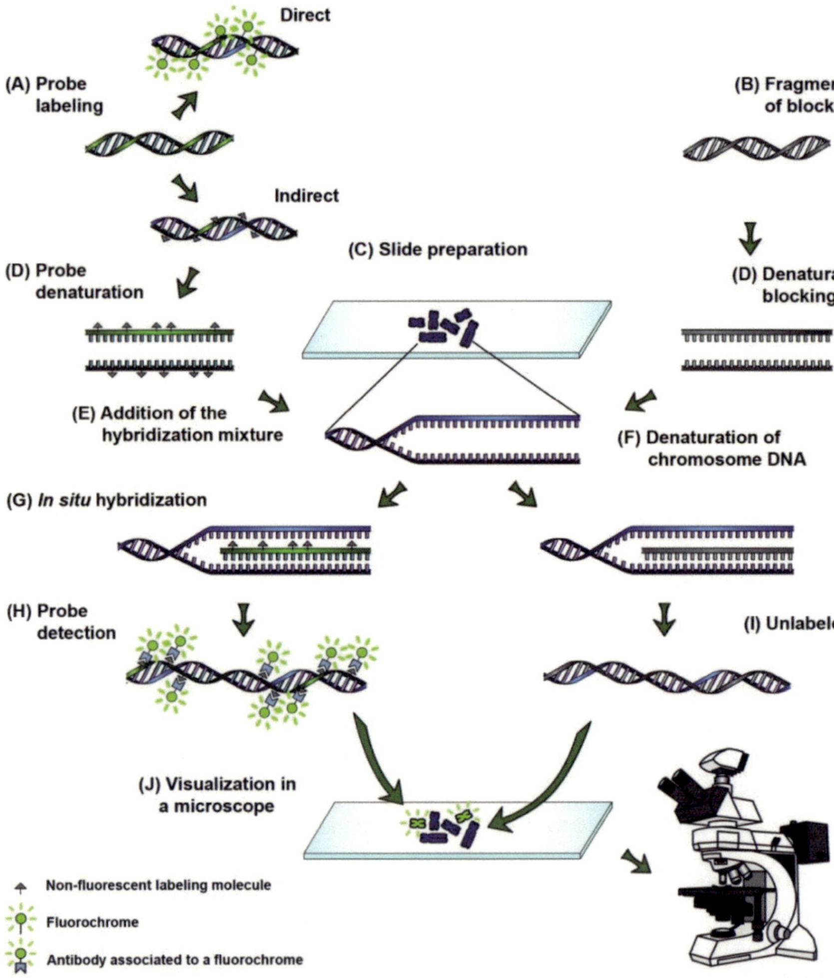

Figure 1. Main steps of the genomic *in situ* hybridization (GISH). (A) Direct and indirect probe labeling. (B) Fragmentation of the blocking DNA. (C) Slide preparation. (D) Probe and blocking DNA denaturation in a hybridization mixture. (E) Addition of the hybridization mixture with the probe and the blocking DNA. (F) Denaturation of the chromosome DNA. (G) *In situ* hybridization of probe and blocking DNA in the target sequence of the chromosome. (H) Detection of the probe in the chromosome DNA of one parent, in an indirect labeling. (I) Chromosome DNA molecule of the second parent associated to the unlabeled blocking DNA. (J) Visualization of hybridization signals associated to a probe (green) in a fluorescence microscope. Unmarked chromosomes are visualized with a counter-staining (blue). When the probe labeling is direct, the detection step of the GISH can be excluded. The fluorochromes are the signaling molecules and can be directly visualized in a fluorescence microscope with the appropriate filter. Santelmo Vasconcelos & Ana C. Brasileiro-Vidal.

The probe labeling can be either direct or indirect (Fig. 1A). In the direct labeling, the marked nucleotides are associated to fluorochromes, which can be directly visualized in a fluorescence microscope with the proper filter, after *in situ* hybridization procedures. On the other hand, in the indirect labeling, the marked nucleotides are associated to marker molecules (Fig. 1A), which cannot be visualized in microscopes. Thus, after *in situ* hybridization procedures, the labeled probes are recognized by antibodies conjugated to fluorochromes, allowing for the probe detection and visualization (Fig. 1J).

The GISH has direct applications on the understanding of the genome evolution of polyploid hybrids, partial allopolyploids and recombinant inbred lines, as well as in detecting the amount of introgressed chromatin during the production of new lineages [11-13]. Therefore, the GISH has efficiently contributed for the analysis on the karyotypic stability of plant materials, indicating the best genotypes, and helping the assisted selection in different phases of crop improvement [9, 14].

Here we describe and discuss the main methodological steps of the GISH process as well as the importance of such an approach for the establishment of successful inbred lines, using as example hybrids between common wheat (*T. aestivum*, $2n = 6x = 42$, AABBDD genome) and rye (*S. cereale*, $2n = 2x = 14$, RR genome), hexaploid ($2n = 6x = 42$, AABBRR genome) and octoploid ($2n = 8x = 56$, AABBDDRR genomes) triticale lines and their derivatives. For this analysis, genomic DNA from rye was used as probe and wheat genomic DNA was used as blocking agent in a proportion of 1:10 (probe:blocking agent). Variations of the technique for other Triticeae species will also be discussed.

2. DNA isolation (probe and blocking DNA)

In a GISH, isolating the genomic DNA of the plant materials is the first step for producing the probe and the blocking DNA, being a critical procedure due to the necessity of obtaining DNA as intact as possible and free of contaminants (such as polysaccharides). For plant materials, the DNA isolation can be affected by several factors, such as the procedures for collecting and storing the plant tissue as well as the method for DNA isolation itself. The leaf tissue is the most common to be used for DNA extraction. However, tissues from other parts, as seeds, roots and cultivated cells in suspension, can also be employed.

2.1. CTAB method from Embrapa Wheat, according to Bonato [15]

1. Weigh approximately 300 mg of leaf tissue and put in a 1.5 mL centrifuge tube.
2. Macerate carefully in liquid nitrogen, avoiding defrosting the tissue.
3. Add 700 µL of preheated (65 °C) isolation buffer [2% CTAB, 100 mM Tris-HCl (pH 8.0), 20 mM EDTA (pH 8.0) and 1.4 M NaCl] and mix well.
4. Incubate the samples for 60 min at 65 °C in a water bath. Mix gently every 10 min.
5. Remove from the water bath and let cool to room temperature (ca. 24 °C) for 5 min.

6. Add 700 μL of CIAA (chloroform:isoamyl alcohol, 24:1, v/v). Mix gently for 10 min.
7. Centrifuge for 7 min (10,000 rpm, room temperature).
8. Transfer the supernatant to new centrifuge tubes and add again 700 μL of CIAA. Mix gently for 10 min.
9. Centrifuge for 7 min (10,000 rpm, room temperature).
10. Transfer the supernatant to new centrifuge tubes and add 500 μL of cold (-20 °C) isopropanol, mix gently to precipitate the DNA and incubate for, at least, 30 min at -20 °C.
11. Centrifuge for 5 min (10,000 rpm, room temperature).
12. Discard the supernatant carefully in order to not lose the pellet.
13. Wash the pellet with 600 μL of cold 70% ethanol. Discard the 70% ethanol.
14. Wash the pellet with 600 μL of cold 96% ethanol. Discard the 96% ethanol and dry the pellet at room temperature.
15. Re-suspend the pellet in 100 μL of 10 mM Tris-HCl (pH 8.0) or ultrapure distilled water.
16. Add 3 μL of 10 mg/mL RNase A, mix and incubate for 1 h at 37 °C.
17. Store samples at -20 °C or -80 °C. For long term conservation, the best results are obtained when pelleted materials are stored in 70% ethanol.

2.2. Selective precipitation of polysaccharides, according to Michaels et al. [16]

1. Add 500 μL of the precipitation solution [10 mM Tris-HCl (pH 8.0) and 250 mM NaCl].
2. Dissolve the pellet by vortexing. The complete dissolution of the pellet is important to not lose DNA. Samples with much polysaccharide contamination tend to dissolve more slowly.
3. Add 180 μL of cold absolute ethanol. Mix the solution by vortexing and put immediately in chopped ice.
4. Put in the refrigerator (10 °C) for 20 min or in the freezer (-20 °C) overnight.
5. Centrifuge for 20 min (10,400 rpm, 4 °C).
6. Transfer the aqueous phase to a new tube. In this step, the DNA is in the aqueous phase and the pellet may be discarded.
7. Add 700 μL of isopropanol and mix gently, inverting the tubes approximately 50 times. Leave the tubes for 15 min at room temperature.
8. Centrifuge for 20 min (10,400 rpm, 4 °C).
9. Discard the supernatant and dry the pellet at room temperature.
10. Add 500 μL of 70% cold ethanol and invert the tube approximately 20 times.

11. Centrifuge for 20 min (10,400 rpm, 4 °C).

12. Discard the supernatant and dry the pellet at room temperature.

13. Re-suspend the pellet in 100 μL of 10 mM Tris-HCl (pH 8.0) or ultrapure distilled water.

3. DNA quantification

After the isolation procedures, the resultant DNA must be quantified prior to probe labeling and preparation of the blocking DNA. Thus, an electrophoresis in agarose gel (0.8%) with an aliquot of each isolated DNA should be performed, using λ-DNA as reference with different amounts (e.g. 50 ng, 100 ng and 150 ng). After the electrophoretic run, a comparison between reference bands and bands of the isolated DNA can be made. In the sample of the rye DNA (Fig. 2A, sample 2), for instance, it is suggested that the band of the sample presents the same fluorescence intensity of the 100 ng reference λ-DNA. Thus, as 1 μL of the rye DNA was loaded in the gel, then concentration of the isolated rye DNA is 100 ng/μL. For the wheat DNA (Fig. 2A sample 1), the band is also similar to the 100 ng reference λ-DNA. However, in this case, only 0.5 μL of the sample where loaded in the gel. Thus, the concentration of the isolated wheat DNA is 200 ng/μL.

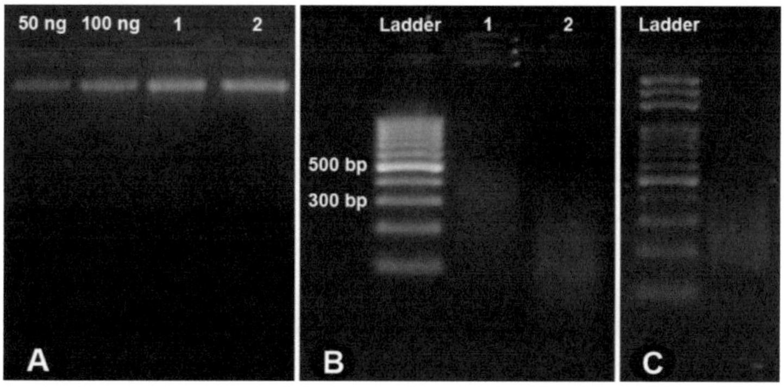

Figure 2. Analysis of genomic DNA by electrophorese in 0.8% agarose. (A) Quantification of genomic DNA of wheat (sample 1; 0.5 μL of DNA) and rye (B; sample 2; 1 μL of DNA). The two first bands are the weight markers with 50 ng and 100 ng (1 μL). (B) Verification of the fragmentation of wheat DNA, which will be used as blocking DNA, by autoclaving and (C) rye DNA after labeling by nick translation. The 100 bp DNA ladder was used as marker. Sandra P. Brammer.

4. Fragmentation of the blocking DNA

In general, the species involved in the production of hybrids are closely related. Therefore, when a GISH is performed with the genomic DNA of one parental species, a non-specific hybridization often happens in chromosomes derived from the second parental species, mainly due to the presence of repetitive DNA that are common between the two parents. In order to avoid this non-specific hybridization, the unlabeled genomic DNA of the second parent should be used in the *in situ* hybridization. As the probe, the blocking DNA should be approximately 300 bp long, or even shorter (50-300 bp) (Fig. 2B, sample 2). In the specific case of the blocking DNA, the exact amount of DNA of the sample has to be known. Considering the total value of the wheat DNA sample as 100 μL, 99.5 μL still remain after the quantification (100 ng/μL). It is important to remember that the DNA should be quantified (total amount in ng or μg) prior to its fragmentation in autoclave (as explained below), in boiling water, in sonicator or by nick translation (without the marked nucleotides). The DNA fragmentation in autoclave can be made as follows:

1. Prepare an aliquot containing 5-50 μg of the previously quantified DNA in 100 μL (diluted in ultrapure distilled water). The sample 1 of the Fig. 2A, for instance, was at 200 ng/μL. Thus, in 100 μL of sample there are 19.9 μg of DNA.
   - Using a 1.5 mL centrifuge microtube of good quality is recommended to avoid breakage of the tube. To avoid evaporation of the sample, the microtubes should be sealed.
2. Put the microtube in a closed flask to avoid both the opening of the microtube and the direct contact of the sample with the autoclave steam. Put the flask in the autoclave.
3. Turn on the autoclave and when the temperature reaches 121 °C, mark 5 min and then turn it off.
4. After removing the microtube from autoclave, expect the microtube to cool and spin down the volume. Run an electrophoresis with the autoclaved DNA and a 100 bp ladder (as reference) in a 0.8% agarose gel (Fig. 2B). The fragmented DNA must be between 100-300 bp.
   - For GISH in wheat × rye hybrids, the blocking DNA (wheat DNA) must be at the concentration of 500 ng/μL due to the concentration of the probe of 50 ng/μL (proportion 1:10, probe:blocking DNA). However, for hybrids between other species, the concentration of the blocking DNA may be higher, if the proportion probe:blocking DNA is different. For instance, if the proportion to be used is 1:20, the blocking DNA should be at 1 μg/μL.
5. Add 2 volumes (vol) of cold absolute ethanol and 0.1 vol of 3 M sodium acetate (or 0.05 vol of 7.5 M sodium acetate) to precipitate the DNA.
6. Mix gently by inverting and store overnight at -20 °C.
7. Centrifuge for 20 min (14,000 rpm, room temperature).
8. Wash the pellet with 1 mL of 70% ethanol.
9. Centrifuge for 5 min (14,000 rpm, room temperature).
10. Dry the pellet at room temperature or at 37 °C.
11. Re-suspend the pellet in 10 mM Tris-HCl (pH 8.0) or in ultrapure distilled water, in order to reach the required concentration (in this case, 500 ng/μL). Take into account that there are losses in the total quantity of DNA during the steps of precipitation and re-suspension.

5. Nick translation

The procedures of probe labeling by nick translation are performed by using 1 μg of DNA. The components that are needed for the labeling reaction are: unmarked nucleotides (dATPs, dCTPs, dGTPs and, in a minor concentration, dTTPs), marked nucleotide (dUTPs) and an enzyme solution with DNase I and DNA polymerase I (Fig. 3A-C). The enzyme DNase I hydrolyzes the DNA by generating random nicks in the double-stranded DNA.

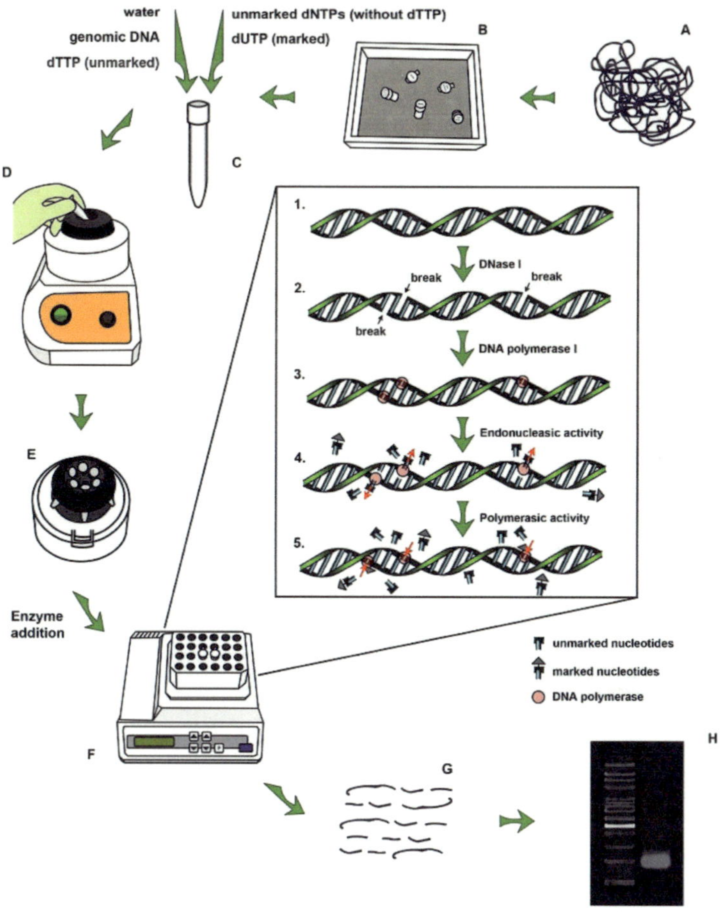

Figure 3. Nick translation reaction. (A) Total genomic DNA to be labeled. (B) Components of the reaction in chopped ice. (C) Preparation of the reaction mixture without the enzymatic solution. (D) The reaction mixture in a vortex. (E) Fast centrifugation of the mixture and addition of the enzymes. (F) Nick translation in a thermoblock at 15-16 °C, according to the manufacturer's recommendation. (G) Fragmented and labeled DNA. (H) Agarose gel showing a fragmented DNA with approximately 200-300 bp. Santelmo Vasconcelos & Ana C. Brasileiro-Vidal.

- A low number of nicks may lead to an inefficient insertion of marked nucleotides, thus generating larger probes. On the other hand, excessive nicks result in very short probes.

The DNA polymerase I has three different activities: 1) an exonuclease function that removes nucleotides from the breakage site in the sense 5′ ▪ 3′; 2) a polymerase function that inserts new nucleotides in the 3′ end, by using the opposite strand as template; and 3) a repair function in the sense 3′ ▪ 5′. Thus, marked and unmarked nucleotides are incorporated by the new synthesized DNA (see Fig. 3F; [17]). Additionally, only part of the thymines may be replaced by marked uracils. If all thymines are changed, the *in situ* hybridization reactions could be impaired.

During the nick translation reaction, the DNA structure becomes extremely fragile, resulting in the breakage of the double-stranded DNA. Besides the incorporation of marked nucleotides, the nick translation also fragments the DNA. Therefore, the longer the reaction lasts, smaller the fragments will be. The ideal size for the probe is around 200-300 bp because if it is above 500 bp, the *in situ* hybridization will not work properly; if the probe is much shorter, it could be washed away during the post-hybridization baths. Thus, the size of the fragments must be checked through electrophoresis in agarose gel before stopping the reaction (Figs. 2C, 3G and 3H).

Nick translation reactions are generally performed with commercial labeling kits, which should be performed according to the manufacturer's recommendations, although always following the procedures below:

1. Prepare the nick translation mixture in centrifuge microtube surrounded by chopped ice without the enzymatic solution (Fig. 3B-C).

2. Vortex the mixture, spin down the volume and add the enzymatic solution rapidly (Fig. 3D-E).

3. Mix gently, spin down the volume and put the microtube either in a thermocycler or in a thermoblock at the recommended temperature (Fig. 3F). To find out if the reaction time recommended by the manufacturer was sufficient for obtaining fragments with 200-300 bp, the labeling process should be temporarily suspended by maintaining the tube in chopped ice. Meanwhile, an electrophoresis in 0.8% agarose gel should be performed with an aliquot of the reaction. If the DNA is sufficiently fragmented (Fig. 3H), add the stop buffer. Otherwise, the reaction must continue as long as necessary for correct DNA fragmentation.

4. After adding the stop buffer, add 2 vol of cold absolute ethanol and 0.1 vol of 3 M sodium acetate, in order to precipitate DNA.

5. Mix gently by inverting and put in the freezer overnight.

6. Centrifuge for 20 min (14,000 rpm, room temperature), discard the supernatant and add 1 mL of 70% ethanol.

7. Centrifuge for 5 min (12,000 rpm, room temperature), discard the supernatant and dry the pellet at room temperature or at 37 °C.

8. Re-suspend the pellet in 15-20 μL of 10 mM Tris-HCl (pH 8.0) and store at -20 °C.

6. Seed germination and collecting, pretreating and fixating root tips

1. Wash seeds in 4% chlorine bleach for 5 min (Fig. 4A).
2. Wash seeds three times with distilled water for 5 min each (Fig. 4A).
3. Put seeds in Petri dishes with cotton and filter paper moistened with distilled water and incubate for 24 h at 25 °C.
4. Transfer the Petri dishes to a refrigerator (4 °C) for 48 h and then incubate again for 24 h at 25 °C. The low temperature promotes cell synchronization. Then, when the cells are restored to 25 °C, the cellular cycle is fully synchronized, thus increasing the amount of metaphases per slide.
5. The following day, collect root tips with a length of 1 to 1.5 times the size of the seed (Fig. 4B). The number of cells obtained during slide preparation is greatly increased when root tips are collected in the morning. Nevertheless, if some roots are still too small, let them grow a little more to collect later.
6. Pretreat the root tips in a 1.5 centrifuge tube containing ultrapure distilled water for 24 h at 4 °C (Fig. 4C). Add no more than six roots per tube. During this step, the tubes must be open because the roots are still alive and they need oxygen. The cold pretreatment is performed to increase the number of cells in metaphase. If there are many cells in anaphase and telophase, it means that the pretreatment did not work properly.
7. Fixate the root tips in Carnoy (absolute ethanol:acetic acid, 3:1, v/v) for 24 h at room temperature (Fig. 4D). Excellent quality products must be used in this step. Maintain the tubes under stirring during the first 90 min for a better fixation.
8. Store the root tips at -20 °C until use. Preferably, use newly fixed root tips.

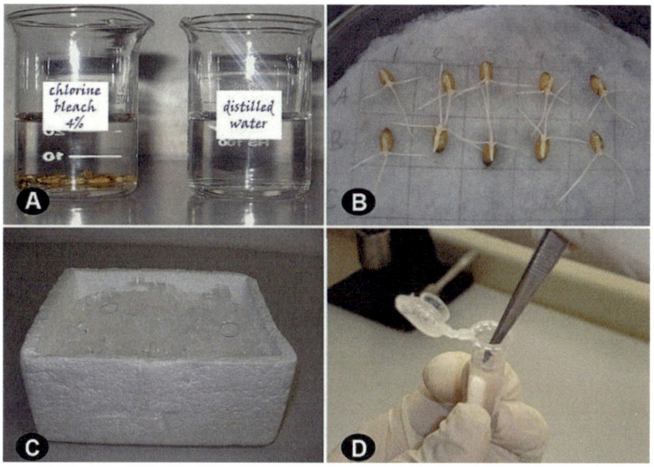

Figure 4. Washing and germinating seeds in (A) and (B); pretreatment and fixation of root tips in (C) and (D). (A) Seed washing in 4% chlorine bleach. (B) Roots with the length of 1 to 1.5 times the size of the seed, adequate for the collection. (C) Cold pretreatment of root tips. (D) Fixation of root tips in absolute ethanol:acetic acid (3:1, v/v). A and C: Ana R. Oliveira & Ana C. Brasileiro-Vidal; B and D: Sandra P. Brammer.

7. Slide preparation

Before starting this step, it is important to treat the slides, as in 6 N HCl for at least 6 h, for instance. Then, wash the slides under flowing water for 15 min, dip in distilled water and store in absolute ethanol until use.

1. Wash fixed root tips twice in a Petri dish with distilled water for 5 min each.
2. Digest the root tips in a 2% cellulase and 20% pectinase solution at 37 °C for 30-90 min, depending on the potential of the enzymatic activity. Digest only one root tip per slide by using high quality enzymes. Use a stereoscopic microscope to remove the root cap, add a drop of the enzymatic solution (ca. 5-10 μL) and incubate at 37 °C.
3. Wash the digested meristems twice with distilled water for 5 min each. For each wash, dry the root tips with filter paper without touching the digested material to avoid damaging it (Fig. 5D). Add a drop of distilled water carefully with a Pasteur pipette.
4. Add a drop of 45% acetic acid for, at least, 20 min (Fig. 5E). Afterwards, remove the acetic acid with filter paper and add a drop of distilled water either for 20 min (at least) at room temperature or overnight in a moisture chamber at 4-10 °C (in the refrigerator). Then, dry the root tips and add again a drop of 45% acetic acid and maintain the slides in a moisture chamber until use. Follow the step 5 for each slide individually.
5. With the aid of a stereoscopic microscope, disrupt completely the meristem with two histological needles, (Fig. 5F). Do not let the material dry. If this starts to happen, add carefully a little more 45% acetic acid. It is important to notice that the quantity of acetic acid used during this step is very critical for obtaining high quality preparations. Too much acid will lead to the loss of material; if too little acid is used, there will be air bubbles, which will negatively affect the quality of the slides.
6. Put an 18×18 mm glass coverslip over the material and tap gently with a blunt tip needle (Fig. 5G-H). While tapping, hold the coverslip with a piece of folded filter paper to avoid cell damage caused by slippage of the coverslip. In a bright field optical microscope, always observe the distribution of the material after and before tapping. This measure is important to determine how intense the tapping must be. A too intense tapping may break drastically the cells and cause chromosome losses. On the other hand, if the tapping is too weak, the material will not spread properly. The ideal condition is when the cells are broken, but all chromosomes are still in a same field of view in the microscope.
7. Heat the preparation in an alcohol Bunsen burner ca. three times, carefully to prevent boiling (Fig. 5I). Fell the temperature with the back of the hand.
8. Then smash the material thoroughly. Put the slide-coverslip set within two sheets of folded filter paper and press with a thumb always taking precaution not to move coverslip (Fig. 5J).
9. Dip the slide-coverslip set in liquid nitrogen for approximately 3 min (Fig. 5K).

10. Quickly remove the coverslip with the aid of a steel blade or a bistoury (Fig. 5L). The liquid nitrogen freezes the slide-coverslip set. Because the slide is thicker, it takes longer to warm up in comparison to the coverslip. Thus, the chromosomes will be attached to the coldest part (the slide) when the coverslip is removed. However, if there is a delay to remove the coverslip, chromosomes may be lost or in two planes in the slide.

11. Let the slides to dry off inclined.

12. Store the slides at -20 °C (or, if possible, at -80 °C) for an indefinite period until the *in situ* hybridization procedures. The results of the GISH will be better when newly prepared slides are used.

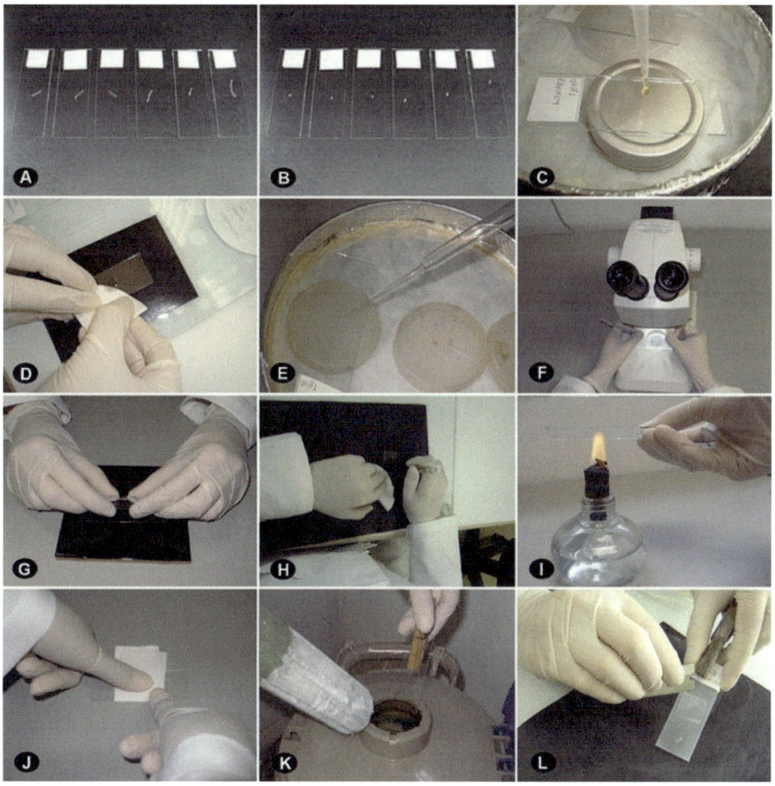

Figure 5. Preparation of slides for genomic *in situ* hybridization. (A) Full length root tips after washing in distilled water. (B) Root meristem to be digested. (C) Enzymatic digestion. (D) Removal of the enzymatic solution. (E) Addition of 45% acetic acid. (F) Disruption of the root meristem, with histological needles in a stereoscopic microscope. (G) Addition of an 18×18 mm coverslip. (H) Gentle tapping with a blunt tip needle. (I) Quick heating of the preparation in an alcohol Bunsen burner. (J) Squashing of the slide-coverslip set with two sheets of filter paper. (K) Dipping the slide-coverslip set in liquid nitrogen. (L) Quick removal of the coverslip. A, B, C, F, H, J, K and L: Sandra P. Brammer; D, E, G and I: Ana R. Oliveira & Ana C. Brasileiro-Vidal.

8. Genomic *in situ* hybridization

8.1. Treatment of slides

Prior to the beginning of the GISH procedures, identify the slides and mark preparation area with a diamond-tipped pen (or similar), along the length of the blade (Fig. 6A). Avoid doing notes with permanent marker or using paper labels.

Slides stored for a long time must be dipped in Carnoy for 15 min, followed by an alcoholic series of 70% and 100% ethanol for 5 min each (Fig. 6B). The Carnoy helps to better fix the chromosome structure. However, this step is not necessary for newly prepared slides.

1. Let the slides to dry off for 30 min at 50-60 °C (Fig. 6C). This drying is important because the grip of the chromosomes to the blade is improved during the process.
   - Paraformaldehyde to be used at step 8 could be prepared during the steps 1-2.
2. Let the slides to cool for 5-10 min at room temperature (Fig. 6D).
3. Add 50 μL of 100 μg/mL RNase A [a 10 mg/mL RNase A solution diluted in 2×SSC (300 mM NaCl and 30 mM $Na_3C_6H_5O_7.2H_2O$) at the proportion of 1:100], cover with a plastic coverslip (made of laboratory film or similar) and incubate in a moisture chamber for 1 h at 37 °C (Fig. 6E-F).
4. Wash the slides three times in 2×SSC for 5 min each (Fig. 6G). After each wash cycle, the used volume of 2×SSC must be replaced by a clean one.
5. Add 50 μL of 10 mM HCl, cover with plastic coverslip and maintain for 5 min (Fig. 6H).
6. Add 50 μL of 15 μg/mL pepsin (a 1 mg/mL pepsin solution diluted in 10 mM HCl at the proportion of 1.5:100), cover with plastic coverslip and incubate at 37 °C for 20 min (Fig. 6I-J). Before adding the pepsin solution, remove the excess of HCl with and absorbing paper as illustrated in Fig. 6M.
7. Wash the slides three times in 2×SSC for 5 min each (Fig. 6K).
8. Fixate the chromosome preparation in 4% paraformaldehyde for 10 min (Fig. 6L). Be extremely cautious when handling paraformaldehyde because it is highly toxic and carcinogenic.
9. Wash the slides three times in 2×SSC for 5 min each (Fig. 6L).
   - In general, for Triticeae species, the procedures from step 3 to 9 may be completely excluded without affecting the *in situ* hybridization.
10. Dehydrate the slides in an alcoholic series of 70% and 100% ethanol for 3 min each (Fig. 6M-N).
11. Let the slides to dry off for, at least, 1 h at room temperature (Fig. 6O).

8.2. *In situ* hybridization according to Heslop-Harrison et al. [18] and Pedrosa et al. [19], with some modifications

The stringency value for the procedures below is 77%. The stringency value refers to the percentage of correct base pairing during the *in situ* hybridization process and is calculated according to formamide and salt (SSC) concentrations in the solution, as well as the reaction temperature [17]. Defrost all components and prepare the hybridization mixture in chopped ice (Fig. 7A).

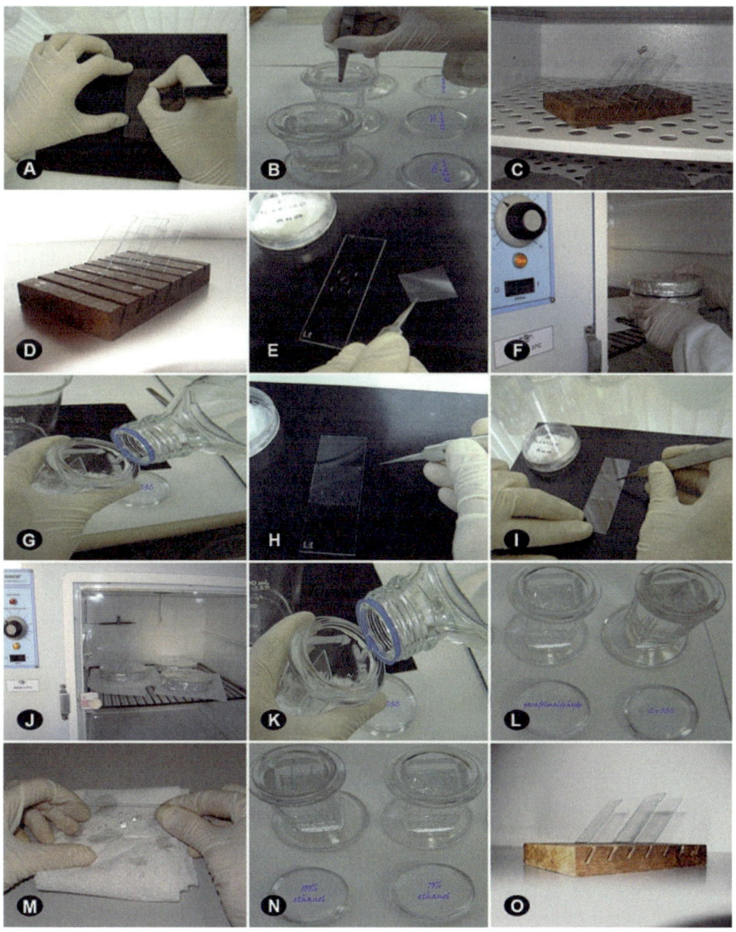

Figure 6. Slide treatment for genomic *in situ* hybridization. (A) Marking the area of the slide that contains the chromosome preparation. (B) Baths in absolute ethanol:acetic acid (3:1, v/v), 70% ethanol and 100% ethanol. (C) Drying slides in an incubation oven at 50-60 °C. (D) Slides in room temperature. (E) Digestion with RNase. (F) Incubation of the slides at 37 °C in a moisture chamber. (G) Washing the slides in 2×SSC to remove the RNase. (H) Addition of 10 mM HCl. (I) Digestion with pepsin. (J) Incubation of the slides at 37 °C in a moisture chamber. (K) Washing the slides in 2×SSC. (L) Treatment with 4% paraformaldehyde and posterior washes in 2×SSC. (M) Removal of the excess of 2×SSC with absorbing paper. (N) Dehydration in an alcoholic series (70% and 100%). (O) Drying the slides at room temperature. A, B, E, F, G, H, I, J, K, L, M and N: Sandra P. Brammer; C, D and O: Ana R. Oliveira & Ana C. Brasileiro-Vidal.

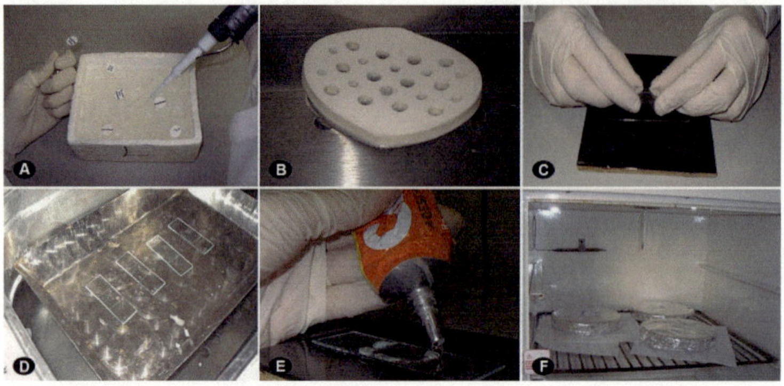

Figure 7. Genomic *in situ* hybridization. (A) Preparation of the hybridization mixture. (B) Denaturation of the probe at 75 °C. (C) Addition of the hybridization mixture in the chromosome preparation and covering with a glass coverslip. (D) Denaturation of the chromosomes in a metal plate inside a water bath at 73 °C. (E) Sealing the coverslip with rubber glue. (F) *In situ* hybridization at 37 °C. A, B, C, D and E: Ana R. Oliveira & Ana C. Brasileiro-Vidal; F: Sandra P. Brammer.

1. Prepare the hybridization mixture (50% formamide, 10% dextran sulfate, 2×SSC, ca. 2.5-5 ng/μL of probe and 25-50 ng/μL of blocking) with a final volume of 10 μL per slide (Table 1). In case of using directly labeled probes, the mixture preparation and all the following steps must be done in partial darkness (avoid direct incidence of light). The formamide destabilizes the DNA molecule, helping in the denaturation. Thus, be careful while handling it due to its high toxicity.

2. For probe denaturing, incubate the mixture at 75 °C for 10 min in a water bath (Figs. 1D and 7B). Immediately put the mixture on ice for at least 5 min to keep the two DNA strands open.

3. Spin down the mixture and then add 10 μL per slide, cover with an 18×18 glass coverslip and denature the slide at 73 °C for 10 min (Figs. 1E-F and 7C).

   - For other plant groups, use 75 °C or above.

4. Seal the coverslip with rubber glue (Fig. 7E) and incubate the slide in a moisture chamber at 37 °C overnight (ca. 16 h) or up to one day and a half (Figs. 1G and 7F).

Component	Quantity	Final concentration
100% formamide	5 μL	50%
50% dextran sulfate	2 μL	10%
20×SSC (saline-sodium citrate)	1 μL	2×
Probe	0.5-1 μL	ca. 2.5-5 ng/μL
Blocking DNA	0.5-1 μL	ca. 25-50 ng/μL
Ultrapure distilled water	Q.s.p. 10 μL	-

Table 1. Components of a 10 μL hybridization mixture.

8.3. Post-hybridization baths and probe detection

In this step, flasks with SSC solutions and the Coplin jar (with the solution of the first wash) must be previously in the water bath at 42 °C (Fig. 8A). Before the temperature of the water bath, the temperature inside the Coplin jar must also be checked. The same jar can be used for all baths by discarding the anterior SSC solution and adding the next one (Fig. 8B-C). Furthermore, the function of the wash procedures is to remove the excess of material from the *in situ* hybridization, mainly non-hybridized probes and incorrectly hybridized ones.

1. Remove the rubber glue with tweezers without moving the coverslip.
2. Dip the slides with the coverslips in the pre-warmed Coplin jar. After dipping the last slide, remove carefully the coverslips to avoid damage to the chromosomes. The time count begins only after the last coverslip is removed.
3. Wash the slides twice in 2×SSC for 5 min each at 42 °C.
4. Wash the slides twice in 0.1×SSC (15 mM NaCl and 1.5 mM $Na_3C_6H_5O_7.2H_2O$) for 5 min (stringency of 73%) at 42 °C.
5. Wash the slides twice in 2×SSC for 5 min each at 42 °C. In the second wash, remove the Coplin jar from the water bath.
6. Wash the slides once in 2×SSC for 5 min at room temperature.
7. Wash the slides once in 4×SSC + 0.1% Tween 20 (600 mM NaCl, 60 mM $Na_3C_6H_5O_7.2H_2O$ and 0.1% Tween 20) at room temperature.

During the washes of slides with directly labeled probes, the procedures must also be done in partial darkness due to the presence of fluorochromes. Moreover, the GISH procedures end after these washes when using this type of probes and the results may be already visualized in an epifluorescence microscope after adding the DAPI-Vectashield, as better explained below in the steps 11-12 (Fig. 1J).

1. Dry the excess of SSC, add the secondary antibody mixture (antibody and 1% BSA in 4×SSC + 0.1% Tween 20, according to the manufacturer's recommendation), cover with a plastic coverslip and incubate at 37 °C for 1 h in a dark moisture chamber.
2. Wash the slides three times for 10 min each in 4×SSC + 0.1% Tween 20 at 42 °C. These washes are needed for removing the excess of antibodies.
3. Dry the excess of SSC, add 8 μL of DAPI (4',6-diamidino-2-phenylindole; 2 μg/mL) and Vectashield anti-fade (1:1, v/v) and mount the slide with a 22×22 glass coverslip (Fig. 8J-K). Seal the coverslip with colorless nail polish and allow it to dry for at least 1h in the dark (Fig. 8L).
4. Analyze the slides in an epifluorescence microscope with the adequate fluorescence filter (Fig. 1J).

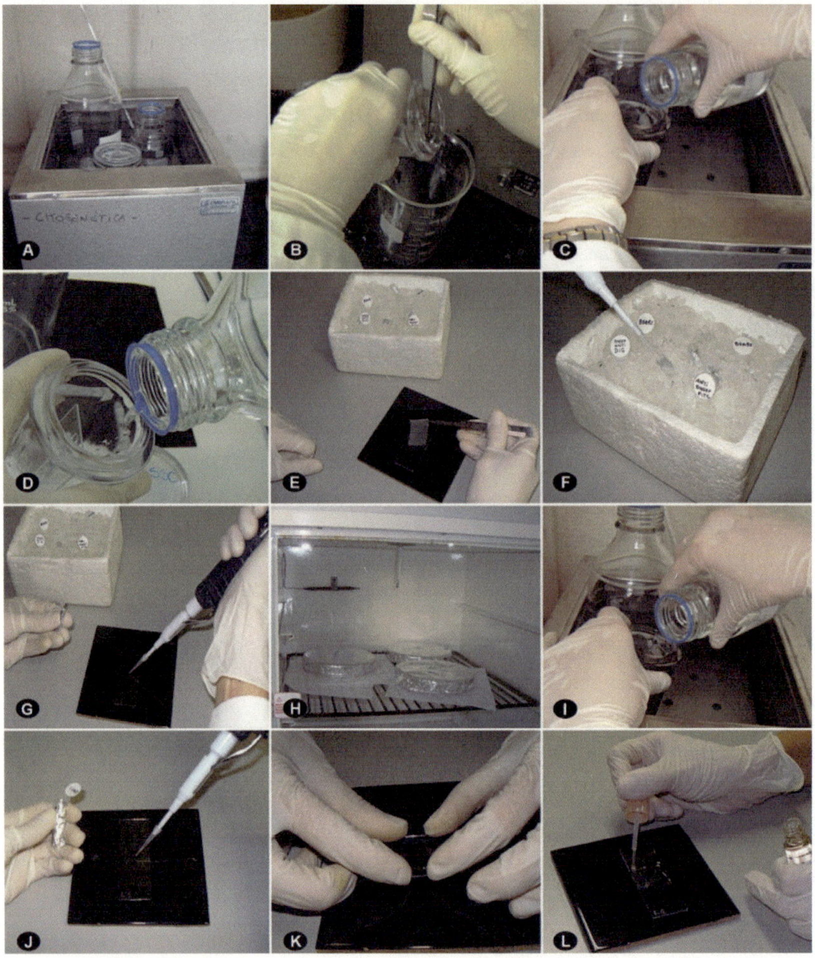

Figure 8. Post-hybridization baths and probe detection. (A) Washing of the slides in a water bath at 42 °C. (B) Disposal of the saline-sodium citrate (SSC) solution. (C) Addition of the next SSC solution. (D) Addition of 4×SSC + 0.1% Tween 20 at room temperature. (E) Addition of 5% bovine serum albumin (BSA) for the blocking step. (F) Preparation of the antibody solution. (G) Addition of the antibody solution and covering with a plastic coverslip. (H) Incubation of the slides during the detection step at 37 °C. (I) Washing the Wash the slides three times for 10 min each in 4×SSC + 0.1% Tween 20 at 42 °C. These washes are needed for removing the excess of antibodies (Fig. 8I). Figures A, B, C, D, H and I: Sandra P. Brammer; E, F, G, J, K and L: Ana R. Oliveira & Ana C. Brasileiro-Vidal.

A metaphase cell of triticale ($2n$ = 56) is shown with the 14 chromosomes from rye detected by GISH in Fig. 9. This cell was hybridized with blocking DNA of wheat and rye DNA probe labeled with digoxigenin and detected with FITC (fluorescein isothiocyanate). The chromosomes are counterstained with DAPI (Fig. 9A). Fig. 9B shows the image capture of the same chromosomes with the fluorescence filter for FITC; and, in Fig. 9C, is shown the superposition of both images.

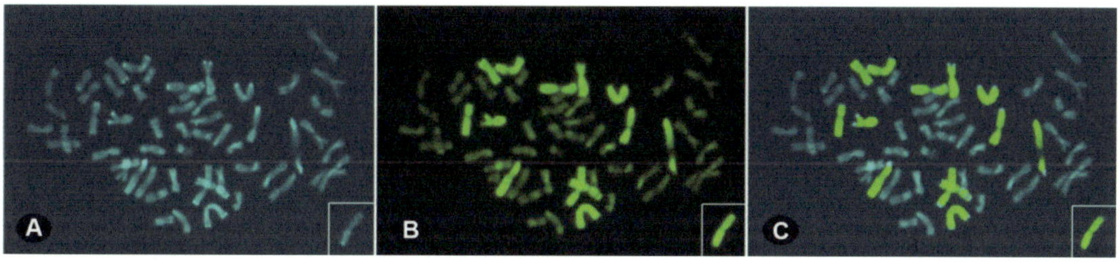

Figure 9. Genomic *in situ* hybridization (GISH) in a triticale cell (2*n* = 56), using rye DNA as probe (green) and wheat DNA as blocking DNA. Chromosomes were counterstained with DAPI (blue). The same cell is represented in A (DAPI), B (FITC) and C (A + B image merging). The detail in A, B and C shows the 14th rye chromosome of the same cell. Ana C. Brasileiro-Vidal.

9. Final considerations

The Triticeae wild relatives continue to be important sources of genes for introducing agronomically desirable traits into common wheat and durum wheat (*Triticum durum*) [20-21]. Thus, alien gene transfer into common wheat via cross-species hybridization makes possible the resistance increasing to biotic and abiotic stresses as well as the quality improving [22-23]. Several species such as of the genera *Aegilops*, *Secale* and *Thinopyrum* have been extensively used in hybridizations with common wheat, thus proving to be a valuable source of genes [3, 24-25].

In all these examples, the genomic *in situ* hybridization methodology can be used to establish the cytogenetic constitution of interspecific or intergeneric hybrids. In addition, this technique allows for a fine-scale characterization of the chromosome structure. Currently, the technique has been used in parallel to different strategies, such as C-banding, high molecular weight (HMW) glutenin subunits, FISH with BACs (bacterial artificial chromosomes), southern blot and molecular markers, in order to confirm the alien gene introgression into the wheat genome [26-29]. Besides, the GISH has been also collaborated in investigations about the evolutionary origin of common wheat and the genome-wide transcriptional dynamics [30].

Acknowledgements

The authors thank the following Brazilian agencies for financial support: Conselho Nacional de Desenvolvimento Científico e Tecnológico (CNPq); Coordenação de Aperfeiçoamento de Pessoal de Nível Superior (CAPES); and Fundação de Amparo à Ciência e Tecnologia do Estado de Pernambuco (FACEPE).

Author details

Sandra Patussi Brammer[1], Santelmo Vasconcelos[2], Liane Balvedi Poersch[3],
Ana Rafaela Oliveira[2,4] and Ana Christina Brasileiro-Vidal[2]

1 Brazilian Agricultural Research Corporation – Embrapa Wheat, Passo Fundo, Brazil

2 Federal University of Pernambuco, Recife, Brazil

3 Federal University of Rio Grande do Sul, Porto Alegre, Brazil

4 Federal Rural University of Pernambuco, Recife, Brazil

References

[1] Oettler G. Crossability and embryo development in wheat-rye hybrids. Euphytica 1983;32(2) 593-600.

[2] Prieto P, Ramírez C, Cabrera A, Ballesteros J, Martín A. Development and cytogenetic characterisation of a double goat grass-barley chromosome substitution in tritordeum. Euphytica 2006;147(3): 337–342.

[3] Molnár-Láng M, Cseh A, Szakács E, Molnár I. Development of a wheat genotype combining the recessive crossability alleles kr1kr1kr2kr2 and the 1BL.1RS translocation, for the rapid enrichment of 1RS with new allelic variation. Theoretical and Applied Genetics 2010;120(8) 1535-1545.

[4] Molnár-Láng M, Kruppa K, Cseh A, Bucsi J, Linc G. Identification and phenotypic description of new wheat: six-rowed winter barley disomic additions. Genome 2012;55(4) 302-311.

[5] Sybenga J. Cytogenetics in Plant Breeding. New York: Springer-Verlag; 1992.

[6] Figueroa DM, Bass HW. A historical and modern perspective on plant cytogenetics. Briefings in Functional Genomics 2010;9(2) 95-102.

[7] Hall BD, Spiegelman S. Sequence complementarity of T2-DNA and T2-specific RNA. Proceedings of the National Academy of Sciences of the United States of America 1961;47(2) 137-146.

[8] Langer PR, Waldrop AA, Ward DC. Enzymatic synthesis of biotin-labeled polynucleotides: novel nucleic acid affinity probes. Proceedings of the National Academy of Sciences of the United States of America 1981;78(11) 6633-6637.

[9] Ohmido N, Fukui K, Kinoshita T. Recent advances in rice genome and chromosome structure research by fluorescence in situ hybridization (FISH). Proceedings of the Japan Academy, Series B 2010;86(2) 103-116.

[10] Singh RJ. Plant Cytogenetics, 2nd edition. Boca Raton: CRC Press; 2003.

[11] Schwarzacher T, Anamthawat-Jonsson K, Harrison GE, Islam A, Jia JZ, King IP, Leitch AR, Miller TE, Reader SM, Rogers WJ, Shi M, Heslop-Harrison JS. Genomic in situ hybridization to identify alien chromosomes and chromosome segments in wheat. Theoretical and Applied Genetics 1992;84(7) 778-786.

[12] Brasileiro-Vidal AC, Cuadrado A, Brammer SP, Benko-Iseppon AM, Guerra M. Molecular cytogenetic characterization of parental genomes in the partial amphidiploid Triticum aestivum × Thinopyrum ponticum. Genetics and Molecular Biology 2005;28(2) 308-313.

[13] Zhou S, Li K, Zhou G. Analysis of endosperm development of allotriploid × diploid/tetraploid crosses in Lilium. Euphytica 2012;184(3) 401-412.

[14] Markova M, Vyskot B. New horizons of genomic in situ hybridization. Cytogenetic and Genome Research 2009;126(4) 368-375.

[15] Bonato ALV. Extração de DNA genômico de cereais de inverno na Embrapa Trigo – comunicado técnico online 235. Passo Fundo: Embrapa Trigo; 2008. http://www.cnpt.embrapa.br/biblio/co/p_co235.htm (accessed 25 July 2012).

[16] Michaels SD, John MC, Amasino RM. Removal of polysaccharides from plant DNA by ethanol precipitation. Biotechniques 1994;17(2) 274-276.

[17] Schwarzacher T, Heslop-Harrison, P. Practical in situ hybridization. Oxford: BIOS Science Publishers; 2000.

[18] Heslop-Harrison JS, Schwazarcher T, Anamthawat-Jónssonn K, Leitch AR, Shi M. In situ hybridization with automated chromosome denaturation. Technique 1991;3(1) 109-115.

[19] Pedrosa A, Jantsch MF, Moscone EA, Ambros PF, Schweizer D. Characterisation of pericentromeric and sticky intercalary heterochromatin in Ornithogalum longibracteatum (Hyacinthaceae). Chromosoma 2001;110(3) 203-213.

[20] Oliver RE, Xu SS, Stack RW, Friesen TL, Jin Y, Cai X. Molecular cytogenetic characterization of four partial wheat-Thinopyrum ponticum amphiploids and their reactions to Fusarium head blight, tan spot, and Stagonospora nodorum blotch. Theoretical and Applied Genetics 2006;112(8) 1473-1479.

[21] Kwiatek M, Błaszczyk L, Wiśniewska H, Apolinarska B. Aegilops-Secale amphiploids: chromosome categorisation, pollen viability and identification of fungal disease resistance genes. Jounal of Applied Genetics 2012;53(1) 37-40.

[22] Sepsi A, Molnár I, Molnár-Láng M. Physical mapping of a 7A.7D translocation in the wheat–Thinopyrum ponticum partial amphiploid BE-1 using multicolour genomic in situ hybridization and microsatellite marker analysis. Genome 2009;52(9) 748-754.

[23] Kang H, Zeng J, Xie Q, Tao S, Zhong M, Zhang H, Fan X, Sha L, Xu L, Zhou Y. Molecular cytogenetic characterization and stripe rust response of a trigeneric hybrid involving Triticum, Psathyrostachys, and Thinopyrum. Genome 2012;55(5) 383-390.

[24] Rawat N, Neelam K, Tiwari VK, Randhawa GS, Friebe B, Gill BS, Dhaliwal HS. Development and molecular characterization of wheat-Aegilops kotschyi addition and substitution lines with high grain protein, iron, and zinc. Genome 2011;54(11) 943-953.

[25] Fu S, Lv Z, Qi B, Guo X, Li J, Liu B, Han F. Molecular cytogenetic characterization of wheat-Thinopyrum elongatum addition, substitution and translocation lines with a novel source of resistance to wheat Fusarium Head Blight. Journal of Genetics and Genomics 2012;39(2) 103-110.

[26] Han F, Liu B, Fedak G, Liu, Z. Genomic constitution and variation in five partial amphiploids of wheat-Thinopyrum intermedium as revealed by GISH, multicolor GISH and seed storage protein analysis. Theoretical and Applied Genetics 2004;109(5) 1070-1076.

[27] Kato A, Vega JM, Jonathan FH, Lamb C, Birchler, JA. Advances in plant chromosome identification and cytogenetic techniques. Current Opinion in Plant Biology 2005; 8(2) 148-154.

[28] Sepsi A, Molnár, I, Szalay, D, Molnár-Láng, M. Characterization of a leaf rust-resistant wheat–Thinopyrum ponticum partial amphiploid BE-1, using sequential multicolor GISH and FISH. Theorical and Applied Genetics 2008;116(6) 825–834.

[29] Wang L, Yuan J, Bie T, Zhou B, Chen P. Cytogenetic and molecular identification of three Triticum aestivum-Leymus racemosus translocation addition lines. Journal of Genetics and Genomics 2009;36(6) 379-385.

[30] Qi B, Huang W, Zhu B, Zhong X, Guo J, Zhao N, Xu C, Zhang H, Pang J, Han F, Liu B. Global transgenerational gene expression dynamics in two newly synthesized allohexaploid wheat (Triticum aestivum) lines. BMC Biology 2012; 10(3).

Chapter 2

SRAP Molecular Marker Technology in Plant Science

Genyi Li, Peter B. E. McVetty and Carlos F. Quiros

Additional information is available at the end of the chapter

http://dx.doi.org/10.5772/54511

1. Introduction

Molecular markers are commonly used in genetic diversity analysis, genetic map construction, gene mapping and cloning, and marker assisted selection in plant breeding. Based on detection procedure, most molecular marker technologies can be classified into hybridization-based or PCR-based systems. Restriction fragment length polymorphism (RFLP) is the first hybridization-based molecular marker system that was intensively used at the beginning of the molecular biology era in life science while hybridization-based marker methods such as microarrays and diversity array technology (DArT) are used currently to detect single nucleotide polymorphisms (SNP). In contrast, many PCR-based molecular marker detection methods have been developed. For example, amplified fragment length polymorphism (AFLP), random amplified polymorphic DNA (RAPD), simple sequence repeats (SSR) and sequence related amplified polymorphism (SRAP), inter-simple sequence repeat (ISSR), sequence tagged site (STS), and sequence characterized amplification region (SCAR), are commonly used in genomic analysis (Jones et al., 2009).

There are advantages and limitations for all molecular marker detection methods. In particular, RFLP probes can be shared in related species so RFLP is advantageous over other molecular markers in comparative genomics. However, the detection procedure in RFLP is complicated and costly. Additionally, RFLP is not easily automated to analyze thousands of individuals for marker assisted selection. AFLP is a commonly used molecular marker system since it can detect multiple genetic loci in a genome. On the other hand, there are many steps in the AFLP detection procedure, which limits its application in marker assisted selection when thousands of individual DNA samples need to be analyzed in a short time. SSRs often have a high level of polymorphism in plant genomes and are commonly used in most genomic applications. Since SSR technology only detects sequence repeats, the number of SSRs in a genome is relatively limited compared with numerous SNPs. RAPD is easily performed in one round of PCR, however, a low level of reproducibility of RAPD amplification limits its wide use in genomic analysis.

As next generation sequencing (NGS) technologies dramatically increase capacity and throughput of DNA sequencing, whole genome sequencing of many plant species has been accomplished and most economically important crop species such as rice, maize, soybean, sorghum, potato, tomato and Chinese cabbage have been fully sequenced. Although it is still challenging to use NGS for assembling a whole complex genome such as barley and wheat, there are thousands of SNPs identified in NGS that can be used to develop molecular markers in species with complex genomes. Furthermore, NGS is directly used in SNP discovery and a few dozen genotypes can be sequenced simultaneously to assemble ultradense genetic maps. Additionally, different strategies are used to produce partial genomes that can be used to directly sequence SNPs using next generation technologies.

2. SRAP technology

We developed and published information on the SRAP marker system in 2001 (Li and Quiros). The original thinking was to simplify the AFLP detection procedure and increase throughput and improve reproducibility compared to RAPD. To produce a simple detection procedure, we skipped restriction enzyme digestion and ligation of target DNA fragments and adapters in the AFLP detection protocol. We designed SRAP primers in sizes similar to those in AFLP, but ran one round of PCR instead of two rounds in AFLP. To detect multiple loci with a pair of SRAP primers, we designed a special PCR running program (94^{0}C for 1 min, 35^{0}C for 1 min and 72^{0}C for 1 min for the first 5 cycles and followed by 30 cycles at the raised annealing temperature of 50^{0}C). At the beginning of PCR, the 35^{0}C annealing temperature allowed SRAP primers to anneal to multiple loci in target DNA so that the multiple loci were amplified to produce a profile that is similar to that in AFLP. Similar to AFLP, most SRAP markers are dominant while most SNPs and SSRs are co-dominant. Compared with RAPD, SRAP used a pair of primers with 16 to 22 nucleotides instead of 10-mer short primers in RAPD, which gives SRAP a big advantage over RAPD so one SRAP primer can combine with unlimited number of other primers. Although SRAP PCR starts at 35^{0}C annealing temperature in the first five cycles, the larger sizes of SRAP primers allowed the increase of annealing temperature to 50^{0}C in the following cycles, which significantly improves the reproducibility in SRAP. In contrast, a low level of reproducibility in RAPD is a limitation factor. In addition, SRAP primers can be fluorescently labelled and combined with unlabeled SRAP primers so SRAP PCR products can be separated in capillary instruments such as ABI genetic analyzers.

In general, there is a difference of GC content between gene coding sequences and other sequences in plant genomes. We used this difference to design two sets of SRAP primers. The forward primers contained a GGCC cassette closing the 3′ end of SRAP primers that might preferentially anneal to the GC-rich regions while the reverse SRAP primer set was incorporated with an AATT cassette that would preferentially anneal SRAP primers to introns and gene spacers so that SRAP could preferentially amplify gene-rich regions in a genome. After sequencing SRAP fragments and constructing a SRAP genetic map in *B. oleracea,* it was found that SRAP indeed amplified more sequences from genes and more SRAP markers fell into chromosome arm regions and produced fewer markers in the centromeres that were filled with AFLP markers.

There is wide flexibility in the design of SRAP primers. After testing the primers we used for gene cloning, we found that most of these primers worked well in SRAP amplification. In the construction of an ultra-dense genetic map in *B. napus,* we used 12 fluorescently labeled forward primers and 442 unlabeled primers to assemble a genetic map with 13,351 molecular markers (Sun et al., 2007). Based on the SRAP markers on the genetic map, the efficiency of each labeled primer was checked by counting the average numbers of SRAP markers produced by individual labeled primers. Some labeled SRAP primers such as FC1, BG23 and SA7 produced more than ten polymorphic loci while EM2 and DC1 produced less than six polymorphic loci. If we checked individual SRAP primer combinations, we found that there was a big difference in the numbers of polymorphic loci detected by individual SRAP primers. Efficient SRAP primer combinations produced over 20 polymorphic loci while less efficient SRAP primer combinations produced one to three mapped loci. Actually, we tested over a thousand SRAP primers in *B. napus* and *B. rapa* and found that most primers produced good profiles with over 30 strong bands (unpublished data). After testing a large set of SRAP primer combinations, we selected a set of SRAP primer combinations that showed the best performance in SRAP amplification in different accessions and populations in various Brassica species. These SRAP primer combinations serve as a standard set and are routinely used in genetic map construction, mapping of quantitative loci (QTL) and gene cloning in our lab. Therefore, if SRAP is frequently used in a lab, it is worthwhile to select a set of SRAP primer combinations which will enhance the effectiveness and efficiency of SRAP marker detection.

To enhance the capacity and effectiveness of SRAP technology, we combined SRAP with Illumina's Solexa sequencing to directly integrate genetic loci on the *B. rapa* genetic map based on paired-end Solexa sequences (Li et al., 2011). To achieve this objective, we used two rounds of PCR to prepare SRAP products that were pooled and sequenced with Illlumina's Solexa sequencing. The first round of PCR produced SRAP fragments using individual DNA samples from a mapping population with the same set of SRAP primer combinations while the second round was used to tail the SRAP PCR products that allowed identifying the original DNA for producing paired-end Solexa sequences. After Illumina's Solexa sequencing, paired-end sequences were sorted using the sequences of tag primers and the numbers of unique paired-end sequences from each DNA samples were obtained. These numbers represent Solexa sequence frequencies in each DNA sample which was used to integrate Solexa sequences onto the SRAP genetic map. To integrate paired-end sequences on the genetic map, we adopted a QTL mapping strategy by using Windows QTL Cartographer software 2.5. When a paired-end sequence was found to have only one significant LOD score in a bin of the genetic map, this sequence was assigned into this bin. In total, 1737 unique paired-end sequences representing the same number of genetic loci were integrated on the genetic map. Eventually, we constructed a high density *B. rapa* genetic map consisting of 1,737 paired-end Solexa sequences, 9,177 SRAP markers and 46 SSR markers.

3. Genetic map construction

Genetic maps are extensively used in gene mapping, QTL mapping and assembly of whole genome sequence. High density molecular markers in genetic maps are advantageous and necessary in most applications. The detection of multiple loci in a SRAP PCR reaction can be automated through fluorescently labelled SRAP primers so it is feasible to construct a high density genetic map using SRAP technology.

In *B. napus*, we used a five-color fluorescent dye set including '6-FAM', 'VIC', 'Pet', 'NED' and 'LIZ' to perform SRAP fragment analysis with the ABI genetic analyzer (Sun et al., 2007). 'LIZ' was used as the internal standard while the other four fluorescent dyes were used to label SRAP primers and combined with unlabeled primers. After obtaining SRAP products with four fluorescently labeled and four unlabeled primers, all the products from four SRAP primer combinations were pooled to increase the detection throughput by four fold. We used 1,634 SRAP primer combinations selected from 12 labeled and 442 unlabeled SRAP primers to produce 13,472 SRAP markers. Together with 79 SSR markers, we assembled currently the most saturated genetic map in *B. napus*.

Using cDNA-SRAP technology, we first constructed a transcriptome map based on *B. oleracea* cDNAs obtained from leaf tissue (Li et al., 2003). In cDNA-SRAP, one step PCR allows the amplification of single strand cDNAs after the first strand cDNA is synthesized using reverse transcriptase. Since most cDNA-SRAP markers come from differences in gene sequence, these markers are considered to be functional markers. SRAP products can be easily isolated from polyacrylamide gels for sequencing so we sequenced 190 fragments that corresponded to 190 polymorphic loci from cDNA-SRAP. Through analysis of sequence similarity, 169 out of 190 cDNA marker sequences were homologous to genes reported in Arabidopsis, which allowed the identification of extensive colinearity between the two genomes according to the gene-for-gene alignment. Later, we developed over 1,000 SRAP markers using genomic DNA from the same mapping population and assembled these SRAP markers from both genomic DNA and cDNA samples on the same genetic map (Gao et al., 2007). In addition, we integrated 10 SCAR markers using sequences of genes with known functions in the biosynthesis of glucosinolates and inflorescence architecture, and one SCAR marker flanking a resistance gene to downy mildew.

SRAP technology can be combined with other markers to construct genetic maps. For example, Yu et al., (2007) constructed a high-density genetic map in a cultivated allotetraploid cotton population using SSR, SRAP, AFLP, and target region amplification polymorphism (TRAP). This high density cotton genetic map consists of 697 SSR, 171 TRAP, 129 SRAP, 98 AFLP, and two morphological markers, covering a genetic distance of 4,536.7 cM with the average genetic distance of 4.1 cM per marker. Gulsen et al., (2010) reported a new citrus linkage map using SRAP, RAPD, SSR, ISSR, peroxidase gene polymorphism (POGP), resistant gene analog (RGA), and a morphological marker, Alternaria brown spot resistance gene. In total, they assembled 385 SRAP, 97 RAPD, 95 SSR, 18 ISSR, 12 POGP, and 2 RGA markers on the citrus genetic map.

In the Cucurbitaceae family, Yeboah et al., (2007) constructed genetic maps in cucumber using SRAP and ISSR markers. They developed pseudo-testcross F1 segregating populations from a cross between two diploid parents and constructed male and female parental genetic maps separately with 164 SSR and 108 SRAP markers. More recently, Zhang et al., (2012) constructed a high density consensus genetic map in an inter-subspecific mapping population in cucumber. The consensus map contained over a thousand molecular markers including 1,152 SSR, 192 SRAP, 21 SCAR and one STS. In another cucurbit species, Levi et al., (2006) constructed an extended genetic map for watermelon using five PCR-based molecular markers SRAP, AFLP, SSR, ISSR and RAPD. As suggested by the authors, low polymorphism is often observed in watermelon cultivars, combining several marker systems is necessary to construct a high density genetic map covering the whole genome.

SRAP markers have been used to construct genetic maps in a wide range of plant species. In Dendrobium plants that are used as Chinese herbs, Xue et al., (2010) constructed two genetic maps in two Dendrobium species, *D. officinale* and *D. hercoglossum* with a double pseudo-testcross strategy using SRAP and RAPD methods. In root plants, Chen et al., (2010) constructed a genetic map in an F_1 population derived from an interspecific cross in cassava by combining AFLP, SSR, SRAP and expressed sequence tag (EST)-SSR markers. In total, they assembled 355 markers into 18 linkage groups covering a genetic distance of 1,707.9 cM, which served as a foundation for QTL mapping in this species. In grass species, Xie et al., (2011) used SSR and SRAP markers to construct two genetic maps of male and female parental lines respectively in diploid orchardgrass (*Dactylis glomerata* L.) using a pseudo-test cross strategy. In total, they assembled 164 SSR markers and 108 SRAP markers on these two genetic maps. In a fruit tree, Luohanguo (*Siraitia grosvenorii* C. Jeffrey), Liu et al., (2011) used SRAP and ISSR markers to assemble a genetic map consisting of 170 SRAP markers and 29 ISSRs in 25 linkage groups. In a fiber crop, Chen et al., (2011) used SRAP, ISSR and RAPD markers to construct a genetic map in Kenaf (*Hibiscus cannabinus* L.) that is one of the most economically important fiber crops globally.

4. QTL mapping

A common application of genetic maps is QTL mapping of complex traits. Since QTL are often underpinned by multiple genes in a genome, it is difficult to tag QTL using procedures for tagging Mendelian loci. In general, if a complex trait is changed into a simple Mendelian trait and the underlying QTL is Mendelized, many strategies are available to map and clone the Mendelized genes. In fact, most cloned QTL have been accomplished through such a Mendelized strategy by developing near-isogenic lines (NILs). However, most QTL are not easily Mendelized, so it is necessary to construct genetic maps first and then perform QTL mapping.

In canola, we used SRAP and SSR to construct a genetic map in a doubled haploid (DH) line population that was developed from a synthetic yellow-seeded line and a conventional canola cultivar through microspore culture (Chen et al., 2009). Data for three complex traits including days to flowering, oil content and seed yield at three locations for three years were collected and used in QTL mapping. For oil content, 27 QTL on 14 linkage groups and for seed yield, 18 QTL on 11 linkage groups were identified while days to flowering was suggested to be controlled by a single genetic locus in this mapping population. In rapeseed, Chen et al., (2007) used 208 SSR and 189 SRAP markers to construct a genetic map for a DH line population and performed QTL mapping of yield-related traits in *B. napus*. They also developed a fixed immortalized population from randomly permutated intermating of these DH lines. They collected data for six yield-related traits, plant height, height of lowest primary effective branch, length of main inflorescence, silique length, number of primary branches and silique density. After QTL mapping in the DH line and immortalized populations, they identified 29 common QTL between the two populations, suggesting that there are some chromosomal regions containing QTL for multiple traits. In another QTL mapping report, Fu et al., (2007) constructed a genetic map in *B. napus* to map gene loci controlling the yellow seeded trait. They developed 420 SSR, RAPD and SRAP markers and assembled two genetic maps, of which one contained 26 linkage groups and another which had 20 linkage groups. After QTL analysis, they identified 19 QTL with one common in the two mapping populations. Further analysis allowed them to identify the collinear genomic region of chromosome 5 in Arabidopsis.

In cotton, Lin et al., (2005) developed a mapping population by crossing *G. hirsutum* and *G. barbadense* and performed QTL mapping with a genetic map constructed with SRAP, SSR and RAPD markers. Using 437 SRAP, 107 RAPD and 205 SSR markers, they constructed a genetic map with 566 markers assembled into 41 linkage groups, of which 28 were assigned to the corresponding known chromosomes. This genetic map was used to perform QTL mapping for fiber traits. In total, 13 QTL for fibre traits including two QTL for fibre strength, four QTL for fibre length and seven QTL for micronaire value were identified, of which six QTL were assigned into the A-subgenome, another six QTL into the D-subgenome while one QTL was not assigned. Three QTL for micronaire value were identified to cluster on linkage group 1, suggesting that the flanking molecular markers of these three QTL might be useful in marker-assisted selection for this trait.

Similarly, Zhang et al., (2009b) reported on QTL mapping in cotton using SRAP and other markers. They assembled a genetic map containing 509 SSR, 58 intron targeted intron/exon splice junction (IT-ISJ), 29 SRAP and 8 morphological loci in 60 linkage groups. Among these 60 linkage groups, 54 were assigned into 26 chromosomes. This genetic map was used to identify QTL for fiber quality traits in five environments. In total, thirteen QTL including four QTL for fiber length, two QTL for fiber strength, two QTL for fiber fineness, three QTL for fiber length uniformity, and two QTL for fiber elongation were identified. Eleven out of 13 QTL were assigned into the A-subgenome and other two QTL, into the D-subgenome.

In chrysanthemum (*Dendranthema morifolium*), Zhang et al., (2011b) performed QTL mapping of inflorescence-related traits using SRAP markers. They constructed two genetic maps in a F_1 segregating population using a double pseudo-testcross mapping strategy. With 500 SRAP primer combinations, they produced 896 polymorphic loci and assembled 333 SRAP markers into 57 linkage groups on one genetic map, 342 SRAP markers into 55 linkage groups on the second genetic map. The results indicated that the distribution of these SRAP markers on these two genetic maps was quite uniform. Using these two genetic maps, they mapped 12 QTL for three inflorescence traits, of which each four QTL underpinned specified flower diameter, ray floret layer number, and ray floret length, respectively.

In radish, Xu et al., (2012) recently constructed a genetic map with 592 molecular markers including 287 SRAP, 135 RAPD, 78 SSR, 49 ISSR, 29 randomly amplified microsatellite polymorphism (RAMP), and 14 resistant gene analogs (RGA). They used this genetic map to analyze QTL that controlled root cadmium accumulation. They mapped four QTL on linkage groups 1. 4. 6 and 9. The QTL on linkage group 9 was a major one that accounted for 48.64% of phenotypic variance, suggesting that this QTL might be applied for marker assisted selection to improve radish root quality by reducing cadmium concentration.

5. Gene tagging and cloning

SRAP technology has several merits for gene tagging. Since SRAP detection uses unlimited primer combinations and there are multiple loci detected in a single SRAP PCR reaction, SRAP technology is advantageous over other molecular marker systems for gene tagging. After many genetic loci in a genome are screened quickly, closely linked SRAP markers to a trait of interest can be identified easily. We intensively used SRAP to perform gene tagging and cloning in Brassica species and worked on several economically important traits such as yellow-seeded canola and rapeseed, disease resistance and glucosinolates.

Yellow-seeded oilseeds in Brassica species are suggested to be related to high oil content so it is worthwhile to characterize the genes controlling seed coat color. Using SRAP technology, we cloned and characterized a gene controlling seed coat color and plant hairiness traits in *B. rapa* (Zhang et al., 2009a). We used 1,100 SRAP primer combinations to screen pooled DNA from yellow-seeded and black-seeded individuals based on the bulk segregant analysis (BSA) strategy and found 48 SRAP primer combinations that produced polymorphic loci in the pooled DNA samples from yellow-seeded and black-seeded individuals. Then we tested more pooled DNA and identified 13 SRAP markers that were linked to the gene of interest. Sequencing these SRAP markers allowed the identification of a chromosomal region that was further used to develop new SCAR markers. With new SCAR markers and chromosome walking, we eventually identified the candidate gene and characterized the gene by complementary transformation of the corresponding mutant in Arabidopsis. The functional copy of the candidate gene recovered the phenotype of the Arabidopsis mutant and the non-functional copy in *B. rapa* mutant did not so the candidate was confirmed to underpin the yellow-seeded mutation in *B. rapa*.

Similarly, we used SRAP to tag other genes controlling the seed-coat color trait in yellow sarson, another yellow-seeded *B. rapa* and also in yellow-seeded *B. napus* canola (Rahman et al., 2007, 2010). Yellow sarson is bright yellow-seeded and there is no color variation under different environments while all yellow-seeded canola accessions developed with yellow sarson are not pure yellow and the seed coat color varies due to differences in maturity and environments. Using SRAP screening, we identified several SRAP markers linked to one seed coat color gene. After extended flanking regions were sequenced, one closely-linked SRAP marker was successfully converted into SNP and SCAR markers. Meanwhile, we analyzed a yellow-seeded canola line that was developed with yellow sarson and found that three genes controlled the yellow-seeded color in this *B. napus* line (Rahman et al., 2010). We identified one SRAP marker that was linked closely to one seed color locus and confirmed that this locus was located on linkage group N9 of our ultradense genetic map of *B. napus*. The second locus was mapped on linkage group N13 of our ultradense genetic map. To identify SRAP markers for the third locus, we screened 768 SRAP primer combinations and eventually found one SRAP that was linked closely to the yellow seeded color locus. These SRAP, SNP and SCAR markers can be used in marker assisted selection of yellow-seeded trait in oilseed crops of *B. rapa* and *B. napus*.

SRAP technology is an effective molecular marker system to analyze qualitative and quantitative resistance to plant diseases. In general, qualitative and quantitative resistances are conferred by oligogenic or multigenic loci, respectively. In canola, blackleg is a major disease and qualitative resistance is available. We used the previously described ultradense genetic map to tag resistance genes to blackleg in *B. napus*. After screening 384 SRAP primer combinations, we identified two SRAP markers that were linked to a blackleg resistance gene. By compared the linked SRAP markers with the molecular markers on the ultradense *B. napus* genetic map that was constructed with another mapping population, we found that one SRAP marker corresponded to a SRAP marker on N10. Therefore we took the flanking SRAP markers of the mapped resistance locus on N10 and identified other SRAP markers on the genetic map that were also polymorphic in the mapping population of the blackleg resistance gene. Eventually, further analysis allowed us to identify two blackleg resistance genes in the region where one resistance gene was suggested by other researchers (Long et al., 2010).

In several reports, SRAP markers were used to map genes controlling resistance to plant diseases in several crop species. For instance, Yi et al., (2008) used SRAP, STS and SSR markers to tag a resistance gene (*Pm4b*) to powdery mildew in wheat. They tested 240 SRAP primer combinations and identified two SRAP markers linked to the *Pm4b* gene. Eventually, they mapped the *Pm4b* gene on chromosome 2AL that was flanked by SRAP, STS and SSR markers. In another study on gene mapping in wheat, Chen et al., (2012) used SSR, SRAP and TRAP markers to tag a wheat strip rust resistance gene. Using 400 SSR, 315 pairs of SRAP primers, and 40 pairs of TRAP primers to screen F_1, F_2 and BC_1 mapping populations, they constructed a fine map flanking the resistance gene locus on chromosome arm 2AS and suggested that the mapped resistance gene should be a novel one.

In rice, Zhao et al., (2010) searched for SSR markers linked to a dominant resistance gene (RSV1) to rice stripe virus and then used the SRAP method to find closely linked markers. They located RSV1 into a region flanked by SSR and SRAP markers. In maize, a new dominant resistance gene to maize head smut was tagged by SSR-BSA and SRAP-BSA methods (Li et al., 2012). Closely linked molecular markers were identified and used to transfer the resistance gene from the resistant source to elite lines via marker assisted selection to breed head smut resistant hybrid cultivars in maize.

In eggplant, Mutlu et al., (2008) tagged a Fusarium wilt resistance gene using SRAP, SRAP-RGA, RAPD, and SCAR markers. They used 2316 primer combinations to identify molecular markers linked to the resistance gene, of which two SRAP markers were closely linked to the resistance gene. The SRAP markers were converted into SCAR markers and used in marker assisted selection of the Fusarium wilt resistance in eggplant.

Besides plant disease resistance, genes underpinning other traits have been tagged using SRAP technology, For instance, genes controlling two important traits, sex determination and tuberculate fruit in cucumber were tagged using SRAP technology (Li et al., 2008; Zhang et al., 2010a). In cucumber, there are three major gene loci, F/f, M/m, and A/a that determine various sex types. Li et al., (2008) analyzed M/m gene locus and identified 8 SRAP markers linked to this gene locus. Additionally, they used SRAP markers to perform chromosome walking and converted some SRAP markers to co-dominant SCAR markers through sequencing SRAP fragments. Eventually they identified very closely linked SRAP markers at a genetic distance of less than one cM. Similarly, Zhang et al., (2010a) performed gene tagging of cucumber tuberculate fruit. They found that the tuberculate fruit (Tu) was controlled by a dominant gene and used a BSA strategy to identify molecular markers linked to this dominant gene. After testing 736 SRAP primer combinations, they found 9 SRAP markers that were linked to the Tu gene and used SSR markers to anchor this gene on chromosome 5, further indicating that they would use the mapping results to clone the Tu gene later.

Male sterility is a commonly used method to produce hybrid seeds for exploiting heterosis in crops. Since genic male sterility is usually controlled by a few genes, SRAP technology is useful to tag the genes underpinning male sterility. For example, Zhang et al., (2011c) used SRAP and SSR markers to tag a dominant genic male sterile gene in *B. oleracea*. They performed BSA analysis with SRAP and SSR markers. By screening polymorphisms between fertile bulks and sterile bulks with 26,417 SRAP primer pairs, they identified 14 SRAP markers that were linked to the male sterility gene MS-cd1. After sequencing the SRAP fragments, three SRAP markers were converted into SCAR markers that were very closely linked to the MS-cd1 gene. Moreover, through comparative genomics with SRAP sequences, they identified a collinear region on chromosome A10 in *B. rapa* corresponding to a collinear genomic region of chromosome 5 in Arabidopsis, which could lead to cloning of this gene in the future.

SRAP technology has also been used to tag quantitative traits using the same approaches as described previously in qualitative traits. In alfalfa, Castonguay et al., (2010) used SRAP to identify polymorphic genetic loci that controlled superior tolerance to freezing. Through BSA analysis, they found four SRAP markers that were associated with freezing tolerance and the frequency of their occurrence reflected changes in response to selection. In another report, SRAP was used to tag a major QTL controlling cadmium accumulation in oat (Tanhuanpaa et al 2007). The concentration of toxic cadmium in oat grains is often over the accepted limit and must be reduced. SRAP, RAPD and retrotransposon-microsatellite amplified polymorphism (REMAP) markers were used to perform BSA analysis in an F2 population and four molecular markers were identified to be associated with cadmium concentration in oat grains. All these four markers were located on the same linkage group, suggesting that this mapped QTL had major effect on grain cadmium concentration in oat.

6. Genetic diversity

Genetic diversity analysis is necessary in plant breeding, plant systematics and evolution, plant pathology. SRAP is an adequate molecular marker system for genetic diversity analysis in plants and fungi. Since SRAP has many features such as simplicity, reliability, flexibility, detection of multiple loci and cost-effectiveness, which allows beginners and experienced people to perform SRAP routinely with limited facilities or in well-established genomics labs. Since genome sequence information is not necessary for SRAP detection, SRAP can be used to perform genetic diversity analysis in a wide range of living organisms. We first used SRAP to analyze the genetic diversity of parental lines that were used to produce hybrid cultivars in *B. napus* (Riaz et al., 2001). As expected, we found that there was a positive correlation of genetic distance and hybrid performance. In celery, we used SRAP to tag a major resistance locus to celery mosaic virus (Ruiz et al., 2001).

In melons, Ferriol et al., (200) used SRAP and AFLP to analyze 69 accessions selected from morphotypes and unclassified types that belong to two subspecies, *Cucurbita pepo* ssp. *pepo* and ssp. *ovifera*. Among these accessions, some commercial cultivars and Spanish landraces represent diversified types in Europe. Their results showed that SRAP markers characterized well the morphological variability and the evolutionary history of these tested accessions better than AFLP markers. Molecular markers were used to identify new types for the development of new cultivars. The genetic diversity in the landraces of *C. pepo* spp. *ovifera* was detected with molecular markers, which is useful for preserving the diversity in this species.

In grasses, Budak et al., (2004a; 2004b; 2005) used SRAP to analyze genetic diversity and ploidy complexity in buffalograss. They found that SRAP markers were abundant and that they could distinguish genetic diversity among closely related cultivars. Their data showed that among several molecular markers (SSRs, ISSRs, SRAPs, and RAPDs), SRAP estimated the highest mean genetic dissimilarities in buffalograss. Additionally, they used SRAP and other markers to analyze ploidy complex and geographic origin of the *Buchloe dactyloides* genome and identified a significant correlation between the ploidy levels such as diploid, tetraploid, pentaploid, and hexaploid and the numbers of alleles detected using nuclear DNA markers. SRAP again was the best one among three molecular markers (ISSR, SSR, and SRAP, r = 0.39, 0.39, and 0.41).

Similarly, Gulsen et al., (2009) used SRAP, peroxidase gene polymorphism (POGP), ISSR and RAPD to study the relationship of ploidy levels, geographic locations and genetic diversity in bermudagrass. They found that there was a significant correlation between ploidy levels in diploids, triploids, tetraploids, pentaploids, and hexaploids and band frequencies of molecular markers ($r = 0.62$, $P < 0.001$), suggesting that ploidy levels resulted in genome variation and genetic diversity. Geographic locations of Cynodon accessions also contributed to genetic diversity based on molecular marker analysis. They suggested that combining several molecular markers would be more efficient to evaluate genetic diversity and genetic structure in bermudagrass and eventually broaden genetic basis for developing new cultivars.

In elephant grass, Xie et al., (2009) used SRAP markers to study the genetic diversity and relationships of commonly used cultivars in China. They generated 1,395 genetic loci with 62 SRAP primer combinations with an average of 22.5 genetic loci per primer combination. They found that SRAP loci were very polymorphic (72.8%) and used these SRAPs to estimate the genetic diversity within and between elephant grass cultivars. The results showed the genetic diversity within cultivars was less than that among tested cultivars and the relationship of those tested cultivars was also estimated.

In cereal crops, Zaefizadeh and Goleiv (2009) analyzed genetic diversity and relationships among durum wheat landraces by SRAP marker and phenotypic differences. They used 65 SRAP markers and 27 traits to perform cluster analysis of 40 subconvars of *Triticum durum* landraces from the region of North West Iran and Azerbaijan. Traits failed to detect any geographic association in durum landraces while 12 combinations of SRAP markers were distinguishable among these landraces, suggesting that SRAP technology is useful for genetic diversity and evolutionary relationship analysis, marker assisted selection and genetic map construction in durum wheat. Yang et al., (2010) used SRAP markers to analyze the genetic diversity of hulless barley cultivars from Sichuan, Gansu, Tibet, Qinghai and Yunnan provinces of the Qinghai-Tibet Plateau in China. With 20 SRAP primer combinations, they detected 153 polymorphic loci and used these SRAP markers to classify 68 hulless barley accessions into four major groups using a unweighted pair-grouping method with arithmetic averages (UPGMA) analysis. They concluded that SRAP was an effective method to perform genetic diversity in hulless barley and develop new cultivars.

In rice, Dai et al., (2012) developed indica- and japonica-specific markers using SRAP, TRAP, and SSR markers and performed genetic diversity analysis of Asian *Oryza sativa* varieties. In general, rice varieties are classified into *O. sativa* ssp. *japonica* kata and ssp. *indica* kata. In this report, they used 45 rice varieties in a cultivated and wild rice collection to study the genetic diversity in rice. By developing 90 indica- and japonica-specific genetic loci, they could easily distinguish typical indica and japonica subspecies and determined whether a domesticated rice variety came from the indica or japonica type.

In alfalfa, Vandemark et al.,(2006) used SRAP markers to analyze genetic relationships among historical sources of alfalfa germplasm in North American. Their results showed that SRAP detected highly polymorphic loci (>90%) in alfalfa, which distinguished nine original sources of Medicago germplasm based on genetic similarity calculated with SRAP markers. They suggested that SRAP technology is an adequate marker system for detecting polymorphisms in alfalfa.

In sesame, Zhang et al., (2010b) performed genetic diversity analysis using SRAP and SSR markers. They analyzed 404 landraces from a sesame collection in China. Using11 SRAP and 3 SSR markers, they produced 175 fragments, of which 126 were polymorphic with an average polymorphism rate of 72%. They calculated several parameters such as Jaccard's genetic similarity coefficients, Nei's gene diversity and Shannon's information index and constructed a dendrogram with all the 404 landraces. According to the dendrogram, landraces from different agro-ecological zones did not cluster together, suggesting that geographical locations did not represent the greater genetic variation among the sesame landraces. They concluded that SRAP and SSR markers would be useful to study sesame genetic diversity and understand the relationship of those indigenous landraces, which would guide the collection, protection and utilization of sesame landraces in breeding purposes.

In banana and plantain, Youssef et al., (2011) used SRAP and AFLP markers to analyze 40 Musa accessions including commercial cultivars and wild species. They developed 353 SRAP and 787 AFLP markers to perform cluster analysis using an unweighted pair-grouping method with arithmetic averages (UPGMA) and principal coordinate (PCO) analysis. They eventually assigned all the 40 accessions into corresponding *Eumusa, Australimusa, Callimusa* and *Rhodochlamys* sections and species. They found that SRAP and AFLP polymorphism amongst sections and species and the relationships within *Eumusa* species and subspecies were not consistent and suggested that SRAP produced threefold more specific and unique loci than AFLP. Therefore, the data showed that SRAP markers were effective to distinguish *M. acuminata, M. balbisiana* and *M. schizocarpa* in the *Eumusa* section, and also triploid plantains and cooking bananas.

In grape, Guo et al., (2012) used SRAP markers to study genetic variability and relationships of cultivated wine-type *Vitis vinifera* and wild *Vitis* species. They selected 76 grape genotypes representing indigenous and new varieties and wild *Vitis* species from China and other countries. After testing 100 SRAP primer combinations, they selected 19 primer combinations based on primer performance to produce 228 genetic loci, of which 78.63% were polymorphic with an average polymorphism information content value of 0.76. The SRAP markers were used to perform cluster analysis to evaluate Nei and Li's similarity coefficients by unweighted pair-group method of arithmetic averages (UPGMA) analysis. Additionally, they performed principal coordinate analysis (PCoA) to plot all 76 grape genotypes which showed a similar cluster pattern to that in the dendrogram, representing their geographical origins and taxonomic classification of these grape varieties. All the results indicated that three main groups including table grape of *V. vinifera,* table grape of Euro-America hybrids and wine grape of *V. vinifera,* wild *Vitis* species were identified and also the table *V. vinifera* group was genetically different from the wine-type *V. vinifera* and wild *Vitis* species originated from America and China. So they suggested that SRAP markers are informative and grape germplasm in China contains abundant genetic diversity.

In medicinal plants, Ortega et al., (2007) analyzed genetic diversity of cultivated and non-cultivated mashua, *Tropaeolum tuberosum* that were grown in six communities in the Cusco region of Perú and selected from the germplasm collection at the International Potato Center (CIP) using SRAP markers. Mashua is used as a medicinal plant, possibly due to a high concentration of glucosinolates in mashua roots. DNA fingerprinting generated by SRAP markers showed that mashua is a genetically variable crop. The genetic analysis also showed that most non-cultivated accessions were likely feral races resulting from escape from cultivation rather than wild relatives. In another medicinal plant, Wang et al., (2012) analyzed the genetic diversity of 35 wild goat's rue accessions (*Galega officinalis* L.) collected from Russia and Europe countries using ISSR and SRAP markers. Although there was some discrepancy between ISSR and SRAP markers, the clustering patterns of genotypes were relatively consistent between these two kinds of molecular markers in this study. They indicated that both markers were useful for goat's rue germplasm characterization, improvement, and conservation.

In ornamental plants, Hao et al., (2008) used SRAP technology to perform genetic diversity analysis of 29 ornamental and medicinal Paeonia. Dendrogram and principle component analysis indicated that SRAP markers well characterized the genetic relationships of these 29 peony cultivars, which is useful to guide parent selection and molecular marker assisted selection in Paeonia breeding. In another ornamental plant, Feng et al., (2009b) performed genetic analysis of diversity and population structure of *Celosia argentea* and related species using SRAP markers. They included 16 populations of *C. argentea.* and 6 populations of *C. cristata.* from China. Using 10 SRAP primer combinations, they produced 507 scored bands, of which 274 were polymorphic. With UPGMA cluster analysis, they constructed a phylogenetic tree and calculated genetic distances of all 22 populations. The results showed that the genetic distances of all populations were coincident with their geographic origins. Additionally, they identified one SRAP marker separating accessions in *C. argentea* from those in *C. cristata* and suggested that the extensive genetic diversity in *C. argentea* populations would be very useful for breeding and conservation of *C. argentea* varieties in the future.

In chrysanthemum, Zhang et al., (2011a) did a genetic diversity study on two flowering traits of chrysanthemum, initial blooming time and the duration of flowering. They identified two pairs of major genes with high levels of inheritance. Using SRAP technology, they performed association mapping of these two traits and identified SRAP markers that were significantly associated with phenotypes, suggesting that SRAP markers might be useful in chrysanthemum breeding. In another report on ornamental plants, Soleimani et al., (2012) used wild, cultivated, and ornamental pomegranates (*Punica granatum* L.) in Iran to perform analysis of genetic diversity and population structure with SRAP molecular markers. They produced 133 SRAP markers with 13 SRAP primer combinations to evaluate the genetic diversity of 63 pomegranate genotypes from five different geographical regions of Iran. Their data showed that the average polymorphism information content value was 0.28 and the genetic distance was 0.10 to 0.37 with an average of 0.24 in all 63 genotypes. Cluster analysis allowed them to identify the relationship between ornamental and wild genotypes. They found that the genetic variation of genotypes from various regions was bigger than that of intra regions. They concluded that SRAP markers could be an effective marker system in the analysis of genetic diversity and population structure in pomegranate.

In woody plants, Li et al., (2010) did genetic diversity analysis of sea buckthorn which is grown as a nutritious berry crop. They produced 191 polymorphic loci using SRAP technology to perform cluster analysis of 77 accessions, of which 73 *Hippophae rhamnoides* were classified into 2 groups and 4 *H. salicifolia,* into 1 group. They associated SRAP markers with dried-shrink disease (DSD) resistance and suggested SRAP markers are useful for breeding new sea buckthorn lines with resistance to DSD. Feng et al., (2009a) reported on the genetic diversity analysis of *Pinus koraiensis* using SRAP markers. They obtained 24 to 33 loci per primer combination and used 143 SRAP markers to analyze 480 samples collected from 24 provinces in China. They found that there was no significant difference in genetic diversity among provinces. However, genetic variation of intra population accounted for 93.355% of the total variation.

In fungi, Sun et al., (2006) used SRAP markers to classify *Ganoderma lucidum* strains. They performed genetic diversity analysis with 31 accessions collected from several countries. Using 75 polymorphic loci, they classified all 31 accessions into five groups. The results showed that *G. lucidum* strains were significantly different from *G. sinense* and *G. lucidum* in China, also different from *G. lucidum* in Yugoslavia. They suggested that SRAP markers are useful in taxonomy and systematics of Ganoderma strains within basidiomycetes. In another fungus, Tang et al., (2010) analyzed Chinese *Auricularia auricula* strains using SRAP and ISSR markers. They found both SRAP and ISSR markers were abundant in *A. auricula* and could be used to effectively distinguish all tested strains. After phylogenetic analysis, they classified 34 *A. auricula* strains into four or five major groups using the UPGMA method. They suggested that genetic diversity information would be used in *A. auricula* breeding programs to develop new medicinal mushroom. Fu et al., (2010) performed genetic diversity analysis in 23 elite *Lentinula edodes* strains from China using RAPD, ISSR and SRAP markers. In total, they used 16 RAPD primers, 5 ISSR primers and 23 SRAP primer combinations to produce 138, 77 and 144 bands, respectively. After UPGMA clustering analysis, they classified all 23 *L. edodes* strains into three or four groups. However, all groups showed high levels of similarity, showing a low level of genetic diversity in all tested strains.

7. Other applications

SRAP amplification is actually a small portion of all possible sampling of a genome. So SRAP can be used to produce a reduced genome samples when multiple SRAP reactions are pooled. As described previously, pooled SRAP produces can be directly sequenced using next generation sequencing technologies. When replacing genomic DNA with cDNA samples, SRAP is adequate to perform gene expression profiling and also construct cDNA genetic maps.

More recently, Yu et al., (2012) used SRAP markers to distinguish fertile somatic hybrids of *G. hirsutum L.* and *G. trilobum* produced by protoplast fusion. They obtained fertile somatic hybrids by symmetric electrofusion of protoplasts of tetraploid upland cotton *G. hirsutum* and wild cotton *G. trilobum.* These hybrids were confirmed using morphological characteristics, flow cytometric analysis, and molecular markers including RAPD, SRAP and AFLP.

In aquaculture, Ding et al., (2010) used SRAP and SCAR markers to differentiate two cultured populations in grass carp (*Ctenopharyngodon idella*). Through cloning and sequencing SRAP fragments, they developed SCAR markers to characterize individuals from the cultured population and the wild population, showing different frequencies of SCAR alleles (87% in the cultured population and 6% in the wild), suggesting that this SCAR might serve as a specific molecular marker for the cultured population. They also identified eight SRAP fragments that shared high similarities to functional genes.

8. Summary remarks

SRAP was first used to construct a genetic map and tag genes in *Brassica oleracea* in 2001 (Li and Quiros, 2001). This molecular marker technology is simply performed with one round PCR to amplify multiple or occasionally over a hundred loci in a genome. In its PCR reaction mixture, two random primers are included, which leads to maximum flexibility in primer designing and primer labelling. There is no limitation on primer combinations and one labelled primer may be combined with any number of unlabelled primers. Most SRAP products fall into a size range of 100 to 1000 base pairs, which can be separated in both polyacrylamide and agarose gels. In automatized detection, one SRAP primer is fluorescently labelled and SRAP products can be analyzed using advanced instruments such as an ABI genetic analyzer, which dramatically increases throughput of SRAP molecular marker detection.

There is a wide range of applications of SRAP technology such as genetic map construction, genetic diversity analysis, gene tagging and cloning. Since SRAP detects multiple loci in one reaction, it is feasible to construct ultradense genetic maps with over 10,000 SRAP molecular markers. SRAP has advantages over other molecular detection techniques in gene tagging and cloning and allows screening thousands of loci shortly to pinpoint the genetic position underlying the trait of interest. Sequencing SRAP products enhances the applications of SRAP technology. In well characterized genomes, SRAP sequences are used to identify the chromosomal region of mapped genes while in species without a known whole genome sequence, sequences of SRAP markers on a genetic map allow arranging sequence contigs and assembly of a whole genome sequence.

SRAP molecular technology is very useful in plant breeding. In QTL mapping, common QTL for the same trait of interest can be effectively identified. Since SRAP has a high throughput feature, multiple mapping populations can be analyzed effectively to construct several genetic maps. In addition, the same set of SRAP primers allows detection of the same genetic loci, which can used to align several genetic maps. SRAP is effective and efficient in marker assisted selection in plant breeding since thousands of samples can be analyzed inexpensively. SRAP technology has been commonly used in analysis of genetic diversity of many plant species. Currently, SRAP are used in most crops, tree species, ornamental and medicinal plants.

Author details

Genyi Li[1], Peter B. E. McVetty[1] and Carlos F. Quiros[2]

1 Department of Plant Science, University of Manitoba, MB, Canada

2 Department of Plant Sciences, University of California, Davis, CA, USA

References

[1] Budak, H. R. C., Shearman, I., Parmaksiz, R. E., Gaussoin, T. P., & Riosdan, D. (2004a). Molecular characterization of Buffalograss germplasm using sequence-related amplified polymorphism markers. *Theor Appl Genet.* , 108, 328-334.

[2] Budak, H., Shearman, R. C., Parmaksiz, I., & Dweikat, I. (2004b). Comparative analysis of seeded and vegetative biotype buffalograsses based on phylogenetic relationship using ISSRs, SSRs, RAPDs, and SRAPs. *Theor Appl Genet.* , 109, 280-8.

[3] Budak, H., Shearman, R. C., Gulsen, O., & Dweikat, I. (2005). Understanding ploidy complex and geographic origin of the *Buchloe dactyloides* genome using cytoplasmic and nuclear marker systems. *Theor Appl Genet.* , 111, 1545-52.

[4] Castonguay, Y., Cloutier, J., Bertrand, A., Michaud, R., & Laberge, S. (2010). SRAP polymorphisms associated with superior freezing tolerance in alfalfa (*Medicago sativa* spp. *sativa*). *Theor Appl Genet.* , 120, 1611-9.

[5] Chen, G., Geng, J., Rahman, M., Liu, X., Tu, J., Fu, T., Li, G., Mc Vetty, P. B. E., & Tahir, M. (2009). Identification of QTL for oil content, seed yield, and flowering time in oilseed rape (*Brassica napus*). *Euphytica* , 142, 161-174.

[6] Chen, M., Wei, C., Qi, J., Chen, X., Su, J., Li, A., Tao, A., & Wu, W. (2011). Genetic linkage map construction for kenaf using SRAP, ISSR and RAPD markers. *Plant Breed.* , 130, 679-687.

[7] Chen, S., Chen, G., Chen, H., Wei, Y., Li, W., Liu, Y., Liu, D., Lan, X., & Zheng, Y. (2012). Mapping stripe rust resistance gene YrSph derived from *Tritium sphaerococcum* Perc. with SSR, SRAP, and TRAP markers. *Euphytica* , 185, 19-26.

[8] Chen, W., Zhang, Y., Liu, X., Chen, B., Tu, J., & Fu, T. (2007). Detection of QTL for six yield-related traits in oilseed rape (*Brassica napus*) using DH and immortalized F(2) populations. *Theor Appl Genet.* , 115, 849-58.

[9] Chen, X., Xia, Z., Fu, Y., Lu, C., & Wang, W. (2010). Constructing a genetic linkage map using an F_1 population of non-inbred parents in cassava (*Manihot esculenta* Crantz). *Plant Molecular Biology Reporter* , 28, 676-683.

[10] Dai, X., Yang, Y., Zhou, L., Ou, L., Liang, M., Li, W., Kang, G., & Chen, B. (2012). Analysis of indica- and japonica-specific markers of *Oryza sativa* and their applications. *Plant Systematics and Evolution* , 298, 287-296.

[11] Ding, W., Cao, Z., & Cao, L. (2010). Molecular analysis of grass carp (*Ctenopharyngodon idella*) by SRAP and SCAR molecular markers. *Aquaculture International* , 18, 575-587.

[12] Feng, F., Chen, M., Zhang, D., Sui, X., & Han, S. (2009a). Application of SRAP in the genetic diversity of *Pinus koraiensis* of different provenances. *African Journal of Biotechnology* , 8, 1000-1008.

[13] Feng, N., Xue, Q., Guo, Q., Zhao, R., & Guo, M. (2009b). Genetic diversity and population structure of *Celosia argentea* and related species revealed by SRAP. *Biochem Genet.* , 47, 521-32.

[14] Ferriol, M., Pico, B., & Nuez, F. (2003). Genetic diversity of a germplasm collection of *Cucurbita pepo* using SRAP and AFLP markers. *Theor Appl Genet.* , 107, 271-282.

[15] Fu, F. Y., Liu, L. Z., Chai, Y., Chen, L., Yang, T., Jin, M., , A., Yan, X., Zhang, Z., & Li, J. (2007). localization of QTLs for seed color using recombinant inbred lines of *Brassica napus* in different environments. *Genome* , 50, 840-854.

[16] Fu, L., Zhang, H., Wu, X., Li, H., Wei, H., Wu, Q., & Wang, L. (2010). Evaluation of genetic diversity in *Lentinula edodes* strains using RAPD, ISSR and SRAP markers. *World Journal of Microbiology and Biotechnology* , 26, 709-716.

[17] Gao, M., Li, G., Yang, B., Qiu, D., Farnham, M., & Quiros, C. F. (2007). High-density *Brassica oleracea* map: Identification of useful new linkages. *Theor Appl Genet.* , 115, 277-287.

[18] Gulsen, O., Sever-Mutlu, S., Mutlu, N., Tuna, M., Karaguzel, O., Shearman, R. C., Riordan, T. P., & Heng-Moss, T. M. (2009). Polyploidy creates higher diversity among *Cynodon* accessions as assessed by molecular markers. *Theor Appl Genet.* , 118, 1309-19.

[19] Gulsen, O., Uzun, A., Canan, I., Seday, U., & Canihos, E. (2010). A new citrus linkage map based on SRAP, SSR, ISSR, POGP, RGA and RAPD markers. *Euphytica* , 173, 265-277.

[20] Guo, D., Zhang, J., Liu, C., Zhang, G., Li, M., & Zhang, Q. (2012). Genetic variability and relationships between and within grape cultivated varieties and wild species based on SRAP markers. *Tree Genetics & Genomes* , 8, 789-800.

[21] Hao, Q., Liu, Z., Shu, Q., Zhang, R., Rick, J. D., & Wang, L. (2008). Studies on *Paeonia* cultivars and hybrids identification based on SRAP analysis. *Hereditas* , 145, 38-47.

[22] Jones, N., Ougham, H., Thomas, H., & Pasakinskiene, I. (2009). Markers and mapping revisited: finding your gene. *New Phytol.* , 183, 935-66.

[23] Levi, A., Thomas, C. E., Trebitsh, T., Salman, A., King, J., Karalius, J., Newman, M., Reddy, O. U. K., Xu, Y., & Zhang, X. (2006). An extended linkage map for watermelon based on SRAP, AFLP, SSR, ISSR, and RAPD markers. *J Am Soc Hortic Sci.* , 131, 393-402.

[24] Li, G., Gao, M., Yang, B., & Quiros, C. F. (2003). Gene to gene alignment between the Arabidopsis and *Brassica oleracea* genomes. *Theor Appl Genet.* , 107, 168-80.

[25] Li, G., & Quiros, C. F. (2001). Sequence-related amplified polymorphism (SRAP), a new marker system based on a simple PCR reaction: Its application to mapping and gene tagging in Brassica. *Theor Appl Genet.* , 103, 455-461.

[26] Li, H., Ruan, C. J., Silva, T., Jaime, A., & Liu, B. Q. (2010). Associations of SRAP markers with dried-shrink disease resistance in a germplasm collection of sea buckthorn (*Hippophae rhamnoides* L.). *Genome* , 53, 447-457.

[27] Li, W., Xu, X., Li, G., Guo, Q., Wu, S., Jiang, Y., Dong, H., Weng, M., Jin, D., Wu, J., Ru, Z., & Wang, B. (2012). Characterization and molecular mapping of RsrR, a resistant gene to maize head smut. *Euphytica* (DOIs10681-012-0747-4, in press).

[28] Li, W., Zhang, J., Mou, Y., Geng, J., Mc Vetty, P. B. E., Hu, S., & Li, G. (2011). Integration of Solexa sequences on an ultradense genetic map in *Brassica rapa* L. *BMC Genomics* 12: 249.

[29] Li, Z., Pan, J., Guan, Y., Tao, Q., He, H., Si, L., & Cai, R. (2008). Development and fine mapping of three co-dominant SCAR markers linked to the M/m gene in the cucumber plant (*Cucumis sativus* L.).*Theor Appl Genet.* , 117, 1253-60.

[30] Lin, Z.., He, D., Zhang, X., Nie, Y., Guo, X., Feng, C., et al. (2005). Linkage map construction and mapping QTL for cotton fiber quality using SRAP, SSR and RAPD. *Plant Breed.* , 124, 180-187.

[31] Liu, L., , X., Wei, J., Qin, J., & Mo, C. (2011). The first genetic linkage map of Luohanguo (*Siraitia grosvenorii*) based on ISSR and SRAP markers. *Genome* , 54, 19-25.

[32] Long, Y., Wang, Z., Sun, Z., Fernando, D. W. G., Mc Vetty, P. B. E., & Li, G. (2010). Identification of two blackleg resistance genes and fine mapping of one of these two genes in a *Brassica napus* canola cultivar 'Surpass 400'. *Theor Appl Genet.* , 122, 1223-1231.

[33] Mutlu, N., Boyaci, F. H., Göçmen, M., & Abak, K. (2008). Development of SRAP, SRAP-RGA, RAPD and SCAR markers linked with a Fusarium wilt resistance gene in eggplant. *Theor Appl Genet.* , 117, 1303-12.

[34] Ortega, O., Duran, E., Arbizu, C., Ortega, R., Roca, W., Potter, D., & Quiros, C. F. (2007). Pattern of genetic diversity of cultivated and non-cultivated mashua, *Tropaeolum tuberosum,* in the Cusco region of Perú. *Genetic Resources and Crop Evolution* , 54, 807-821.

[35] Rahman, M., Li, G., Schroeder, D., & Mc Vetty, P. B. E. (2010). Inheritance of seed coat color genes in *Brassica napus* (L.) and tagging the genes using SRAP, SCAR and SNP molecular markers. *Molecular Breed.*, 26, 439-453.

[36] Rahman, M., Sun, Z., Mc Vetty, P. B. E., & Li, G. (2007). Development of SRAP, SNP and SCAR molecular markers for the major seed coat color gene in *Brassica rapa*. *Theor Appl Genet.*, 115, 1101-7.

[37] Riaz, A., Li, G., Quresh, Z., Swati, M., & Quiros, C. F. (2001). Genetic diversity of oilseed *Brassica napus* inbred lines based on sequence-related amplified polymorphism and its relation to hybrid performance. *Plant Breed.*, 120, 1-5.

[38] Ruiz, J. J., Pico, B., Li, G., D'Antonio, V., Falk, B., & Quiros, C. F. (2001). Identification of markers linked to a Celery Mosaic Virus resistance gene in celery. *J Amer Soc for Hortic Sci.*, 126(4), 432-435.

[39] Soleimani, M. H., Talebi, M., & Sayed-Tabatabaei, B. E. (2012). Use of SRAP markers to assess genetic diversity and population structure of wild, cultivated, and ornamental pomegranates (Punica granatum L.) in different regions of Iran. *Plant Systematics and Evolution*, 298, 1141-1149.

[40] Sun, S., Gao, W., Lin, S., Zhu, J., Xie, B., & Lin, Z. (2006). Analysis of genetic diversity in Ganoderma population with a novel molecular marker SRAP. *Applied Microbiology and Biotechnology*, 72, 537-543.

[41] Sun, Z., Wang, Z., Tu, J., Zhang, J., Yu, F., Mc Vetty, P. B. E., & Li, G. (2007). An ultradense genetic recombination map for *Brassica napus*, consisting of 13551 SRAP markers. *Theor Appl Genet.*, 114(8), 1305-17.

[42] Tang, L., Xiao, Y., Li, L., Guo, Q., & Bian, Y. (2010). Analysis of genetic diversity among Chinese *Auricularia auricula* cultivars using combined ISSR and SRAP markers. *Current Microbiology*, 61, 132-140.

[43] Tanhuanpää, P., Kalendar, R., Schulman, A. H., & Kiviharju, E. (2007). A major gene for grain cadmium accumulation in oat (*Avena sativa* L.). *Genome*, 50, 588-94.

[44] Vandemark, G. J., Ariss, J. J., Bauchan, G. A., Larsen, R. C., & Hughes, T. J. (2006). Estimating genetic relationships among historical sources of alfalfa germplasm and selected cultivars with sequence related amplified polymorphisms. *Euphytica*, 152, 9-16.

[45] Wang, Z., Wang, J., Wang, X., Gao, H., Dzyubenko, N. I., & Chapurin, V. F. (2012). Assessment of genetic diversity in *Galega officinalis* L. using ISSR and SRAP markers. *Genetic Resources and Crop Evolution*, 59, 865-873.

[46] Xie, W., Zhang, X., Cai, H., Huang, L., Peng, Y., & , X. (2011). Genetic maps of SSR and SRAP markers in diploid orchardgrass (*Dactylis glomerata* L.) using the pseudo-testcross strategy. *Genome*, 54, 212-221.

[47] Xie, X., Zhou, F., Zhang, X., & Zhang, J. (2009). Genetic variability and relationship between MT-1 elephant grass and closely related cultivars assessed by SRAP markers. *Journal of Genetics* , 88, 281-290.

[48] Xu, L., Wang, L., Gong, Y., Dai, W., Wang, Y., Zhu, X., Wen, T., & Liu, L. (2012). Genetic linkage map construction and QTL mapping of cadmium accumulation in radish (*Raphanus sativus* L.).*Theor Appl Genet.* , 125, 659-70.

[49] Xue, D., Feng, S., Zhao, H., Jiang, H., Shen, B., Shi, N., Lu, J., Liu, J., & Wang, H. (2010). The linkage maps of *Dendrobium* species based on RAPD and SRAP markers. *Journal of Genetics and Genomics* , 37, 197-204.

[50] Yang, P., Liu, X., Liu, X., Yang, W., & Feng, Z. (2010). Diversity analysis of the developed qingke (hulless barley) cultivars representing different growing regions of the Qinghai-Tibet Plateau in China using sequence related amplified polymorphism (SRAP) markers. *African Journal of Biotechnology* , 9, 8530-8538.

[51] Yeboah, M. A., Xuehao, C., Feng, C., Liang, G., & Gu, M. (2007). A genetic linkage map of cucumber (*Cucumis sativus* L.) combining SRAP and ISSR markers. *African Journal of Biotechnology* , 6, 2784-2791.

[52] Yi, Y., Liu, H., Huang, X., An, L., Wang, F., & Wang, X. (2008). Development of molecular markers linked to the wheat powdery mildew resistance gene *Pm4b* and marker validation for molecular breeding. *Plant Breed.* , 127, 116-120.

[53] Youssef, M., James, A. C., Rivera-Madrid, R., Ortiz, R., & Escobedo-Gracia, Medrano. R. M. (2011). Musa genetic diversity revealed by SRAP and AFLP. *Molecular Biotechnology* , 47, 189-199.

[54] Yu, J., Yu, S., Lu, C., Wang, W., Fan, S., Song, M., Lin, Z., Zhang, X., & Zhang, J. (2007). High-density linkage map of cultivated allotetraploid cotton based on SSR, TRAP, SRAP and AFLP markers. *Journal of Integrative Plant Biology* , 49, 716-724.

[55] Yu, X., Chu, B., Liu, R., Sun, J., Brian, J. J., Wang, H., Shuijin, Z., & Sun, Y. (2012). Characteristics of fertile somatic hybrids of *G. hirsutum* L. and *G. trilobum* generated via protoplast fusion. *Theor Appl Genet.* 2012 Jul 10.

[56] Zaefizadeh, M., & Goleiv, R. (2009). Diversity and relationships among durum wheat landraces (subconvars) by SRAP and phenotypic marker polymorphism. *Research Journal of Biological Sciences* , 4, 960-966.

[57] Zhang, F., Chen, S., Chen, F., Fang, W., Deng, Y., Chang, Q., & Liu, P. (2011a). Genetic analysis and associated SRAP markers for flowering traits of chrysanthemum (*Chrysanthemum morifolium*). *Euphytica* , 177, 15-24.

[58] Zhang, F., Chen, S., Chen, F., Fang, W., Chen, Y., & Li, F. (2011b). SRAP-based mapping and QTL detection for inflorescence-related traits in chrysanthemum (Dendranthema morifolium). *Molecular Breed.* 27: 11-23,

[59] Zhang, J., Lu, Y., Yuan, Y., Zhang, X., Geng, J., Chen, Y., Cloutier, S., Mc Vetty, P. B. E., & Li, G. (2009a). Map-based cloning and characterization of a gene controlling hairiness and seed coat color traits in *Brassica rapa*. *Plant Molecular Biol.* , 69, 553-563.

[60] Zhang, W., He, H., Guan, Y., Du, H., Yuan, L., Li, Z., Yao, D., Pan, J., & Cai, R. (2010a). Identification and mapping of molecular markers linked to the tuberculate fruit gene in the cucumber (*Cucumis sativus* L.). *Theor Appl Genet.* , 120, 645-654.

[61] Zhang, W., Pan, J., He, H., Zhang, C., Li, Z., Zhao, J., Yuan, X., Zhu, L., Huang, S., & Cai, R. (2012). Construction of a high density integrated genetic map for cucumber (*Cucumis sativus* L.) *Theor Appl Genet.* , 124, 249-259.

[62] Zhang, Y., Zhang, X., Hua, W., Wang, L., & , Z. (2010b). Analysis of genetic diversity among indigenous landraces from sesame (*Sesamum indicum* L.) core collection in China as revealed by SRAP and SSR markers. *Genes & Genomics* , 32, 207-215.

[63] Zhang, X., Wu, J., Zhang, H., , Y., Guo, A., & Wang, X. (2011c). Fine mapping of a male sterility gene MS-cd1 in *Brassica oleracea*. *Theor Appl Genet.* , 123, 231-8.

[64] Zhang, Z., Hu, M., Zhang, J., Liu, D., Zheng, J., Zhang, K., Wang, W., & Wan, Q. (2009b). Construction of a comprehensive PCR-based marker linkage map and QTL mapping for fiber quality traits in upland cotton (*Gossypium hirsutum* L.) *Molecular Breed.* , 24, 49-61.

[65] Zhao, F., Cai, Z., Hu, T., Yao, H., Wang, L., Dong, N., Wang, B., Ru, Z., & Zhai, W. . (2010). Genetic analysis and molecular mapping of a novel gene conferring resistance to rice stripe virus. *Plant Molecular Biology Reporter* , 28, 512-518.

Chapter 3

Molecular Markers and Marker-Assisted Breeding in Plants

Guo-Liang Jiang

Additional information is available at the end of the chapter

http://dx.doi.org/10.5772/52583

1. Introduction

Molecular breeding (MB) may be defined in a broad-sense as the use of genetic manipulation performed at DNA molecular levels to improve characters of interest in plants and animals, including genetic engineering or gene manipulation, molecular marker-assisted selection, genomic selection, etc. More often, however, molecular breeding implies molecular marker-assisted breeding (MAB) and is defined as the application of molecular biotechnologies, specifically molecular markers, in combination with linkage maps and genomics, to alter and improve plant or animal traits on the basis of genotypic assays. This term is used to describe several modern breeding strategies, including marker-assisted selection (MAS), marker-assisted backcrossing (MABC), marker-assisted recurrent selection (MARS), and genome-wide selection (GWS) or genomic selection (GS) (Ribaut et al., 2010). In this article, we will address general principles and methodologies of marker-assisted breeding in plants and discuss some issues related to the procedures and applications of this methodology in practical breeding, including marker-assisted selection, marker-based backcrossing, marker-based pyramiding of multiple genes, etc., beginning with a brief introduction to molecular markers as a powerful tool for plant breeding.

2. Genetic markers in plant breeding: Conceptions, types and application

Genetic markers are the biological features that are determined by allelic forms of genes or genetic loci and can be transmitted from one generation to another, and thus they can be used as experimental probes or tags to keep track of an individual, a tissue, a cell, a nucleus, a chromosome or a gene. Genetic markers used in genetics and plant breeding can be classified into two categories: classical markers and DNA markers (Xu, 2010). Classical markers include morphological markers, cytological markers and biochemical markers. DNA markers have developed into many systems based on different polymorphism-detecting techniques or methods (southern blotting – nuclear acid hybridization, PCR – polymerase chain reaction, and DNA sequencing) (Collard et al., 2005), such as RFLP, AFLP, RAPD, SSR, SNP, etc.

2.1. Classical markers

Morphological markers: Use of markers as an assisting tool to select the plants with desired traits had started in breeding long time ago. During the early history of plant breeding, the markers used mainly included visible traits, such as leaf shape, flower color, pubescence color, pod color, seed color, seed shape, hilum color, awn type and length, fruit shape, rind (exocarp) color and stripe, flesh color, stem length, etc. These morphological markers generally represent genetic polymorphisms which are easily identified and manipulated. Therefore, they are usually used in construction of linkage maps by classical two- and/or three-point tests. Some of these markers are linked with other agronomic traits and thus can be used as indirect selection criteria in practical breeding. In the green revolution, selection of semi-dwarfism in rice and wheat was one of the critical factors that contributed to the success of high-yielding cultivars. This could be considered as an example for successful use of morphological markers to modern breeding. In wheat breeding, the dwarfism governed by gene *Rht10* was introgressed into Taigu nuclear male-sterile wheat by backcrossing, and a tight linkage was generated between *Rht10* and the male-sterility gene *Ta1*. Then the dwarfism was used as the marker for identification and selection of the male-sterile plants in breeding populations (Liu, 1991). This is particularly helpful for implementation of recurrent selection in wheat. However, morphological markers available are limited, and many of these markers are not associated with important economic traits (e.g. yield and quality) and even have undesirable effects on the development and growth of plants.

Cytological markers: In cytology, the structural features of chromosomes can be shown by chromosome karyotype and bands. The banding patterns, displayed in color, width, order and position, reveal the difference in distributions of euchromatin and heterochromatin. For instance, Q bands are produced by quinacrine hydrochloride, G bands are produced by Giemsa stain, and R bands are the reversed G bands. These chromosome landmarks are used not only for characterization of normal chromosomes and detection of chromosome mutation, but also widely used in physical mapping and linkage group identification. The physical maps based on morphological and cytological markers lay a foundation for genetic linkage mapping with the aid of molecular techniques. However, direct use of cytological markers has been very limited in genetic mapping and plant breeding.

Biochemical/protein markers: Protein markers may also be categorized into molecular markers though the latter are more referred to DNA markers. Isozymes are alternative forms or structural variants of an enzyme that have different molecular weights and electrophoretic mobility but have the same catalytic activity or function. Isozymes reflect the products of different alleles rather than different genes because the difference in electrophoretic mobility is caused by point mutation as a result of amino acid substitution (Xu, 2010). Therefore, isozyme markers can be genetically mapped onto chromosomes and then used as genetic markers to map other genes. They are also used in seed purity test and occasionally in plant breeding. There are only a small number of isozymes in most crop species and some of them can be identified only with a specific strain. Therefore, the use of enzyme markers is limited.

Another example of biochemical markers used in plant breeding is high molecular weight glutenin subunit (HMW-GS) in wheat. Payne et al. (1987) discovered a correlation between the presence of certain HMW-GS and gluten strength, measured by the SDS-sedimentation volume test. On this basis, they designed a numeric scale to evaluate bread-making quality as a function of the described subunits (*Glu-1* quality score) (Payne et al., 1987; Rogers et al., 1989). Assuming the effect of the alleles to be additive, the Bread-making quality was predicted by adding the scores of the alleles present in the particular line. It was established that the allelic variation at the *Glu-D1* locus have a greater influence on bread-making quality than the variation at the others *Glu-1* loci. Subunit combination 5+10 for locus *Glu-D1* (*Glu-D1* 5+10) renders stronger dough than *Glu-D1* 2+12, largely due to the presence of an extra cysteine residue in the Dx-5 subunit compared to the Dx-2 subunit, which would promote the formation of polymers with larger size distribution. Therefore, breeders may enhance the bread-making quality in wheat by selecting subunit combination Glu-D1 5+10 instead of Glu-D1 2+12. Of course, the variation of bread-making quality among different varieties cannot be explained only by the variation in HMW-GS composition, because the low molecular weight glutinen subunit (LMW-GS) (as well as the gliadins in a smaller proportion) and their interactions with the HMW-GS also play an important role in the gluten strength and bread-making quality.

2.2. DNA markers

DNA markers are defined as a fragment of DNA revealing mutations/variations, which can be used to detect polymorphism between different genotypes or alleles of a gene for a particular sequence of DNA in a population or gene pool. Such fragments are associated with a certain location within the genome and may be detected by means of certain molecular technology. Simply speaking, DNA marker is a small region of DNA sequence showing polymorphism (base deletion, insertion and substitution) between different individuals. There are two basic methods to detect the polymorphism: Southern blotting, a nuclear acid hybridization technique (Southern 1975), and PCR, a polymerase chain reaction technique (Mullis, 1990). Using PCR and/or molecular hybridization followed by electrophoresis (e.g. PAGE – polyacrylamide gel electrophoresis, AGE – agarose gel electrophoresis, CE – capillary electrophoresis), the variation in DNA samples or polymorphism for a specific region of DNA sequence can be identified based on the product features, such as band size and mobility. In addition to Sothern blotting and PCR, more detection systems have been also developed. For instance, several new array chip techniques use DNA hybridization combined with labeled nucleotides, and new sequencing techniques detect polymorphism by sequencing. DNA markers are also called molecular markers in many cases and play a major role in molecular breeding. Therefore, molecular markers in this article are mainly referred to as DNA markers except specific definitions are given, although isozymes and protein markers are also molecular markers. Depending on application and species involved, ideal DNA markers for efficient use in marker-assisted breeding should meet the following criteria:

- High level of polymorphism
- Even distribution across the whole genome (not clustered in certain regions)
- Co-dominance in expression (so that heterozygotes can be distinguished from homozygotes)
- Clear distinct allelic features (so that the different alleles can be easily identified)
- Single copy and no pleiotropic effect
- Low cost to use (or cost-efficient marker development and genotyping)
- Easy assay/detection and automation
- High availability (un-restricted use) and suitability to be duplicated/multiplexed (so that the data can be accumulated and shared between laboratories)
- Genome-specific in nature (especially with polyploids)
- No detrimental effect on phenotype

Since Botstein et al. (1980) first used DNA restriction fragment length polymorphism (RFLP) in human linkage mapping, substantial progress has been made in development and improvement of molecular techniques that help to easily find markers of interest on a large-scale, resulting in extensive and successful uses of DNA markers in human genetics, animal genetics and breeding, plant genetics and breeding, and germplasm characterization and management. Among the techniques that have been extensively used and are particularly promising for application to plant breeding, are the restriction fragment length polymorphism (RFLP), amplified fragment length polymorphism (AFLP), random amplified polymorphic DNA (RAPD), microsatellites or simple sequence repeat (SSR), and single nucleotide polymorphism (SNP). According to a causal similarity of SNPs with some of these marker systems and fundamental difference with several other marker systems, the molecular markers can also be classified into SNPs (due to sequence variation, e.g. RFLP) and non-SNPs (due to length variation, e.g. SSR) (Gupta et al., 2001). The marker techniques help in selection of multiple desired characters simultaneously using F_2 and back-cross populations, near isogenic lines, doubled haploids and recombinant inbred lines. In view of page limitation, only five marker systems mentioned above are briefly addressed here according to published literatures. The details about the technical methods how to develop DNA markers and the procedures how to detect in practice have been described in the recently published reviews and books in this area (Farooq and Azam, 2002a, 2002b; Gupta et al., 2001; Semagn et al., 2006a; Xu, 2010).

RFLP markers: RFLP markers are the first generation of DNA markers and one of the important tools for plant genome mapping. They are a type of Southern-Boltting-based markers. In living organisms, mutation events (deletion and insertion) may occur at restriction sites or between adjacent restriction sites in the genome. Gain or loss of restriction sites resulting from base pair changes and insertions or deletions at restriction sites within the restriction fragments may cause differences in size of restriction fragments. These variations may cause alternation or elimination of the recognition sites for restriction enzymes. As a consequence, when homologous chromosomes are subjected to restriction enzyme digestion, different restriction products are produced and can be detected by electrophoresis and DNA probing techniques.

RFLP markers are powerful tools for comparative and synteny mapping. Most RFLP markers are co-dominant and locus-specific. RFLP genotyping is highly reproducible, and the methodology is simple and no special equipment is required. By using an improved RFLP technique, i.e., cleaved amplified polymorphism sequence (CAPS), also known as PCR-RFLP, high-throughput markers can be developed from RFLP probe sequences. Very few CAPS are developed from probe sequences, which are complex to interpret. Most CAPS are developed from SNPs found in other sequences followed by PCR and detection of restriction sites. CAPS technique consists of digesting a PCR-amplified fragment and detecting the polymorphism by the presence/absence of restriction sites (Konieczny and Ausubel, 1993). Another advantage of RFLP is that the sequence used as a probe need not be known. All that a researcher needs is a genomic clone that can be used to detect the polymorphism. Very few RFLPs have been sequenced to determine what sequence variation is responsible for the polymorphism. However, it may be problematic to interpret complex RFLP allelic systems in the absence of sequence information. RFLP analysis requires large amounts of high-quality DNA, has low genotyping throughput, and is very difficult to automate. Radioactive autography involving in genotyping and physical maintenance of RFLP probes limit its use and share between laboratories. RFLP markers were predominantly used in 1980s and 1990s, but since last decade fewer direct uses of RFLP markers in genetic research and plant breeding have been reported. Most plant breeders would think that RFLP is too laborious and demands too much pure DNA to be important for plant breeding. It was and is, however, central for various types of scientific studies.

RAPD markers: RAPD is a PCR-based marker system. In this system, the total genomic DNA of an individual is amplified by PCR using a single, short (usually about ten nucleotides/bases) and random primer. The primer which binds to many different loci is used to amplify random sequences from a complex DNA template that is complementary to it (maybe including a limited number of mismatches). Amplification can take place during the PCR, if two hybridization sites are similar to one another (at least 3000 bp) and in opposite directions. The amplified fragments generated by PCR depend on the length and size of both the primer and the target genome. The PCR products (up to 3 kb) are separated by agarose gel electrophoresis and imaged by ethidium bromide (EB) staining. Polymorphisms resulted from mutations or rearrangements either at or between the primer-binding sites are visible in the electrophoresis as the presence or absence of a particular RAPD band.

RAPD predominantly provides dominant markers. This system yields high levels of polymorphism and is simple and easy to be conducted. First, neither DNA probes nor sequence information is required for the design of specific primers. Second, the procedure does not involve blotting or hybridization steps, and thus it is a quick, simple and efficient technique.

Third, relatively small amounts of DNA (about 10 ng per reaction) are required and the procedure can be automated, and higher levels of polymorphism also can be detected compared with RFLP. Fourth, no marker development is required, and the primers are non-species specific and can be universal. Fifth, the RAPD products of interest can be cloned, sequenced and then converted into or used to develop other types of PCR-based markers, such as sequence characterized amplified region (SCAR), single nucleotide polymorphism (SNP), etc. However, RAPD also has some limitations/disadvantages, such as low reproducibility and incapability to detect allelic differences in heterozygotes.

AFLP markers: AFLPs are PCR-based markers, simply RFLPs visualized by selective PCR amplification of DNA restriction fragments. Technically, AFLP is based on the selective PCR amplification of restriction fragments from a total double-digest of genomic DNA under high stringency conditions, i.e., the combination of polymorphism at restriction sites and hybridization of arbitrary primers. Because of this AFLP is also called selective restriction fragment amplification (SRFA). An AFLP primer (17-21 nucleotides in length) consists of a synthetic adaptor sequence, the restriction endonuclease recognition sequence and an arbitrary, non-degenerate 'selective' sequence (1-3 nucleotides). The primers used in this technique are capable of annealing perfectly to their target sequences (the adapter and restriction sites) as well as a small number of nucleotides adjacent to the restriction sites. The first step in AFLP involves restriction digestion of genomic DNA (about 500 ng) with two restriction enzymes, a rare cutter (6-bp recognition site, *Eco*RI, *Pts*I or *Hind*III) and a frequent cutter (4-bp recognition site, *Mse*I or *Taq*I). The adaptors are then ligated to both ends of the fragments to provide known sequences for PCR amplification. The double-stranded oligonucleotide adaptors are designed in such a way that the initial restriction site is not restored after ligation. Therefore, only the fragments which have been cut by the frequent cutter and rare cutter will be amplified. This property of AFLP makes it very reliable, robust and immune to small variations in PCR amplification parameters (e.g., thermal cycles, template concentration), and it also can produce a high marker density. The AFLP products can be separated in high-resolution electrophoresis systems. The fragments in gel-based or capillary DNA sequencers can be detected by dye-labeling primers radioactively or fluorescently. The number of bands produced can be manipulated by the number of selective nucleotides and the nucleotide motifs used.

A typical AFLP fingerprint (restriction fragment patterns generated by the technique) contains 50-100 amplified fragments, of which up to 80% may serve as genetic markers. In general, AFLP assays can be conducted using relatively small DNA samples (1-100 ng per individual). AFLP has a very high multiplex ratio and genotyping throughput, and is relatively reproducible across laboratories. Another advantage is that it does not require sequence information or probe collection prior to generating the fingerprints, and a set of primers can be used for different species. This is especially useful when DNA markers are rare. However, AFLP assays have some limitations also. For instance, polymorphic information content for bi-allelic markers is low (the maximum is 0.5). High quality DNA is required for complete restriction enzyme digestion. AFLP markers usually cluster densely in centromeric regions in some species with large genomes (e.g., barley and sunflower). In addition, marker development is complicated and not cost-efficient, especially for locus-specific markers. The applications of AFLP markers include biodiversity studies, analysis of germplasm collections, genotyping of individuals, identification of closely linked DNA markers, construction of genetic DNA marker maps, construction of physical maps, gene mapping, and transcript profiling.

SSR markers: SSRs, also called microsatellites, short tandem repeats (STRs) or sequence-tagged microsatellite sites (STMS), are PCR-based markers. They are randomly tandem repeats of short nucleotide motifs (2-6 bp/nucleotides long). Di-, tri- and tetra-nucleotide repeats, e.g. (GT)n, (AAT)n and (GATA)n, are widely distributed throughout the genomes of plants and animals. The copy number of these repeats varies among individuals and is a source of polymorphism in plants. Because the DNA sequences flanking microsatellite regions are usually conserved, primers specific for these regions are designed for use in the PCR reaction. One of the most important attributes of microsatellite loci is their high level of allelic variation, thus making them valuable genetic markers. The unique sequences bordering the SSR motifs provide templates for specific primers to amplify the SSR alleles via PCR. SSR loci are individually amplified by PCR using pairs of oligonucleotide primers specific to unique DNA sequences flanking the SSR sequence. The PCR-amplified products can be separated in high-resolution electrophoresis systems (e.g. AGE and PAGE) and the bands can be visually recorded by fluorescent labeling or silver-staining.

SSR markers are characterized by their hyper-variability, reproducibility, co-dominant nature, locus-specificity, and random genome-wide distribution in most cases. The advantages of SSR markers include that they can be readily analyzed by PCR and easily detected by PAGE or AGE. SSR markers can be multiplexed, have high throughput genotyping and can be automated. SSR assays require only very small DNA samples (~100 ng per individual) and low start-up costs for manual assay methods. However, SSR technique requires nucleotide information for primer design, labor-intensive marker development process and high start-up costs for automated detections. Since the 1990s SSR markers have been extensively used in constructing genetic linkage maps, QTL mapping, marker-assisted selection and germplasm analysis in plants. In many species, plenty of breeder-friendly SSR markers have been developed and are available for breeders. For instance, there are over 35,000 SSR markers developed and mapped onto all 20 linkage groups in soybean, and this information is available for the public (Song et al., 2010).

SNP markers: An SNP is a single nucleotide base difference between two DNA sequences or individuals. SNPs can be categorized according to nucleotide substitutions either as transitions (C/T or G/A) or transversions (C/G, A/T, C/A or T/G). In practice, single base variants in cDNA (mRNA) are considered to be SNPs as are single base insertions and deletions (indels) in the genome. SNPs provide the ultimate/simplest form of molecular markers as a single nucleotide base is the smallest unit of inheritance, and thus they can provide maximum markers. SNPs occur very commonly in animals and plants. Typically, SNP frequencies are in a range of one SNP every 100-300 bp in plants (Edwards et al., 2007; Xu, 2010). SNPs may present within coding sequences of genes, non-coding regions of genes or in the intergenic regions between genes at different frequencies in different chromosome regions.

Based on various methods of allelic discrimination and detection platforms, many SNP genotyping methods have been developed. A convenient method for detecting SNPs is RFLP (SNP-RFLP) or by using the CAPS marker technique. If one allele contains a recognition site for a restriction enzyme while the other does not, digestion of the two alleles will produce different fragments in length. A simple procedure is to analyze the sequence data stored in the major databases and identify SNPs. Four alleles can be identified when the complete base sequence of a segment of DNA is considered and these are represented by A, T, G and C at each SNP locus in that segment. There are several SNP genotyping assays, such as allele-specific hybridization, primer extension, oligonucleotide ligation and invasive cleavage based on the molecular mechanisms (Sobrino et al., 2005), and different detection methods to analyze the products of each type of allelic discrimination reaction, such as gel electrophoresis, mass spectrophotometry, chromatography, fluorescence polarization, arrays or chips, etc. At the present, SNPs are also widely detected by sequencing. Detailed procedures are described in the review by Gupta at el. (2001) and the book Molecular Plant Breeding by Xu (2010).

SNPs are co-dominant markers, often linked to genes and present in the simplest/ultimate form for polymorphism, and thus they have become very attractive and potential genetic markers in genetic study and breeding. Moreover, SNPs can be very easily automated and quickly detected, with a high efficiency for detection of polymorphism. Therefore, it can be expected that SNPs will be increasingly used for various purposes, particularly as whole DNA sequences become available for more and more species (e.g., rice, soybean, maize, etc.). However, high costs for start-up or marker development, high-quality DNA required and high technical/equipment demands limit, to some extent, the application of SNPs in some laboratories and practical breeding programs.

The features of the widely used DNA markers discussed above are compared in Table 1. The advantages or disadvantages of a marker system are relevant largely to the purposes of research, available genetic resources or databases, equipment and facilities, funding and personnel resources, etc. The choice and use of DNA markers in research and breeding is still a challenge for plant breeders. A number of factors need to be considered when a breeder chooses one or more molecular marker types (Semagn et al., 2006a). A breeder should make an appropriate choice that best meets the requirements according to the conditions and resources available for the breeding program.

Feature and description	**RFLP**	**RAPD**	**AFLP**	**SSR**	**SNP**
Genomic abundance	High	High	High	Moderate to high	Very high
Genomic coverage	Low copy coding region	Whole genome	Whole genome	Whole genome	Whole genome
Expression/inheritance	Co-dominant	Dominant	Dominant / co-dominant	Co-dominant	Co-dominant

Feature and description	RFLP	RAPD	AFLP	SSR	SNP
Number of loci	Small (<1,000)	Small (<1,000)	Moderate (1,000s)	High (1,000s – 10,000s)	Very high (>100,000)
Level of polymorphism	Moderate	High	High	High	High
Type of polymorphism	Single base changes, indels	Single base changes, indels	Single base changes, indels	Changes in length of repeats	Single base changes, indels
Type of probes/primers	Low copy DNA or cDNA clones	10 bp random nucleotides	Specific sequence	Specific sequence	Allele-specific PCR primers
Cloning and/or sequencing	Yes	No	No	Yes	Yes
PCR-based	Usually no	Yes	Yes	Yes	Yes
Radioactive detection	Usually yes	No	Yes or no	Usually no	No
Reproducibility/ reliability	High	Low	High	High	High
Effective multiplex ratio	Low	Moderate	High	High	Moderate to high
Marker index	Low	Moderate	Moderate to high	High	Moderate
Genotyping throughput	Low	Low	High	High	High
Amount of DNA required	Large (5 – 50 µg)	Small (0.01 – 0.1 µg)	Moderate (0.5 – 1.0 µg)	Small (0.05 – 0.12 µg)	Small (≥ 0.05 µg)
Quality of DNA required	High	Moderate	High	Moderate to high	High
Technically demanding	Moderate	Low	Moderate	Low	High
Time demanding	High	Low	Moderate	Low	Low
Ease of use	Not easy	Easy	Moderate	Easy	Easy
Ease of automation	Low	Moderate	Moderate to high	High	High
Development/start-up cost	Moderate to high	Low	Moderate	Moderate to high	High
Cost per analysis	High	Low	Moderate	Low	Low
Number of polymorphic loci per analysis	1.0 – 3.0	1.5 – 5.0	20 – 100	1.0 – 3.0	1.0
Primary application	Genetics	Diversity	Diversity and genetics	All purposes	All purposes

Table 1. Comparison of most widely used DNA marker systems in plants; Adapted from Collard et al. (2005), Semagn et al. (2006a), Xu (2010), and others.

3. Pre-requisites and general activities of marker-assisted breeding

3.1. Prerequisites for an efficient marker-assisted breeding program

Compared with conventional breeding approaches, molecular breeding, mainly referred to as DNA marker-assisted breeding, needs more complicated equipment and facilities. In general, the pre-requisites listed below are essential for marker-assisted breeding (MAB) in plants.

a. Appropriate marker system and reliable markers: For a plant species or crop, a suitable marker system and reliable markers available are critically important to initiate a marker-assisted breeding program. As discussed above, suitable markers should have following attributes:

- Ease and low-cost of use and analysis;
- Small amount of DNA required;
- Co-dominance;
- Repeatability/reproducibility of results;
- High levels of polymorphism; and
- Occurrence and even distribution genome wide

In addition, another important desirable attribute for the markers to be used is close association with the target gene(s). If the markers are located in close proximity to the target gene or present within the gene, selection of the markers will ensure the success in selection of the gene. Although they can also be used in plant breeding programs, the number of classical markers possessing these features is very small. DNA markers for polymorphism are available throughout the genome, and their presence or absence is not affected by environments and usually do not directly affect the phenotype. DNA markers can be detected at any stage of plant growth, but the detection of classical markers is usually limited to certain growth stages. Therefore, DNA markers are the predominant types of genetic markers for MAB. Each type of markers has advantages and disadvantages for specific purposes. Relatively speaking, SSRs have most of the desirable features and thus are the current marker of choice for many crops. SNPs require more detailed knowledge of the specific, single nucleotide DNA changes responsible for genetic variation among individuals. However, more and more SNPs have become available in many species, and thus they are also considered an important type for marker-assisted breeding.

b. Quick DNA extraction and high throughput marker detection: For most plant breeding programs, hundreds to thousands of plants/individuals are usually screened for desired marker patterns. In addition, the breeders need the results instantly to make selections in a timely manner. Therefore, a quick DNA extraction technique and a high throughput marker detection system are essentially required to handle a large number of tissue samples and a large-scale screening of multiple markers in breeding programs. Extracting DNA from small tissue samples in 96- or 384-well plates and streamlined operations are adopted in many labs and programs. High throughput PAGE and AGE systems are commonly used for marker detection. Some labs also provide marker detection services using automated detection systems, e.g. SNP chips based on thousands to ten thousands of markers.

c. Genetic maps: Linkage maps provide a framework for detecting marker-trait associations and for choosing markers to use in marker-assisted breeding. Therefore, a genetic linkage map, particularly high-density linkage map is very important for MAB. To use markers and select a desired trait present in a specific germplasm line, a proper population of segregation for the trait is required to construct a linkage map. Once a marker or a few markers are found to be associated with the trait in a given population, a dense molecular marker map in a standard reference population will help identify makers that are close to (or flank) the target gene. If a region is found associated with the desired traits of interest, fine mapping also can be done with additional markers to identify the marker(s) tightly linked to the gene controlling the trait. A favorable genetic map should have an adequate number of evenly-spaced polymorphic markers to accurately locate desired QTLs/genes (Babu et al., 2004).

d. Knowledge of marker-trait association: The most crucial factor for marker-assisted breeding is the knowledge of the associations between markers and the traits of interest. Only those markers that are closely associated with the target traits or tightly linked to the genes can provide sufficient guarantee for the success in practical breeding. The more closely the markers are associated with the traits, the higher the possibility of success and efficiency of use will be. This information can be obtained in various ways, such as gene mapping, QTL analysis, association mapping, classical mutant analysis, linkage or recombination analysis, bulked segregant analysis, etc. In addition, it is also critical to know the linkage situation, i.e. the markers are linked in cis/trans (coupling or repulsion) with the desired allele of the trait. Even if some markers have been reported to be tightly linked with a QTL, a plant breeder still needs to determine the association of alleles in his own breeding material. This makes QTL information difficult to directly transfer between different materials.

e. Quick and efficient data processing and management: In addition to above-mentioned pre-requisites, quick and efficient data process and management may provide timely and useful reports for breeders. In a marker-assisted breeding program, not only are large numbers of samples handled, but multiple markers for each sample also need to be screened at the same time. This situation requires an efficient and quick system for labeling, storing, retrieving, processing and analyzing large data sets, and even integrating data sets available from other programs. The development of bioinformatics and statistical software packages provides a useful tool for this purpose.

3.2. Activities of marker-assisted breeding

Marker-assisted breeding involves the following activities provided the prerequisites are well equipped or available:

a. Planting the breeding populations with potential segregation for traits of interest or polymorphism for the markers used.

b. Sampling plant tissues, usually at early stages of growth, e.g. emergence to young seedling stage.

c. Extracting DNA from tissue sample of each individual or family in the populations, and preparing DNA samples for PCR and marker screening.

d. Running PCR or other amplifying operation for the molecular markers associated with or linked to the trait of interest.

e. Separating and scoring PCR/amplified products, by means of appropriate separation and detection techniques, e.g. PAGE, AGE, etc.

f. Identifying individuals/families carrying the desired marker alleles.

g. Selecting the best individuals/families with both desired marker alleles for target traits and desirable performance/phenotypes of other traits, by jointly using marker results and other selection criteria.

h. Repeating the above activities for several generations, depending upon the association between the markers and the traits as well as the status of marker alleles (homozygous or heterozygous), and advancing the individuals selected in breeding program until stable superior or elite lines that have improved traits are developed.

4. Marker-assisted selection

4.1. MAS procedure and theoretical and practical considerations

Marker-assisted selection (MAS) refers to such a breeding procedure in which DNA marker detection and selection are integrated into a traditional breeding program. Taking a single cross as an example, the general procedure can be described as follow:

a. Select parents and make the cross, at least one (or both) possesses the DNA marker allele(s) for the desired trait of interest.

b. Plant F_1 population and detect the presence of the marker alleles to eliminate false hybrids.

c. Plant segregating F_2 population, screen individuals for the marker(s), and harvest the individuals carrying the desired marker allele(s).

d. Plant $F_{2:3}$ plant rows, and screen individual plants with the marker(s). A bulk of F_3 individuals within a plant row may be used for the marker screening for further confirmation in case needed if the preceding F_2 plant is homozygous for the markers. Select and harvest the individuals with required marker alleles and other desirable traits.

e. In the subsequent generations (F_4 and F_5), conduct marker screening and make selection similarly as for $F_{2:3}$s, but more attention is given to superior individuals within homozygous lines/rows of markers.

f. In $F_{5:6}$ or $F_{4:5}$ generations, bulk the best lines according to the phenotypic evaluation of target trait and the performance of other traits, in addition to marker data.

g. Plant yield trials and comprehensively evaluate the selected lines for yield, quality, resistance and other characters of interest.

A frequently asked question about marker-assisted selection is that "how many QTLs should be selected for MAS?" Theoretically, all the QTLs contributing to the trait of interest could be taken into account. For a quantitatively-inherited character like yield, numerous QTLs or genes are usually involved. It is almost impossible to select all QTLs or genes simultaneously so that the selected individuals incorporate all the desired QTLs due to the limitation of resources and facilities. The number of individuals in the population increases exponentially with the increase of target loci involved. The relative efficiency of MAS decreases as the number of QTLs increases and their heritability decreases (Moreau et al., 1998). In other words, MAS will be less effective for a highly complex character governed by many genes than for a simply inherited character controlled by a few genes. The number of genes/QTLs not only impacts the efficiency of MAS, but also the breeding design and implement scheme (detail will be discussed below). Typically no more than three QTLs are regarded as an appropriate and feasible choice (Ribaut and Betran, 1999), although five QTLs were used in improvement of fruit quality traits in tomato via marker-assisted introgression (Lecomte et al., 2004). With development of SNP markers (especially rapid automated detection and genotyping technologies), selection of more QTLs at the same time might be preferred and practicable (Kumpatla et al., 2012).

For MAS for multiple genes/QTLs, it was suggested to limit the number of genes undergoing selection to three to four if they are QTLs selected on the basis of linked markers, and to five to six if they are known loci selected directly (Hospital, 2003). Only the multi-environmentally verified QTLs that possess medium to large effects are selected. The first priority should be given to the major QTLs that can explain greatest proportion of phenotypic variation and/or can be consistently detected across a range of environments and different populations. In addition, an index for selection that weights markers differently could be constructed, depending on their relative importance to the breeding objectives. Flint-Garcia et al. (2003) presented an example of such an index used to select for QTLs with different effect magnitudes.

Another question that is commonly asked also is that "how many markers should be used in MAS?" The more markers associated with a QTL are used, the greater opportunity of success in selecting the QTL of interest will be ensured. However, efficiency is also important for a breeding program, especially when the resources and facilities are limited. From the point of both effectiveness and efficiency, for a single QTL it is usually suggested to use two markers (i.e. flanking markers) that are tightly linked to the QTL of interest. The markers to be used should be close enough to the gene/QTL of interest (<5cM) in order to ensure that only a minor proportion of the selected individuals will be recombinants. If a marker (e.g. the peak marker) is found to be located within the region of gene sequence of interest or in such a close proximity to the QTL/gene that no recombination occurs between the marker and the QTL/gene, such a marker only should be preferable. However, if a marker is not tightly linked to a gene of interest, recombination between the marker and gene may reduce the efficiency of MAS because a single crossover may alternate the linkage association and leads to selection errors. The efficiency of MAS decreases as the recombination frequency (genetic distance) between the marker and gene increases. Use of two flanking markers rather than one may decrease the chance of such errors due to homologous recombination and increase the efficiency of MAS. In this case, only a double crossover (i.e. two single crossovers occurring simultaneously on both sides of the gene/QTL in the region) may result in selection errors, but the frequency of a double crossover is considerably rare. For instance, if two flanking markers with an interval of 20cM or so between them are used, there will be higher probability (99%) for recovery of the target gene than only one marker used.

In practical MAS, a breeder is also concerned about how the markers should be detected, how many generations of MAS have to be conducted, and how large size of the population is needed. In general, detection of marker polymorphism is performed at early stages of plant growth. This is true especially for marker-assisted backcrossing and marker-assisted recurrent selection, because only the individuals that carry preferred marker alleles are expected to be used in backcrossing to the recurrent parent and/or inter-mating between selected individuals/progenies. The generations of MAS required vary with the number of markers used, the degree of association between the markers and the QTLs/genes of interest, and the status of marker alleles. In many cases, marker screening is performed for two to four consecutive generations in a segregating population. If fewer markers are used and the markers are in close proximity to the QTL or gene of interest, fewer generations are needed. If homozygous status of marker alleles of interest is detected in two consecutive generations, marker screening may not be performed in their progenies. Bonnett et al. (2005) discussed the strategies for efficient implementation of MAS involving several issues, e.g. breeding systems or schemes, population sizes, number of target loci, etc. Their strategies include F_2 enrichment, backcrossing, and inbreeding.

In MAS, phenotypic evaluation and selection is still very helpful if conditions permit to do so, and even necessary in cases when the QTLs selected for MAS are not so stable across environments and the association between the selected markers and QTLs is not so close. Moreover, one should also take the impact of genetic background into consideration. The presence of a QTL or marker does not necessarily guarantee the expression of the desired trait. QTL data derived from multiple environments and different populations help a better understanding of the interactions of QTL x environment and QTL x QTL or QTL x genetic background, and thus help a better use of MAS. In addition to genotypic (markers) and phenotypic data for the trait of interest, a breeder often pays considerable attention to other important traits, unless the trait of interest is the only objective of breeding.

There are several indications for adoption of molecular markers in the selection for the traits of interest in practical breeding. The situations favorable for MAS include:

- The selected character is expressed late in plant development, like fruit and flower features or adult characters with a juvenile period (so that it is not necessary to wait for the plant to become fully developed before propagation occurs or can be arranged)
- The target gene is recessive (so that individuals which are heterozygous positive for the recessive allele can be selected and/or crossed to produce some homozygous offspring with the desired trait)
- Special conditions are required in order to invoke expression of the target gene(s), as in the case of breeding for disease and pest resistance (where inoculation with the disease or subjection to pests would otherwise be required), or the expression of target genes is highly variable with the environments.
- The phenotype of a trait is conditioned by two or more unlinked genes. For example, selection for multiple genes or gene pyramiding may be required to develop enhanced or durable resistance against diseases or insect pests.

4.2. MAS for major genes or improvement of qualitative traits

In crop plants, many economically important characteristics are controlled by major genes/ QTLs. Such characteristics include resistance to diseases/pests, male sterility, self-incompatibility and others related to shape, color and architecture of whole plants and/or plant parts. These traits are often of mono- or oligogenic inheritance in nature. Even for some quality traits, one or a few major QTLs or genes can account for a very high proportion of the phenotypic variation of the trait (Bilyeu et al., 2006; Pham et al., 2012). Transfer of such a gene to a specific line can lead to tremendous improvement of the trait in the cultivar under development. The marker loci which are tightly linked to major genes can be used for selection and are sometimes more efficient than direct selection for the target genes. In some cases, such advantages in efficiency may be due to higher expression of the marker mRNA in such cases that the marker is actually within a gene. Alternatively, in such cases that the target gene of interest differs between two alleles by a difficult-to-detect SNP, an external marker of which polymorphism is easier to detect, may present as the most realistic option.

Soybean cyst nematode (SCN) (*Heterodera glycines* Inchinoe) may be taken as an example of MAS for major genes. This pathogen is the most economically significant soybean pest. The principal strategy to reduce or eliminate damage from this pest is the use of resistant cultivars (Cregan et al., 1999). However, identifying resistant segregants in breeding populations is a difficult and expensive process. A widely used phenotypic assay takes five weeks, requires a large greenhouse space, and about 5 to 10 h of labor for every 100 plant samples processed (Young, 1999). Fortunately, the SSR marker Satt309 has been identified to be located only 1–2 cM away from the resistance gene *rhg1* (Cregan et al., 1999), which forms the basis of many public and commercial breeding efforts. In a direct comparison, genotypic selection with Satt309 was 99% accurate in predicting lines that were susceptible in subsequent greenhouse assays for two test populations, and 80% accurate in a third population, each with a different source of SCN resistance (Young, 1999). In soybean, Shi et al. (2009) reported that using molecular markers in a cross J05 x V94-5152, they developed five $F_{4:5}$

lines that were homozygous for all eight marker alleles linked to the genes/loci of resistance to soybean mosaic virus (SMV). These lines exhibited resistance to SMV strains G1 and G7 and presumably carried all three resistance genes (*Rsv1, Rsv3* and *Rsv4*) that would potentially provide broad and durable resistance to SMV.

4.3. MAS for improvement of quantitative traits

Most of the important agronomic traits are polygenic or controlled by multiple QTLs. MAS for the improvement of such traits is a complex and difficult task because it is related to many genes or QTLs involved, QTL x E interaction and epistasis. Usually, each of these genes has a small effect on the phenotypic expression of the trait and expression is affected by environmental conditions. Phenotyping of quantitative traits becomes a complex endeavor consequently, and determining marker-phenotype association becomes difficult as well. Therefore, repeated field tests are required to accurately characterize the effects of the QTLs and to evaluate the stability across environments. The QTL x E interaction reduces the efficiency of MAS and epistasis can result in a skewed QTL effect on the trait.

Despite a tremendous amount of QTL mapping experiments over the past decade, application and utilization of the QTL mapping information in plant breeding has been constrained by a number of factors (Collard and Mackill, 2008):

1. Strong QTL-environmental interaction which make phenotyping difficult since expression may vary from one location/year to another;

2. Lack of universally valid QTL-marker associations applicable across populations. The notion that QTL mapping to identify new QTL markers whenever a new germplasm is used, puts some people off and they lose interest in MAS;

3. Deficiencies in QTL statistical analysis which lead to either overestimation or underestimation of the number of QTLs involved and their effect on the trait;

4. Often times, there are no QTLs with major effects on the trait and this means a large number of QTLs have to be identified and in many cases this becomes a tough goal to achieve and further complicates identification of marker-QTL association.

In order to improve the efficiency of MAS for quantitative traits, appropriate field experimental designs and approaches have to be employed. Attention should be given to replications both over time and space, consistency in experimental techniques, samplings and evaluations, robust data processing and statistical analysis. For example, composite interval mapping (CIM) allows the integration of data from different locations for joint analysis to estimate QTL-environment interaction so that stable QTLs across environments can be identified. A saturated linkage map enables accurate identification of both targeted QTLs as well as linked QTLs in coupling and repulsion linkage phases. In practical breeding for improvement of a quantitative trait, usually not many minor QTLs are considered but only a few major QTLs are used in MAS. In case many QTLs especially minor-effect QTLs are involved, a breeder would prefer to consider the strategy of gene pyramiding (see the later section).

Fusarium head blight (FHB) caused by *Fusarum* species is one of the most destructive diseases in wheat and barley worldwide. To combat this disease, a great effort from multiple fields, including plant breeding and genetics, molecular genetics and genomics, plant pathology, and integrated management, has been dedicated since 1990s. Resistance to HFB in both wheat and barley is quantitatively inherited, and many QTLs have been identified from different resources of germplasm (Buerstmayr et al., 2009). Use of MAS to improve the resistance has become a choice for many breeding programs. In wheat, a major QTL designated as *Fhb1* was consistently detected across multiple environments and populations, and explained 20-40% of phenotypic variation in most cases (Buerstmayr et al., 2009; Jiang et al., 2007a, 2007b). Thus wheat breeders would especially prefer to use this major QTL to develop new cultivars with FHB resistance. Pumphrey et al. (2007) compared 19 pairs of NIL for *Fhb1* derived from an ongoing breeding program and found that the average reduction in disease severity between NIL pairs was 23% for disease severity and 27% for kernel infection. Later investigation from the group also demonstrated successful implementation of MAS for this QTL (Anderson et al. 2007).

In addition, researchers also tried to incorporate multiple QTLs by MAS. Miedaner et al. (2006) demonstrated that MAS for three FHB resistance QTLs simultaneously was highly effective in enhancing FHB resistance in German spring wheat. FHB resistance was the highest in recombinant lines with multiple QTLs combined, especially 3B plus 5A. Jiang et al. (2007a) made a comparison of multiple-locus combinations in a RIL population derived from the cross "Veery x CJ 9306". For three loci, the average levels of resistance from low to high in genotypes were: no favorable allele – one favorable allele – two favorable alleles – three favorable alleles, except for the non-reciprocal comparisons. When four or five loci carrying favorable alleles from the resistant parent CJ 9306 were considered simultaneously, the coefficients of determination between the accumulated effects of alleles for different combinations and the averages of number or percentage of diseased spikelets for the corresponding RILs were 0.33-0.41 ($P<0.01$) (Jiang et al., 2007a). Therefore, the authors concluded that the effects of FHB resistance QTLs could be accumulated and the resistance could be feasibly enhanced by selection of favorable marker alleles for multiple loci in breeding programs.

In the U.S., the Coordinated Agricultural Projects (CAPs) with aims to encourage collaborative efforts in applied plant genomics and molecular research have been implemented in several crops, such as rice, wheat, barley, beans, potato, tomato, etc. An important strategy CAPs take is applying marker-assisted selection to plant breeding and efficiently using genetic resources and facilities available, including thousands and ten thousands of DNA markers and plant introductions, to facilitate development of crop cultivars with improved yield, resistance and quality.

5. Marker-assisted backcrossing

5.1. MABC procedure and theoretical and practical considerations

Marker-assisted or marker-based backcrossing (MABC) is regarded as the simplest form of marker-assisted selection, and at the present it is the most widely and successfully used method in practical molecular breeding. MABC aims to transfer one or a few genes/QTLs of interest from one genetic source (serving as the donor parent and maybe inferior agronomically or not good enough in comprehensive performance in many cases) into a superior cultivar or elite breeding line (serving as the recurrent parent) to improve the targeted trait. Unlike traditional backcrossing, MABC is based on the alleles of markers associated with or linked to gene(s)/QTL(s) of interest instead of phenotypic performance of target trait. The general procedure of MABC is as follow, regardless of dominant or recessive nature of the target trait in inheritance:

a. Select parents and make the cross, one parent is superior in comprehensive performance and serves as recurrent parent (RP), and the other one used as donor parent (DP) should possess the desired trait and the DNA markers allele(s) associated with or linked to the gene for the trait.

b. Plant F_1 population and detect the presence of the marker allele(s) at early stages of growth to eliminate false hybrids, and cross the true F_1 plants back to the RP.

c. Plant BCF_1 population, screen individuals for the marker(s) at early growth stages, and cross the individuals carrying the desired marker allele(s) (in heterozygous status) back to the RP. Repeat this step in subsequent seasons for two to four generations, depending upon the practical requirements and operation situations as discussed below.

d. Plant the final backcrossing population (e.g. BC_4F_1), and screen individual plants with the marker(s) for the target trait and discard the individuals carrying homozygous markers alleles from the RP. Have the individuals with required marker allele(s) selfed and harvest them.

e. Plant the progenies of backcrossing-selfing (e.g. BC_4F_2), detect the markers and harvest individuals carrying homozygous DP marker allele(s) of target trait for further evaluation and release.

Theoretically, the proportion of the RP genome after n generations of backcrossing is given by $1 - (1/2)^{n+1}$ for a single locus and $[1 - (1/2)^{n+1}]^k$ for k loci, respectively, for a population large enough in size (or with adequate individuals) and no selection being made during backcrossing (i.e. "blind" backcrossing only). The percentage of the RP genome is the average of the population, with some individuals possessing more of the RP genome than others. To fully recover the genome of the RP, 6-8 generations of backcrossing is needed typically in case no selection is made for the RP. However, this process is usually slower than expected for the target gene-carrier chromosome, i.e. linkage drag, especially in case a linkage exists between the target gene and other undesirable traits. On the other hand, the process of introgression of QTLs/genes and recovery of the RP genome may be accelerated by selection using markers flanking QTLs and evenly spaced markers from other chromosomes (i.e. unlinked to QTLs) of the RP (Collard et al., 2005) or selection for the performance of the RP conducted simultaneously. For MABC program, therefore, there are two types of selection recognized: Foreground selection and background selection (Hospital, 2003).

In foreground selection, the selection is made only for the marker allele(s) of donor parent at the target locus to maintain the target locus in heterozygous state until the final backcrossing is completed. Then the selected plants are selfed and the progeny plants with homozygous DP allele(s) of selected markers are harvested for further evaluation and release. As described above, this is the general procedure of MABC. The effectiveness of foreground selection depends on the number of genes/loci involved in the selection, the marker-gene/QTL association or linkage distance and the undesirable linkage to the target gene/QTL.

In background selection, the selection is made for the marker alleles of recurrent parent in all genomic regions of desirable traits except the target locus, or selection against the undesirable genome of donor parent. The objective is to hasten the restoration of the RP genome and eliminate undesirable genes introduced from the DP. The progress in recovery of the RP genome depends on the number of markers used in background selection. The more markers evenly located on all the chromosomes are selected for the RP alleles, the faster recovery of the RP genome will be achieved but larger population size and more genotyping will be required as well. In addition, the linkage drag also can be efficiently addressed by background selection using DNA markers, although it is difficult to overcome in a traditional backcrossing program.

Foreground selection and background selection are two respective aspects of MABC with different foci of selection. In practice, however, both foreground and background selection are usually conducted in the same program, either simultaneously or successively. In many cases, they can be performed alternatively even in the same generation. The individuals that have the desired marker alleles for target trait are selected first (foreground selection). Then the selected individuals are screened for other marker alleles again for the RP genome (background selection). It is understandable to do so because selection of the target gene/QTL is the essential and only critical point for backcrossing program, and the individuals that do not have the allele of target gene will be discarded and thus it is not necessary to genotype them for other traits.

The efficiency of MABC depends upon several factors, such as the population size for each generation of backcrossing, marker-gene association or the distance of markers from the target locus, number of markers used for target trait and RP background, and undesirable linkage drag. Based on simulations of 1000 replicates, Hospital (2003) presented the expected results of a typical MABC program, in which heterozygotes were selected at the target locus in each generation, and RP alleles were selected for two flanking markers on target chromosome each located 2 cM apart from the target locus and for three markers on non-target chromosomes. As shown in Table 2, a faster recovery of the RP genome could be achieved by MABC with combined foreground and background selection, compared to traditional backcrossing. Therefore, using markers can lead to considerable time savings compared to conventional backcrossing (Frisch et al., 1999; Collard et al., 2005).

Backcross generation	Number of individuals	% homozygosity of recurrent parent alleles at selected markers		% recurrent parent genome	
		Chromosome with target locus	All other chromosomes	Marker-assisted backcross	Conventional backcross
BC_1	70	38.4	60.6	79.0	75.0
BC_2	100	73.6	87.4	92.2	87.5
BC_3	150	93.0	98.8	98.0	93.7
BC_4	300	100.0	100.0	99.0	96.9

Table 2. Expected results of a MABC program with combined foreground and background selection used; Adapted from Hospital (2003).

In a MABC program, the population to be analyzed should contain at least one genotype that has all favorable alleles for a particular QTL. Later, the number of QTLs may be increased progressively, but not beyond six QTLs in most cases because of prohibitive difficulty in handling all QTLs (Hospital, 2003). In addition, the more QTLs/genes are transferred, the larger the proportion of unwanted genes would be due to linkage drag. In general, most of the unwanted genes are located on non-target chromosomes in early BC generations, and are rapidly removed in subsequent BC generations. On the contrary, the quantity of DP genes on the target chromosome decreases much more slowly, and even after generation BC_6 many of the unwanted donor genes are still located on the target chromosome in segregating state (Newbury, 2003). Given a total genome length is 3000 cM, 1% donor DNA fragments after six backcrosses represents a 30 cM chromosomal segment or region, which may host many unwanted genes, especially if the DP is a wild genetic resource. Young and Tanksley (1989) genotyped a collection of tomato varieties in which the resistance gene was previously transferred at the *Tm*-2 locus with RLFP markers. Their data indicated that the size of chromosomal segment retained around the *Tm*-2 locus during backcross breeding was very variable, with one line exhibiting a donor segment of 50 cM after 11 backcrosses and other one possessing 36 cM donor segment after 21 backcrosses. This clearly demonstrates the need for background selection.

As discussed above, linkage drag can be reduced by performing background selection. Typically, two markers flanking the target gene are used, and the individuals (or double recombinants) that are heterozygous at the target locus and homozygous for the recipient (RP) alleles at both flanking markers are selected. Use of closer flanking markers leads to more effective and faster reduction of linkage drag compared to distant markers. However, less distance between two flanking markers implies less probability of double recombination, and thus larger populations and more genotyping are needed. In order to optimize genotyping effort (i.e. the cost of the program), therefore, it is important to determine the minimal population sizes necessary to ensure the desired genotypes can be obtained. Hospital and Decoux (2002) developed a statistical software for determining the minimum population size required in BC program to identify at least one individual that is double-recombinant with heterozygosity at target locus and homozygosity for recurrent parent alleles at flanking marker loci. In addition, for closely-linked flanking markers, it is unlikely to obtain double recombinant genotypes through only one generation of backcrossing. Therefore, additional backcrossing should be conducted. For instance, in one BC generation (e.g. BC_1) single recombination on one side of the target gene is selection, and single recombination on the other side may be selected in another BC generation (e.g. BC_2) (Young and Tanksley 1989). In this way, individuals with desired RP alleles at two flanking markers and donor allele at target locus can be finally obtained.

To accelerate the recovery of RP genome on non-target chromosomes, scientists suggested using markers in backcrossing and discussed how many makers should be used (Tanksley et al., 1989; Hospital et al. 1992; Visscher et al. 1996). In background selection, the approaches involve selecting individuals that are of homozygous recipient type at a collection of markers located on non-carrier chromosomes. From a point of both effectiveness and efficiency, it is important to determine an appropriate number of markers to be used. More markers do not necessarily mean better benefits in practice. Generally, several markers are involved and MABC should be performed over two or more generations. It is unlikely that the selection objective can be realized in a single BC generation.

Dense marker coverage of non-target chromosomes is not mandatory to increase the overall proportion of recurrent parent genome, unless fine-mapping of specific chromosome regions is highly important. An appropriate number of markers and optimal position on chromosomes are important. Computer simulation suggested that for a chromosome of 100 cM, two to four markers are sufficient, and selection based on markers would be most efficient if the markers are optimally positioned along the chromosomes (Servin and Hospital, 2002). In practice, at least two or three markers per chromosome are needed, and every chromosome should be involved. In such a MABC scheme, three to four generations of backcrossing is generally enough to achieve more than 99% of the recurrent parent genome. With respect to the time necessary to release new varieties, the gain due to background selection can be economically valuable. In addition, background selection is more efficient in late BC generations than in early BC generations. For example, if a BC breeding scheme is conducted over three successive BC generations and yet the preference is to genotype individuals only once, then it is more efficient to genotype and select the individuals in BC_3 generation rather than in the BC_1 generation (Hospital et al. 1992, Ribaut et al. 2002).

5.2. Application of MABC

Success in integrating MABC as a breeding approach lies in identifying situations in which markers offer noticeable advantages over conventional backcrossing or valuable complements to conventional breeding effort. MABC is essential and advantageous when:

1. Phenotyping is difficult and/or expensive or impossible;
2. Heritability of the target trait is low;
3. The trait is expressed in late stages of plant development and growth, such as flowers, fruits, seeds, etc.;

4. The traits are controlled by genes that require special conditions to express;
5. The traits are controlled by recessive genes; and
6. Gene pyramiding is needed for one or more traits.

Among the molecular breeding methods, MABC has been most widely and successfully used in plant breeding up to date. It has been applied to different types of traits (e.g. disease/pest resistance, drought tolerance and quality) in many species, e.g. rice, wheat, maize, barley, pear millet, soybean, tomato, etc. (Collard et al., 2005; Dwivedi et al., 2007; Xu, 2010). In maize, for example, *Bacillus thuringiens* is a bacterium that produces insecticidal toxins, which can kill corn borer larvae when they ingest the toxins in corn cells (Ragot et al. 1995). The integration of the *Bt* transgene into various corn genetic backgrounds has been achieved by using MABC. Aroma in rice is controlled by a recessive gene which is due to an eight base-pair deletion and three single nucleotide polymorphism in a gene that codes for betaine aldehyde dehydrgenase 2 (Bradbury et al., 2005a). This discovery allows identification of the aromatic and non-aromatic rice varieties and discriminates homozygous recessive and dominant as well as heterozygous individuals in segregating population for the trait. MABC has been used to select for aroma in rice (Bradbury et al. 2005b). High lysine *opaque2* gene in corn was incorporated using MABC (Babu et al. 2005). However, the rate of success decreases when large numbers of QTL_s are targeted for introgression. Sebolt et al. (2000) used MABC for two QTL for seed protein content in soybeans. However, only one QTL was confirmed in $BC_3F_{4:5}$. When that QTL was introduced in three different genetic backgrounds, it had no effect in one background. In tomato, Tanksley and Nelson (1996) proposed a MABC strategy, called advanced backcross-QTL (AB-QTL), to transfer resistance genes from wild relative/unadapted genotype into elite germplasm. The strategy has proven effective for various agronomically important traits in tomato, including fruit quality and black mold resistance (Tanksley and Nelson, 1996; Bernacchi et al., 1998; Fulton et al., 2002). In addition, AB-QTL has been used in other crop species, such as rice, barley, wheat, maize, cotton and soybean, collectively demonstrating that this strategy is effective in transferring favorable alleles from the wild/unadapted germplasm to elite germplasm (Wang and Chee, 2010; Concibido et al., 2003).

In barley, a marker linked (0.7 cM) to the *Yd2* gene for resistance to barley yellow dwarf virus was successfully used to select for resistance in a backcrossing scheme (Jefferies et al., 2003). Compared to lines without the marker, the BC_2F_2-derived lines carrying the linked marker had lighter leaf symptoms and higher yield when infected by the virus. In maize, marker-facilitated backcrossing was also successfully employed to improve complex traits such as grain yield. Using MABC, six chromosomal segments each in two elite lines, Tx303 and Oh43, were transferred into two widely used inbred lines, B73 and Mo17, through three generations of backcrossing followed by two selfing generations. Then the enhanced lines with better performance were selected based on initial evaluations of testcross hybrids. The single-cross hybrids of enhanced B73 x enhanced Mo17 out-yielded the check hybrids by 12-15% (Stuber et al., 1999). Zhao et al. (2012) reported that a major quantitative trait locus (named *qHSR1*) for resistance to head smut in maize was successfully integrated into ten high-yielding inbred lines (susceptible to head smut). Each of the ten high-yielding lines was crossed with a donor parent Ji 1037 that contains *qHSR1* and is completely resistant to head smut, followed by five generations of backcrossing to the respective recurrent parents. In BC_1 through BC_3 only phenotypic selection was conducted to identify highly resistant individuals after artificial inoculation. In BC_4phenotypic selection, foreground selection and recombinant selection were conducted to screen for resistant individuals with the shortest *qHSR1* donor regions. In BC_5, phenotypic selection, foreground selection and background selection were performed to identify resistant individuals with the highest proportion of the recurrent parent genome, followed by one generation of self-pollination to obtain homozygous genotypes at the *qHSR1* locus. The ten improved inbred lines all showed substantial resistance to head smut, and the hybrids derived from these lines also showed a significant increase in the resistance. Semagn et al. (2006b) provided a detail review on the progress and prospects of MABC in crop breeding.

Currently, a cooperative marker-based backcrossing project for high-oleic acid in soybean has been initiated among multiple U.S. land-grant universities and USDA-ARS. Backcrossing and selection will be performed using the markers tightly linked to the high-oleic genes/loci. Hopefully, the high-oleic (80% or higher) traits will be successfully transferred from mutant lines or derived lines into other locally superior cultivars/lines, or combined with other unique traits like low linolenic acid (Pham et al., 2012).

6. Marker-assisted gene pyramiding and marker-assisted recurrent selection

Marker-assisted gene pyramiding (MAGP) is one of the most important applications of DNA markers to plant breeding. Gene pyramiding has been proposed and applied to enhance resistance to disease and insects by selecting for two or more than two genes at a time. For example in rice such pyramids have been developed against bacterial blight and blast (Huang et al., 1997; Singh et al., 2001; Luo et al., 2012). Castro et al. (2003) reported a success in pyramiding qualitative gene and QTLs for resistance to stripe rust in barley. The advantage of using markers in this case allows selecting for QTL-allele-linked markers that have the same phenotypic effect. To enhance or improve a quantitatively inherited trait in plant breeding, pyramiding of multiple genes or QTLs is recommended as a potential strategy (Richardson et al., 2006). The cumulative effects of multiple-QTL pyramiding have been proven in crop species like wheat, barley and soybean (Richardson et al., 2006; Jiang et al., 2007a, 2007b; Li et al., 2010; Wang et al., 2012). Pyramiding of multiple genes/QTLs may be achieved through different approaches: multiple-parent crossing or complex crossing, backcrossing, and recurrent selection. A suitable breeding scheme for MAGP depends on the number of genes/QTLs required for improvement of traits, the number of parents that contain the required genes/QTLs, the heritability of traits of interest, and other factors (e.g. marker-gene association, expected duration to complete the plan and relative cost). Assuming three or four desired genes/QTLs exist separately in three or four lines, pyramiding of them can be realized by three-way, four-way or double crossing. They may also be integrated by convergent backcrossing or stepwise backcrossing. However, if there are more than four genes/QTLs to be pyramided, complex or multiple crossing and/or recurrent selection may be often preferred.

For MABC-based gene pyramiding, in general, there may be three strategies or breeding schemes: stepwise, simultaneous/synchronized and convergent backcrossing or transfer. Supposing one cultivar W is superior in comprehensive performance but lack of a trait of interest, and four different genes/QTLs contributing to the trait have been identified in four germplasm lines (e.g. P1, P2, P3 and P4). Three MABC schemes for pyramiding the genes/QTLs can be described as follow.

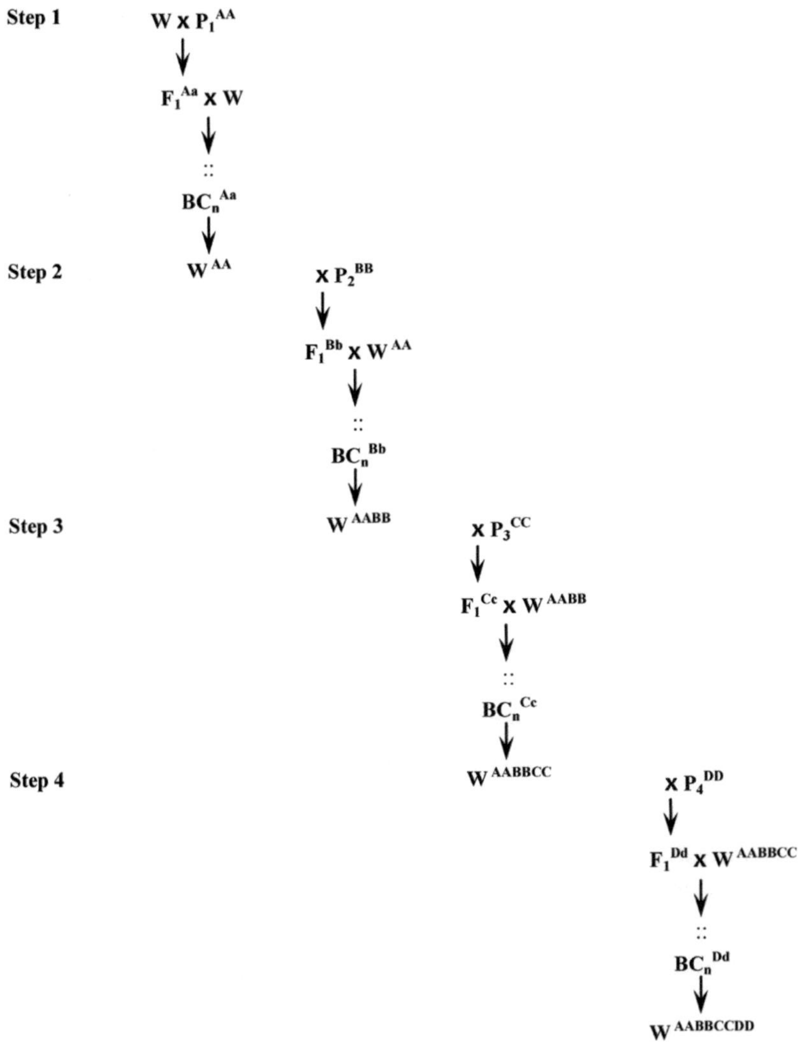

Scheme 1. Stepwise Backcrossing

http://dx.doi.org/10.5772/52583

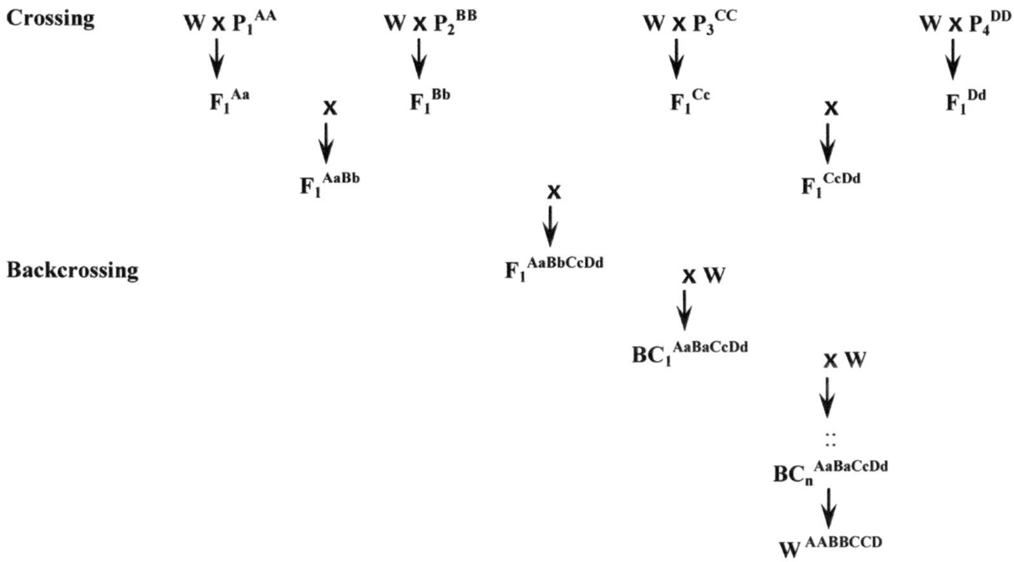

Scheme 2. Simultaneous/Synchronized Backcrossing

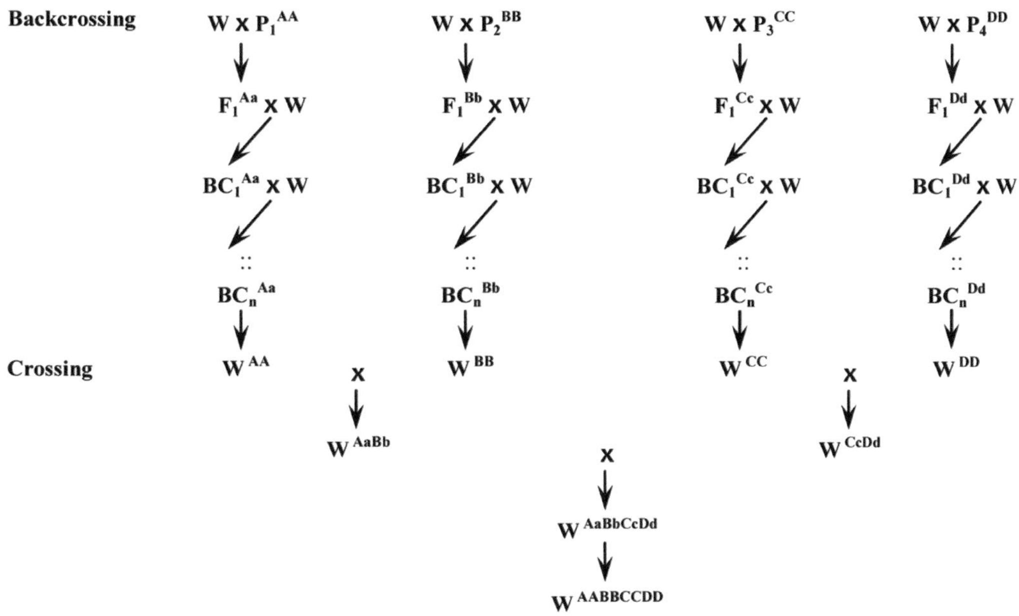

Scheme 3. Convergent Backcrossing

In the stepwise backcrossing, four target genes/QTLs are transferred into the recurrent parent W in order. In one step of backcrossing, one gene/QTL is targeted and selected, followed by next step of backcrossing for another gene/QTL, until all target genes/QTLs have been introgressed into the RP. The advantage is that gene pyramiding is more precise and easier to implement as it involves only one gene/QTL at one time and thus the population size and genotyping amount will be small. The improved recurrent parent may be released before the final step as long as the integrated genes/QTLs (e.g. two or three) meet the requirement at that time. The disadvantage is that it takes a longer time to complete. In the simultaneous or synchronized backcrossing, the recurrent parent W is first crossed to each of four donor parents to produce four single-cross F_1s. Two of the four single-cross F_1s are crossed with each other to produce two double-cross F_1s, and these two double-cross F_1s are crossed again to produce a hybrid integrating all four target genes/QTLs in heterozygous state. The hybrid and/or progeny with heterozygous markers for all four target genes/QTLs is subsequently crossed back to the RP W until a satisfactory recovery of the RP genome, and finalized by one generation of selfing. The advantage of this method is that it takes the shortest time to complete. However, in the backcrossing all target genes/QTLs are involved at the same time and thus it requires a large population and more genotyping. Convergent backcrossing is a strategy combining the advantages of stepwise and synchronized backcrossing. First the four target gene/QTLs are transferred separately from the donors into the recurrent parent W by single crossing followed by backcrossing based on markers linked to the target genes/QTLs, to produce four improved lines (W^{AA}, W^{BB}, W^{CC}, and W^{DD}). Two of the improved lines are crossed with each other and the two hybrids are then intercrossed to integrate all four genes/QTLs together and develop the final improved line with all four genes/QTLs pyramided (i.g. $W^{AABBCCDD}$). Relatively speaking, convergent backcrossing is more acceptable because in this scheme not only is time reduced (compared to stepwise transfer) but gene fixation and/or pyramiding is also more easily assured (compared to simultaneous transfer).

Theoretical issues and efficiency of MABC for gene pyramiding have been investigated through computer simulations (Ribaut et al., 2002; Servin et al., 2004; Ye and Smith, 2008). Practical application of MABC to gene pyramiding has been reported in many crops, including rice, wheat, barley, cotton, soybean, common bean and pea, especially for developing durable resistance to stresses in crops. However, there is very limited information available about the release of commercial cultivars resulted from this strategy. Somers et al. (2005) implemented a molecular breeding strategy to introduce multiple pest resistance genes into Canadian wheat. They used high throughput SSR genotyping and half-seed analysis to process backcrossing and selection for six FHB resistance QTLs, plus orange blossom wheat midge resistance gene *Sm1* and leaf rust resistance gene *Lr21*. They also used 45-76 SSR markers to perform background selection in backcrossing populations to accelerate the restoration of the RP genetic background. This strategy resulted in 87% fixation of the elite genetic background at the BC_2F_1 on average and successfully introduced all (up to 4) of the chromosome segments containing FHB, *Sm1* and *Lr21* resistance genes in four separate crosses(Somers et al., 2005). Joshi and Nayak (2010) and Xu (2010) recently reviewed the techniques and practical cases in marker-based gene pyramiding.

Similar to the simultaneous/synchronized backcrossing scheme, marker-assisted complex or convergent crossing (MACC) can be undertaken to pyramid multiple genes/QTLs. In particular, MACC is a proper option of breeding schemes for gene pyramiding if all the parents are improved cultivars or lines with good comprehensive performance and have different or complementary genes or favorable alleles for the traits of interest. The difference from simultaneous backcrossing is that selfing hybrid and progenies replaces backcrossing hybrid to the recurrent parent. In MACC, the hybrid of convergent crossing is subsequently self-pollinated and marker-based selection for target traits is performed for several consecutive generations until genetically stable lines with desired marker alleles and traits have been developed. In order to reduce population size and to avoid loss of most important genes/QTLs, different markers may be used and selected in different generations, depending on their relative importance. The markers for the most important genes/QTLs can be detected and selected first in early generations and less important markers later. Once homozygous alleles of the markers for a gene/locus are detected, they may not be necessarily detected again in the subsequent generations. Instead, phenotypic evaluation should be conducted if conditions permit.

Using markers to select or pyramid for multiple genes/QTLs is more complex and less proven. Recurrent selection is widely regarded as an effective strategy for the improvement of polygenic traits. However, the effectiveness and efficiency of selection are not so satisfactory in some cases because phenotypic selection is highly dependent upon environments and genotypic selection takes a longer time (2-3 crop seasons at least for one cycle of selection). Marker-assisted recurrent selection (MARS) is a scheme which allows performing genotypic selection and intercrossing in the same crop season for one cycle of selection (Fig. 1). Therefore, MARS could enhance the efficiency of recurrent selection and accelerate the progress of the procedure (Jiang et al., 2007a), particularly helps in integrating multiple favorable genes/QTLs from different sources through recurrent selection based on a multiple-parental population.

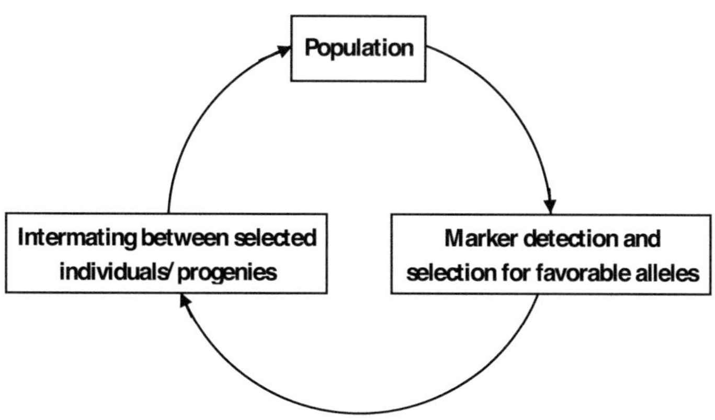

Figure 1. General procedure of marker-assisted recurrent selection (MARS)

For complex traits such as grain yield, biotic and abiotic resistance, MARS has been proposed for "forward breeding" of native genes and pyramiding multiple QTLs (Ragot et al., 2000; Ribaut et al., 2000, 2010; Eathington, 2005; Crosbie et al., 2006). As defined by Ribaut et al. (2010), MARS is a recurrent selection scheme using molecular markers for the identification and selection of multiple genomic regions involved in the expression of complex traits to assemble the best-performing genotype within a single or across related populations. Johnson (2004) presented an example to demonstrate the efficiency of MARS for quantitative traits. In their maize MARS programs, a large-scale use of markers in biparental populations, first for QTL detection and then for MARS on yield (i.e. rapid cycles of recombination and selection based on associated markers for yield), could allow increased efficiency of long-term selection by increasing the frequency of favorable alleles (Johnson, 2004). Eathington (2005) and Crosbie et al. (2006) also indicated that the genetic gain achieved through MARS in maize was about twice that of phenotypic selection (PS) in some reference populations. In upland cotton, Yi et al. (2004) reported significant effectiveness of MARS for resistance to *Helicoverpa armigera*. The mean levels of resistance in improved populations after recurrent selection were significantly higher than those of preceding populations.

7. Genomic selection

Genomic selection (GS) or genome-wide selection (GWS) is a form of marker-based selection, which was defined by Meuwissen (2007) as the simultaneous selection for many (tens or hundreds of thousands of) markers, which cover the entire genome in a dense manner so that all genes are expected to be in linkage disequilibrium with at least some of the markers. In GS genotypic data (genetic markers) across the whole genome are used to predict complex traits with accuracy sufficient to allow selection on that prediction alone. Selection of desirable individuals is based on genomic estimated breeding value (GEBV) (Nakaya and Isobe, 2012), which is a predicted breeding value calculated using an innovative method based on genome-wide dense DNA markers (Meuwissen et al., 2001). GS does not need significant testing and identifying a subset of markers associated with the trait (Meuwissen et al., 2001). In other words, QTL mapping with populations derived from specific crosses can be avoided in GS. However, it does first need to develop GS models, i.e. the formulae for GEBV prediction (Nakaya and Isobe, 2012). In this process (training phase), phenotypes and genome-wide genotypes are investigated in the training population (a subset of a population) to predict significant relationships between phenotypes and genotypes using statistical approaches. Subsequently, GEBVs are used for the selection of desirable individuals in the breeding phase, instead of the genotypes of markers used in traditional MAS. For accuracy of GEBV and GS, genome-wide genotype data is necessary and require high marker density in which all quantitative trait loci (QTLs) are in linkage disequilibrium with at least one marker.

GS can be possible only when high-throughput marker technologies, high-performance computing and appropriate new statistical methods become available. This approach has become feasible due to the discovery and development of large number of single nucleotide polymorphisms (SNPs) by genome sequencing and new methods to efficiently genotype large number of SNP markers. As suggested by Goddard and Hayes (2007), the ideal method to estimate the breeding value from genomic data is to calculate the conditional mean of the breeding value given the genotype at each QTL. This conditional mean can only be calculated by using a prior distribution of QTL effects, and thus this should be part of the research to implement GS. In practice, this method of estimating breeding values is approximated by using the marker genotypes instead of the QTL genotypes, but the ideal method is likely to be approached more closely as more sequence and SNP data are obtained (Goddard and Hayes, 2007).

Since the application of GS was proposed by Meuwissen et al. (2001) to breeding populations, theoretical, simulation and empirical studies have been conducted, mostly in animals (Goddard and Hayes, 2007; Jannink et al., 2010). Relatively speaking, GS in plants was less studied and large-scale empirical studies are not available in public sectors for plant breeding (Jannink et al., 2010), but it has attracted more and more attention in recent years (Bernardo, 2010; Bernardo and Yu, 2007; Guo et al., 2011; Heffner et al., 2010, 2011; Lorenzana and Bernardo, 2009; Wong and Bernardo, 2008; Zhong et al., 2009). Studies indicated that in all cases, accuracies provided by GS were greater than might be achieved on the basis of pedigree information alone (Jannink et al., 2010). In oil palm, for a realistic yet relatively small population, GS was superior to MARS and PS in terms of gain per unit cost and time (Wong and Bernardo, 2008). The studies have demonstrated the advantages of GS, suggesting that GS would be a potential method for plant breeding and it could be performed with realistic sizes of populations and markers when the populations used are carefully chosen (Nakaya and Isobe, 2012).

GS has been highlighted as a new approach for MAS in recent years and is regarded as a powerful, attractive and valuable tool for plant breeding. However, GS has not become a popular methodology in plant breeding, and there might be a far way to go before the extensive use of GS in plant breeding programs. The major reason might be the unavailability of sufficient knowledge of GS for practical use (Nakaya and Isobe, 2012). Statistics and simulation discussed in terms of formulae in GS studies are most likely too specific and hard for plant breeders to understand and to use in practical breeding programs. From a plant breeder's point of view, GS can be practicable for a few breeding populations with a specific purpose, but may be impractical for a whole breeding program dealing with hundreds and thousands of crosses/populations at the same time. Therefore, GS must shift from theory to practice, and its accuracy and cost effectiveness must be evaluated in practical breeding programs to provide convincing empirical evidence and warrant a practicable addition of GS to a plant breeder's toolbox (Heffner et al., 2009). Development of easily understandable formulae for GEBVs and user-friendly software packages for GS analysis is helpful in facilitating and enhancing the application of GS in plant breeding. Kumpatla et al. (2012) recently presented an overall review on the GS for plant breeding.

8. Marker-based breeding and conventional breeding: Challenges and perspectives

Marker-assisted breeding became a new member in the family of plant breeding as various types of molecular markers in crop plants were developed during the 1980s and 1990s. The extensive use of molecular markers in various fields of plant science, e.g. germplasm evaluation, genetic mapping, map-based gene discovery, characterization of traits and crop improvement, has proven that molecular technology is a powerful and reliable tool in genetic manipulation of agronomically important traits in crop plants. Compared with conventional breeding methods, MAB has significant advantages:

a. MAB can allow selection for all kinds of traits to be carried out at seedling stage and thus reduce the time required before the phenotype of an individual plant is known. For the traits that are expressed at later developmental stages, undesirable genotypes can be quickly eliminated by MAS. This feature is particularly important and useful for some breeding schemes such as backcrossing and recurrent selection, in which crossing with or between selected individuals is required.

b. MAB can be not affected by environment, thus allowing the selection to be performed under any environmental conditions (e.g. greenhouse and off-season nurseries). This is very helpful for improvement of some traits (e.g. disease/pest resistance and stress tolerance) that are expressed only when favorable environmental conditions present. For low-heritability traits that are easily affected by environments, MAS based on reliable markers tightly linked to the QTLs for traits of interest can be more effective and produce greater progress than phenotypic selection.

c. MAB using co-dominance markers (e.g. SSR and SNP) can allow effective selection of recessive alleles of desired traits in the heterozygous status. No selfing or test crossing is needed to detect the traits controlled by recessive alleles, thus saving time and accelerating breeding progress.

d. For the traits controlled by multiple genes/QTLs, individual genes/QTLs can be identified and selected in MAB at the same time and in the same individuals, and thus MAB is particularly suitable for gene pyramiding. In traditional phenotypic selection, however, to distinguish individual genes/loci is problematic as one gene may mask the effect of additional genes.

e. Genotypic assays based on molecular markers may be faster, cheaper and more accurate than conventional phenotypic assays, depending on the traits and conditions, and thus MAB may result in higher effectiveness and higher efficiency in terms of time, resources and efforts saved.

The research and use of MAB in plants has continued to increase in the public and private sectors, particularly since 2000s. However, MAS and MABC were and are primarily constrained to simply-inherited traits, such as monogenic or oligogenic resistance to diseases/ pests, although quantitative traits were also involved (Collard and Mackill, 2008; Segmagn et al., 2006; Wang and Chee, 2010). The application of molecular markers in plant breeding has not achieved the results as expected previously in terms of extent and success (e.g. release of commercial cultivars). Collard and Mackill (2008) listed ten reasons for the low impact of MAS and MAB in general. Improvement of most agronomic traits that are of complicated inheritance and economic importance like yield and quality is still a great challenge for MAB including the newly developed GS. From the viewpoint of a plant breeder, MAB is not universally or necessarily advantageous. The application of molecular technologies to plant breeding is still facing the following drawbacks and/or challenges:

a. Not all markers are breeder-friendly. This problem may be solved by converting of non-breeder-friendly markers to other types of breeder-friendly markers (e.g. RFLP to STS, sequence tagged site, and RAPD to SCAR, sequence characterized amplified region).

b. Not all markers can be applicable across populations due to lack of marker polymorphism or reliable marker-trait association. Multiple mapping populations are helpful in understanding marker allelic diversity and genetic background effects. In addition, QTL positions and effects also need to be validated and re-estimated by breeders in their specific germplasm (Heffner et al., 2009).

c. False selection may occur due to recombination between the markers and the genes/QTLs of interest. Use of flanking markers or more markers for the target gene/QTL can help.

d. Imprecise estimates of QTL locations and effects result in slower progress than expected. The efficiency of QTL detection is attributed to multiple factors, such as algorithms, mapping methods, number of polymorphic markers, and population type and size (Wang et al., 2012). High marker density fine mapping with large populations and well-designed phenotyping across multiple environments may provide more accurate estimates of QTL location and effects.

e. A large number of breeding programs have not been equipped with adequate facilities and conditions for a large-scale adoption of MAB in practice.

f. The methods and schemes of MAB must be easily understandable, acceptable and implementable for plant breeders, unless they are not designed for a large scale use in practical breeding programs.

g. Higher startup expenses and labor costs.

With a long history of development, especially since the fundamental principles of inheritance were established in the late 19th and early 20th centuries, plant breeding has become an important component of agricultural science, which has features of both science and arts. Conventional breeding methodologies have extensively proven successful in development of cultivars and germplasm. However, subjective evaluation and empirical selection still play a considerable role in conventional breeding. Scientific breeding needs less experience and more science. MAB has brought great challenges, opportunities and prospects for conventional breeding. As a new member of the whole family of plant breeding, however, MAB, as transgenic breeding or genetic manipulation does, cannot replace conventional breeding but is and only is a supplementary addition to conventional breeding. High costs and technical or equipment demands of MAB will continue to be a major obstacle for its large-scale use in the near future, especially in the developing countries (Collard and Mackill, 2008; Ribaut et al., 2010). Therefore, integration of MAB into conventional breeding programs will be an optimistic strategy for crop improvement in the future. It can be expected that the drawbacks of MAB will be gradually overcome, as its theory, technology and application are further developed and improved. This should lead to a wide adoption and use of MAB in practical breeding programs for more crop species and in more countries as well.

Author details

Guo-Liang Jiang

Plant Science Department, South Dakota State University, Brookings, USA

References

[1] Anderson, J.A., S. Chao, and S. Liu, 2007: Molecular breeding using a major QTL for Fusarium head blight resistance in wheat. Crop Sci. 47, S-112–119.

[2] Babu, R., S.K. Nair, B.M. Prasanna, and H.S. Gupta. 2004. Integrating marker-assisted selection in crop breeding – Prospects and challenges. Current Science 87: 607-619.

[3] Babu, R., S.K. Nair, A. Kumar, S. Venkatesh, J.C. Sekhar, N.N Singh, G. Srinivasan, and H.S. Gupta. 2005. Two-generation marker-aided backcrossing for rapid conversion of normal maize lines to quality protein maize (QPM). Theor. Appl. Genet. 111: 888-897.

[4] Bernacchi, D., T. Beck-Bunn, D. Emmatty, Y. Eshed, S. Inai, J. Lopez, V. Petiard, H. Sayama, J. Uhlig, D. Zamir, and S.D. Tanksley. 1998. Advanced backcross QTL analysis of tomato: II. Evaluation of near-isogenic lines carrying single-donor introgressions for desirable wild QTL-alleles derived from *Lycopersicon hirsutum* and *L. pimpinellifolium*. Theor. Appl. Genet. 97: 170-180.

[5] Bernardo, R. 2010. Genomewide selection with minimal crossing in self-pollinated crops. Crop Sci. 50: 624-627.

[6] Bernardo, R., and J. Yu. 2007. Prospects for genomewide selection for quantitative traits in maize. Crop Sci. 47: 1082-1090.

[7] Bilyeu, K., L. Palavalli, D.A. Sleper, and P. Beuselinck. 2006. Molecular genetic resources for development of 1% linolenic acid soybeans. Crop Sci. 46: 1913-1918.

[8] Bonnett, D.G., G.J. Rebetzke, and W. Spielmeyer. 2005. Strategies for efficient implementation of molecular markers in wheat breeding. Mol. Breeding 15: 75-85.

[9] Botstein, D., R.L. White, M. Skolnick, and R.W. Davis. 1980. Construction of a genetic linkage map in man using restriction fragment length polymorphisms. Am. J. Hum. Genet. 32: 314-331.

[10] Bradbury, L.M.T., T.L. Fitzgerald, R.J. Henry, Q. Jin, and Waters, D.L.E. (2005a). The gene for fragrance in rice. Plant Biotech. J. 3: 363–370.

[11] Bradbury, L.M.T., R.J. Henry, Q. Jin, R.F. Reinke, and Waters, D.L.E. (2005b). A perfect marker for fragrance genotyping in rice. Mol. Breeding 16:279-283.

[12] Buerstmayr, H., T. Ban, and J.A. Anderson. 2009. QTL mapping and marker-assisted selection for Fusarium head blight resistance in wheat: a review. Plant Breeding 128: 1-26.

[13] Castro, A.J., F. Capettini, A.E. Corey, T. Filichkina, P.M. Hayes, A. Kleinhofs, D. Kudrna, K. Richardson, S. Sandoval-Islas, C. Rossi, and H. Vivar. 2003. Mapping and pyramiding of qualitative and quantitative resistance to stripe rust in barley. Theor. Appl. Genet. 107: 922-930.

[14] Collard, B.C.Y., and D.J. Mackill. 2008. Marker-assisted selection: an approach for precision plant breeding in the twenty-first century. Phil. Trans. R. Soc. B 363: 557-572.

[15] Collard, B.C.Y., M.Z.Z. Jahufer, JB Brouwer, and E.C.K. Pang. 2005. An introduction to markers, quantitative trait loci (QTL) mapping and marker-assisted selection for crop improvement: the basic concepts. Euphytica 142: 169-196.

[16] Concibido, V.C., B. La Vallee, P. Mclaird, N. Pineda, J. Meyer, L. Hummel, J. Yang, K. Wu, and X. Delannay. 2003. Introgression of a quantitative trait locus for yield from *Glycine soja* into commercial soybean cultivars. Theor. Appl. Genet. 106: 575-582.

[17] Cregan, P.B., J. Mudge, E.W Fickus, D. Danesh, R. Denny, and N.D. Young. 1999. Two simple sequence repeat markers to select for soybean cyst nematode resistance conditioned by the *rhg1* locus. Theor. Appl. Genet. 99: 811-818.

[18] Crosbie, T.M., S.R. Eathington, G.R. Johnson, M. Edwards, R. Reiter, S. Stark, R.G. Mohanty, M. Oyervides, R.E. Buehler, A.K. Walker, R. Dobert, X. Delannay, J.C. Pershing, M.A. Hall, and K.R. Lamkey. 2006. Plant breeding: past, present and future. In: K.R. Lamkey and M. Lee (eds.), Plant Breeding: the Arnel R. Hallauer International Symposium, Blackwell Publishing, Oxford, UK, pp. 3-50.

[19] Dwivedi, S.L., J.H. Crouch, D.J. Mackill, Y. Xu, M.W. Blair, M. Ragot, H.D. Upadhyaya, and R. Oritiz. 2007. The molecularization of public sector crop breeding: progress, problems and prospects. Advances in Agronomy 95: 163-318.

[20] Eathington, S.R. 2005.Practical applications of molecular technology in the development of commercial maize hybrids. In: Proceedings of the 60th Annual Corn and Sorghum Seed Research Conferences, American Seed Trade Association, Washington, D.C.

[21] Edwards, D., J.W. Forster, D. Chagne, and J. Batley. 2007. What is SNPs? In: N.C. Oraguzie, E.H.A. Rikkerink, S.E. Gardiner and H.N. de Silva (eds.), Association Mapping in Plants. Springer, Berlin, pp 41-52.

[22] Farooq, S., and F. Azam. 2002a. Molecular markers in plant breeding-I: Concepts and characterization. Pakistan J Biol. Sci. 5: 1135-1140.

[23] Farooq, S., and F. Azam. 2002b. Molecular markers in plant breeding-II: Some prerequisites for use. Pakistan J Biol. Sci. 5: 1141-1147.

[24] Flint-Garcia, S.A., L.L. Darrah, M.D. McMullen, and B.E. Hibbard. 2003. Phenotypic versus marker-assisted selection for stalk strength and second-generation European corn borer resistance in maize. Theor. Appl. Genet. 107: 1331-1336.

[25] Frisch, M., M. Bohn, and A.E. Melchinger. 1999. Comparison of selection strategies for marker-assisted backcrossing of a gene. Crop Sci. 39: 1295-1301 (See also Errata, Frisch et al., 1999. Crop Sci. 39: 1903).

[26] Fulton, T.M., P. Bucheli, E. Voirol, J. Lopez, V. Peetiard, and S.D. Tanksley. 2002. Quantitative trait loci (QTL) affecting sugars, organic acids and other biochemical properties possibly contributing to flavor, identified in four advanced backcross populations of tomato. Euphytica 127: 163-177.

[27] Goddard, M.E., and B.J. Hayes. 2007. Genomic selection. J. Anim. Breed. Genet..124: 323-330.

[28] Guo, Z., D.M. Tucker, J. Liu, V. Kishore, and G. Gay. 2011. Evaluation of genome-wide selection efficiency in maize nested association mapping populations. Theor. Appl. Genet. 124: 261-275.

[29] Gupta, P.K., J.K. Roy, and M. Prasad. 2001. Single nucleotide polymorphisms: a new paradigm for molecular marker technology and DNA polymorphism detection with emphasis on their use in plants. Current Science 80: 524-535.

[30] Heffner, E.L., M.E. Sorrells, and Jannink, J.-L. 2009. Genomic selection for crop improvement. Crop Sc. 49: 1-12.

[31] Heffner, E.L., A.J. Lorenz, Jannink, J.-L. and M.E. Sorrells. 2010. Plant breeding with genomic selection: gain per unit time and cost. Crop Sci. 50: 1681-1690.

[32] Heffner, E.L., Jannink, J.-L., H. Iwata, E. Souza, and M.E. Sorrells. 2011. Genomic selection accuracy for grain quality traits in biparental wheat populations. Crop Sci. 51: 2597-2606.

[33] Hospital, F. 2003.Marker-assisted breeding. In: H.J. Newbury (ed.), Plant molecular breeding. Blackwell Publishing and CRC Press, Oxford and Boca Raton, pp. 30-59.

[34] Hospital, F., C. Chevalet, and P. Mulsant. 1992. Using markers in gene introgression breeding programs. Genetics 231: 1199-1210.

[35] Hospital, F., and G. Decoux. 2002. Popmin: a program for the numerical optimization of population sizes in marker-assisted backcross breeding programs. Journal of Heredity 93: 383-384.

[36] Huang, N., E.R. Angeles, J. Domingo, G. Magpantay, S. Singh, G. Zhang, N. Kumaravadivel, J. Bennet, and G.S. Khush. 1997. Pyramiding of bacterial blight resistance genes in rice: marker-assisted selection using RFLP and PCR. Theor. Appl. Genet. 95: 313-320.

[37] Jannink, J.-L., A.J. Lorenz, and H. Iwata. 2010. Genomic selection in plant breeding: from theory to practice. Briefings in Functional Genomics 9: 166-177.

[38] Jefferies, S.P., B.J. King, A.R. Barr, P. Warner, S.J. Logue, and P. Langridge. 2003. Marker-assisted backcross introgression of the *Yd2* gene conferring resistance to barley yellow dwarf virus in barley. Plant Breeding 122: 52-56.

[39] Jiang, G.-L., Shi, J., & Ward, R. W. (2007a). QTL analysis of resistance to Fusarium head blight in the novel wheat germplasm CJ 9306. I. Resistance to fungal spread. Theor. Appl. Genet. 116: 3-13.

[40] Jiang, G.-L., Dong, Y., Shi, J., & Ward, R. W. (2007b). QTL analysis of resistance to *Fusarium* head blight in the novel wheat germplasm CJ 9306. II. Resistance to deoxynivalenol accumulation and grain yield loss. Theor. Appl. Genet. 115: 1043-1052.

[41] Johnson, R. 2004. Marker assisted selection. In: J. Jannick (Ed.), Plant Breed. Rev. Vol. 24, Part 1, 293-309.

[42] Joshi, R.K., and S. Nayak. 2010. Gene pyramiding – A broad spectrum technique for developing durable stress resistance in crops. Biotechol. Mol. Biol. Rev. 5: 51-60.

[43] Konieczny, A., and F. Ausubel. 1993. A procedure for mapping Arabidopsis mutations using co-dominant ecotype-specific PCR based markers. The Plant Journal 4: 403-410.

[44] Kumpatla, S.P., R. Buyyarapu, I.Y. Abdurakhmonov, and J.A. Mammadov. 2012. Genomics-assisted plant breeding in the 21st century: technological advances and progress. In: I.Y. Abdurakhmonov (ed.), Plant Breeding, InTech, pp 131-184.

[45] Lecomte, L., P. Duffé, M. Buret, B. Servin, F. Hospital, and M. Causse. 2004. Marker-assisted introgression of five QTLs controlling fruit quality traits into three tomato lines revealed interactions between QTLs and genetic backgrounds. Theor. Appl. Genet. 109: 568-668.

[46] Li, X., Y. Han, W. Teng, S. Zhang, K. Yu, V. Poysa, T. Anderson, J. Ding, and W. Li. 2010. Pyramided QTL underlying tolerance to Phytophthora root rot in mega-environment from soybean cultivar 'Conrad' and 'Hefeng 25'.Theor. Appl. Genet. 121: 651-658.

[47] Liu, B.-H. 1991. Development and prospects of dwarf male-sterile wheat. Chinese Science Bulletin, 36(4), 306.

[48] Lorenzana, R.F., and R. Bernardo. 2009. Accuracy of genotypic predictions for marker-based selection in biparental plant populations. Theor. Appl. Genet. 120: 151-161.

[49] Luo, Y., J.S. Sangha, S. Wang, Z. Li, J. Yang, and Z. Yin. 2012. Marker-assisted breeding of *Xa4, Xa21* and *Xa27* in the restorer lines of hybrid rice for broad-spectrum and enhanced disease resistance to bacterial blight. Mol. Breeding DOI 10.1007/s11032-012-9742-7.

[50] Meuwissen, T. 2007. Genomic selection: marker assisted selection on a genome wide scale. J. Anim. Breed. Genet. 124: 321-322.

[51] Meuwissen, T.H.E., B.J. Hayes, and M.E. Goddard. 2001. Prediction of total genetic value using genome wide dense marker maps. Genetics 157: 1819-1829.

[52] Miedaner, T., F. Wilde, B. Steiner, H. Buerstmayr, V. Korzun, and E. Ebmeyer, 2006. Stacking quantitative trait loci (QTL) for Fusarium head blight resistance from non-adapted sources in an European elite spring wheat background and assessing their effects on deoxynivalenol (DON) content and disease severity. Theor. Appl. Genet. 112: 562-569.

[53] Moreau, L., A. Charcosset, F. Hospital, and A. Gallais. 1998. Marker-assisted selection efficiency in populations of finite size. Genetics 148: 1353-1365.

[54] Mullis, K. 1990. The unusual origin of the polymerase chain reaction. Scientific American 262 (4): 56–61, 64–65.

[55] Nakaya, A., and S.N. Isobe. 2012. Will genomic selection be a practical method for plant breeding? Annals of Botany, DOI:10.1093/aob/mcs109.

[56] Newbury, H.J. 2003. Plant Molecular Breeding. Blackwell Publishing, CRC Press, Birmingham, UK.

[57] Payne, P.I., M.A. Nigtingale, A.F. Krattiger, and L.M. Holt. 1987. The relationship between HMW glutenin subunit composition and the bread-making quality of British-grown wheat varieties. Journal of the Science of Food and Agriculture 40: 51-65.

[58] Pham, A.-T., J.G. Shannon, and K.D. Bilyeu. 2012. Combinations of mutant FAD2 and FAD3 genes to produce high oleic acid and low linolenic acid soybean oil. Theor. Appl. Genet. 125: 503–515.

[59] Pumphrey, M. O., R. Bernardo, and J. A. Anderson, 2007: Validating the *Fhb1* QTL for Fusarium head blight resistance in near-isogenic wheat lines developed from breeding populations. Crop Sci. 47: 200-206.

[60] Ragot, M., M. Biasiolli, M.F. Dekbut, A. Dell'orco, L. Margarini, P. Thevenin, J. Vernoy, J. Vivant, R. Zimmermann, and G. Gay. 1995. Marker-assisted backcrossing: a practical example. In: A. Berville and M. Tersac (eds.), Les Colloques, No. 72, INRA, Paris, 45-46.

[61] Ragot, M., G. Gay, J.P. Muller, and J. Durovray. 2000. Efficient selection for the adaptation to the environment through QTL mapping and manipulation in maize. In: J.M.

Ribaut and D. Poland (eds.), Molecular Approaches for the Genetic Improvement of Cereals for Stable Production in Water-limited Environments. CIMMYT, Mexico, pp 128-130.

[62] Ribaut, J.M., and J. Betran. 1999. Single large-scale marker-assisted selection (SLS-MAS). Mol. Breeding 5: 531-541.

[63] Ribaut, J.M., G. Edmeades, E. Perotti, and D. Hoisington. 2000. QTL analysis, MAS results and perspectives for drought-tolerance improvement in tropical maize. In: J.M. Ribaut and D. Poland (eds.), Molecular Approaches for the Genetic Improvement of Cereals for Stable Production in Water-limited Environments. CIMMYT, Mexico, pp 131-136.

[64] Ribaut, J.M., C. Jiang, and D. Hoisington. 2002. Simulation experiments on efficiencies of gene introgression by backcrossing. Crop Sci. 42: 557-565.

[65] Ribaut, J.M., M.C. de Vicente, and X. Delannay. 2010. Molecular breeding in developing countries: challenges and perspectives. Current Opinion in Plant Biology 13: 1-6.

[66] Richardson, K.L., M.I. Vales, J.G. Kling, C.C. Mundt, and P.M. Hayes. 2006. Pyramiding and dissecting disease resistance QTL to barley stripe rust. Theor. Appl. Genet. 113: 485-495.

[67] Rogers, W.J., P.I. Payne, and Harinder K. (1989). The HMW glutenin subunit and gliadin compositions of German-Grown wheat varieties and their relationship with bread-making quality. Plant Breeding 103: 89-100.

[68] Sebolt, A.M., R.C. Shoemaker, and B.W. Diers. 2000. Analysis of a quantitative trait locus allele from wild soybean that increases seed protein concentration in soybean. Crop Sci. 40: 1438-1444.

[69] Semagn, K., A. Bjornstad, and M.N. Ndjiondjop. (2006a). An overview of molecular marker methods for plants. Afr. J. Biotechnol. 5: 2540-2568.

[70] Semagn, K., A. Bjornstad, and M.N. Ndjiondjop. (2006b). Progress and prospects of marker assisted backcrossing as a tool in crop breeding programs. Afr. J. Biotechnol. 5: 2588-2603.

[71] Servin, B., and F. Hospital. 2002. Optimal positioning of markers to control genetic background in marker-assisted backcrossing. The Journal of Heredity 93: 214-217.

[72] Servin, B., O.C. Martin, M. Mezard, and F. Hospital. 2004. Toward a theory of marker-assisted gene pyramiding. Genetics 168: 513-523.

[73] Shi, A., P. Chen, D. Li, C. Zheng, B. Zhang, and A. Hou. 2009. Pyramiding multiple genes for resistance to soybean mosaic virus in soybean using molecular markers. Mol. Breeding 23: 113-124.

[74] Singh, S., J.S. Sidhu, N. Huang, Y. Vikal, Z. Li, D.S. Brar, H.S. Dhaliwal, and G.S Khush. 2001. Pyramiding three bacterial blight resistance genes (*xa5*, *xa13* and *Xa21*)

using marker-assisted selection into indica rice cultivar PR106. Theor. Appl. Genet. 102: 1011-1015.

[75] Sobrino, B., M. Briona, and A. Carracedoa. 2005. SNPs in forensic genetics: a review on SNP typing methodologies. Forensic Science International 154: 181-194.

[76] Somers, D.J., J. Thomas, R. DePauw, S. Fox, G. Humphreys, and G. Fedak. 2005. Assembling complex genotypes to resist *Fusarium* in wheat (*Triticum aestivum* L.). Theor. Appl. Genet. 111: 1623-1631.

[77] Song, Q., G. Jia, Y. Zhu, D. Grant, R.T. Nelson, , Hwang, E.-Y., D.L. Hyten, and P.B. Cregan. 2010. Abundance of SSR motifs and development of candidate polymorphic SSR markers (BARCSOYSSR_1.0) in soybean. Crop Sci. 50: 1950-1960.

[78] Southern, E. M. (1975). Detection of specific sequences among DNA fragments separated by gel electrophoresis. Journal of Molecular Biology 98: 503-517.

[79] Stuber, C.W., M. Polacco, and M.L. Senior. 1999. Synergy of empirical breeding, marker-assisted selection and genomics to increase crop yield potential. Crop Sci. 39: 1571-1583.

[80] Tanksley, S.D., and J.C. Nelson. 1996. Advanced backcross QTL analysis: a method for the simultaneous discovery and transfer of valuable QTLs from unadapted germplasm into elite breeding lines. Theor. Appl. Genet. 92: 191-203.

[81] Tanksley, S.D., N.D. Young, A.H. Paterson, and M.W. Bonierbale. 1989. RFLP mapping in plant breeding: new tools for an old science. Bio. Technology 7: 257-263.

[82] Visscher, P.M., R. Thompson, and C.S. Haley. 1996. Confidence intervals in QTL mapping by booststrapping. Genetics 143: 1013-1020.

[83] Wang, B., and P.W. Chee. 2010. Application of advanced backcross quantitative trait locus (QTL) analysis in crop improvement. Journal of Plant Breeding and Crop Science 2: 221-232.

[84] Wang, X., Jiang, G.-L., M. Green, R.A. Scott, D.L. Hyten, and P.B. Cregan. 2012. Quantitative trait locus analysis of saturated fatty acids in a population of recombinant inbred lines of soybean. Mol. Breeding, DOI 10.1007/s11032-012-9704-0.

[85] Wong, C.K., and R. Bernardo. 2008. Genome wide selection in oil palm: increasing selection gain per unit time and cost with small populations. Theor. Appl. Genet. 116: 815-824.

[86] Xu, Y. 2010. Molecular plant breeding. CAB International.

[87] Ye, G., and K.F. Smith. 2008. Marker-assisted gene pyramiding for inbred line development: Basic principles and practical guidelines. Intern. J. Plant Breed. 2: 1-10.

[88] Yi, C., W. Guo, X. Zhu, L. Min, and T. Zhang. 2004. Pyramiding breeding by marker-assisted recurrent selection in upland cotton II. Selection effects on resistance to *Helicoverpa armigera*. Scientia Agricultura Sinica 37: 801-807.

[89] Young, N.D. 1999. A cautiously optimistic vision for marker-assisted breeding. Mol. Breeding 5: 505-510.

[90] Young, N.D., and S.D. Tanksley. 1989. RFLP analysis of the size of chromosomal segments retained around the *Tm-2* locus of tomato during backcross breeding. Theor. Appl. Genet. 77: 353-359.

[91] Zhao, X., G. Tan, Y. Xing, L. Wei, Q. Chao, W. Zuo, T. Lübberstedt, and M. Xu. 2012. Marker-assisted introgression of *qHSR1* to improve maize resistance to head smut. Mol. Breeding, DOI 10.1007/s11032-011-9694-3

[92] Zhong, S., J.C.M. Dekkers, R.L. Fernando, and Jannink, J.-L. (2009). Factors affecting accuracy from genomic selection in populations derived from multiple inbred lines: a barley case study. Genetics 182: 355-364.

Chapter 4

Genetic Dissection of Blackleg Resistance Loci in Rapeseed (*Brassica napus* L.)

Harsh Raman, Rosy Raman and Nick Larkan

Additional information is available at the end of the chapter

http://dx.doi.org/10.5772/53611

1. Introduction

Blackleg disease caused by the heterothallic ascomycete fungus *Leptosphaeria maculans* (Desm.) Ces. et de Not. (anamorph: *Phoma lingam* Tode ex Fr.), is the major disease of Brassica crops such as turnip rape (*Brassica rapa* L. syn. *B. campestris;* 2n = 2x = 20, genome AA), cabbage (*B. oleracea* L.; 2n = 2x = 18, genome CC), rapeseed (syn. canola or oilseed rape *B. napus* L.; 2n = 4x = 38, genome AACC), and *B. juncea* L. (Indian or brown mustard; 2n = 4x = 36, genome AABB) grown in temperate regions of the world. It was recorded for the first time on stems of red cabbage [1]. *B. napus* originated as a result of natural interspecific hybridization and genome doubling between the monogenomic diploid species, *B. rapa* and *B. oleracea,* in southern Europe approximately 10,000–100,000 years ago [2, 3]. However, it was selected and grown as an oilseed crop only 300-500 years ago [4, 5]. *B. napus* originally evolved as a spring or semi-winter type under the Mediterranean climates, and spread rapidly from southern to northern Europe after the development of winter *B. napus* varieties [6]. Both spring and winter types are affected by blackleg disease, particularly in Australia, Europe and North America. Currently *B. napus* is the world's third most important oilseed crop, grown on an area of over 23 million hectares and produce almost 53.3 million tonnes annually [7]. Increase in *B. napus* production has been attributed to the development and release of high yielding superior varieties including hybrids having traits such as high oil content, improved protein quality and herbicide resistance for better crop management.

Among the bacterial, fungal, viral and phytoplasmic-like diseases, blackleg is the most important global disease of *B. napus* crops and causes annual yield losses of more than $900 million in Europe, North America and Australia [8-10]. *L. maculans* has an ability to kill plants even at the seedling stage, infecting cotyledons, leaves, stems, roots and pods. Under epiphytotic conditions, this disease can cause yield losses of up to 90 per cent [11 - 13]. Therefore, control of blackleg disease has been one of the major objectives of many *B. napus* breeding programs.

2. Symptoms

Blackleg disease causes two distinct symptoms; leaf lesions and stem canker. Outbreak of the fungus is characterised by dirty-whitish spots on leaves with small dark fruiting bodies (pycnidia). Black lesions are generally also seen on the leaves and deep brown lesions with a dark margin can be seen on the base of stem [11]. In severe epidemic conditions fungus girdles the stem at the crown, leading to lodging of the plant and possible severance of the stem. Typical lesions of blackleg can also occur on pods. Pod infection may leads to premature pod shatter and seed infection.

3. Biology of the pathogen and epidemiology of the *L. maculans*

The pathogen can infect several crucifers, including cruciferous weeds. Up to 28 crucifer species have been reported as hosts [14]. During infection, the pathogen grows systemically down towards the tap root of the plant, producing severe disease symptoms at the adult plant stage characterised by stem cankers. *L. maculans* reproduces both asexually and sexually on host species and can complete several disease cycles during a single growing season. The fungus survives as mycelium, pycnidia and pseudothecia on crop residues, mainly on stubble [15, 16] subsisting from one season to the next. Sexual mating occurs on crop residues, resulting in the production of ascospores which can travel up to 8 km [17]. High humidity and moderate temperatures during vegetative growth promote disease development [18].

In Australia and most parts of Europe, *L. maculans* infection generally occurs during the seedling stage from infected seed and wind-dispersed ascospores (sexual spores), released from pseudothecia. In western Canada and Poland, asexual pycnidospores are the primary source of inoculum [19], dispersed largely by rain-splash. Under high humidity conditions, ascospores and pycnidiospores adhere to cotyledons or young leaves and germinate to produce hyphae which penetrate through stomata and wounds [9, 20, 21] and grow into sub-stomatal cavities without forming appressoria [22]. After entering into substomatal cavities, the fungus grows between the epidermis and palisade layer and then into intercellular spaces in the mesophyll of lamina. The fungus then reaches the vascular strands and grows within the plant asymptomatically, until eventually invading and killing cells of the stem cortex and causing the stem canker symptom [22-24]. Variability for virulence in *L. maculans* for the first time was reported in 1927 [25]. Australian populations of *L. maculans* have a high level of genetic variability as compared to European and North American isolates [26], along with a high diversity of avirulence genes [27]. Molecular analyses of populations of *L. maculans* have shown high gene flow within and between populations. Isolates of *L. maculans* are usually classified either on the basis of their aggressiveness or into pathogenicity groups [28].

4. Management of the *L. maculans*

Various practices such as crop rotation, stubble management, time of sowing, seed dressing and foliar application of fungicide, and deployment of genetic resistance have been employed to control this disease and subsequently reduce yield losses [9, 29]. Deployment of host resistance has been used as the most cost-effective and environmentally sound measure for disease control in various crops including in rapeseed. This strategy has been extensively used to manage blackleg disease especially in Australia, Canada, France, and Germany.

5. Evaluation of germplasm for *L. maculans* resistance

An efficient and reliable method for phenotyping resistance to *L. maculans* is required for germplasm evaluation and predictive breeding including molecular mapping and gene cloning research. Various criteria are used to assess disease severity, such as severity of cotyledon or stem canker lesions, which rely principally on scales or estimates of the percent of diseased leaf tissue at either seedling (intact and detached leaf) or at adult plant stages. Symptom expression can vary with the environmental conditions, test locations (glasshouse, environment chamber and field conditions), and the method of inoculations (cotyledon, leaf and stem).

Resistance of *B. napus* germplasm to *L. maculans* is tested on the basis of disease reaction under glasshouse and/or field conditions. Cotyledon inoculations, performed under controlled conditions in either a growth chamber or glasshouse, allow for large scale and efficient screening of germplasm. Various environmental conditions such as temperature, light intensity and humidity can be reliably controlled, expediting the development of suitable resistant cultivars [30] as selections can be performed at early stages of plant development. This method also overcomes some of the uncertainties inherent in field testing with its dependence upon growing environment and further reduce the genotype by environment (G x E) interactions. Growth conditions are typically maintained with at 18°C to and 22°C. For uniform infection, a spore suspension is used to inoculate wounded cotyledons of 7 to 15 day-old seedlings [31-33]. Alternatively, seedlings can be sprayed with a spore suspension at up to the third leaf stage and kept at 100 % humidity for 48-72 hr. Spore suspensions of *L. maculans* are generally raised from single-spore isolate cultures grown on different media such as V8-agar, malt-agar and rapeseed leaf extract-agar [21, 22, 34]. Published studies used spore concentrations in the range from 4 x 10^6 to 1x10^8 spores per ml [31 - 33].

Doubled haploid (DH) populations were screened for resistance to *L. maculans* in the glass-house at three plant growth stages: cotyledon, true leaf and adult plant, as well as under field conditions and reported a high correlation ($r \geq 0.82$) for disease severity between glasshouse and field grown lines [33]. Similar observations were also made by McNabb et al [35]. High correlation coefficient values suggest that the resistance to *L. maculans* can be evaluated at all three stages [33]. However among three stages, cotyledon stage was the most promising as inoculum-droplets can be kept at the inoculation site as compared to true leaves.

Assessment of adult plants for resistance to *L. maculans* populations under field conditions is considered very important for the selection of resistant germplasm by the rapeseed breeders. Inoculum is provided by either spreading infected stubble in a disease nursery or spraying plants with fungal spore suspension. Two measures; disease severity and disease incidence are commonly used for evaluating resistance to *L. maculans*. However, disease severity is much more difficult to estimate than disease incidence, due to the G x E interactions and unreliable and inconsistent estimation of canker lesions, even within the same genotype, particularly when infection is not uniform. The use of increased sample size (25 to 50 plants/genotype) and reliable and congenial growing conditions for the disease development will allow better estimation of canker lesions.

Assessment of blackleg resistance under field conditions is usually performed by exposing the plants to a mixed population of *L. maculans* races, which can make the detection of race-specific *R*-genes difficult. No relationship between the degree of cotyledon-lesion development at the seedling stage and crown canker development in mature plants was observed in the intercross population derived from Maluka/Niklas [36]. This study concluded the limited value of the cotyledon test in screening for adult plant blackleg resistance. Similarly a lack of correlation between cotyledon (seedling) resistance and stem (adult plant) resistance in *B. napus* and B genome sources has also been reported [37]. Recently, a poor correlation between seedling and field reactions was reported in the DH from Skipton/Ag-Spectrum which could have been due to the prevalence of different pathotypes under field conditions as contrary to cotyledon test, where often a specific isolate is used for phenotyping [32]. In order to mimic field conditions and increase reliability of disease development, an ascospore shower test [38] has been used for germplasm evaluation and varietal release in Australia. In this test, stubble with mature pseudothecia is sprayed with distilled water until run-off, producing 'ascospore shower'. The infected plants can then be assessed for resistance at both the cotyledon and adult plant stages. This method has shown a high correlation with canker lesions scored under field conditions [39].

6. Natural genetic variation for resistance to *L. maculans*

The introgression of blackleg resistance (*R*) genes into *B. napus* germplasm for blackleg disease management is one of the major objectives of breeding programs aiming to release cultivars in disease-prone areas. Genetic variation for resistance to *L. maculans* exists within *B. napus* germplasm [39, 40, 41]. Some other Brassica species such as *B. rapa, B. juncea, B. nigra* (black mustard; 2n = 2x = 16, genome BB) and *B. carinata* (Abyssinian or Ethiopian mustard; 2n = 34, genome BBCC), as well as other crucifers such as *Sinapis arvensis* have been reported to carry resistance [42-53]. Some of these sources were utilised in transferring resistance into *B. napus* breeding lines and cultivars. A continuous variation for blackleg resistance in a world-wide collection of *B. rapa* genotypes was reported [54]. None of genotypes were completely susceptible or completely resistant to either *L. maculans* pathotypes used. However, some *B. rapa* accessions that were either highly resistant or completely susceptible were identified (Raman et al., unpublished) in a set of differential cultivars currently being used in Australia [39].

It has been reported that all B genome Brassica species; *B. nigra, B. carinata* and *B. juncea* carry complete resistance to *L. maculans* which remains effective throughout the life of the plant [40], however susceptible *B. juncea* cultivars have also been identified [55] demonstrating that complete resistance is not a feature of all B genomes. Some B genome resistance genes have been introgressed into *B. napus* lines. [47, 56-59]. Earlier studies have shown that C genome species of the *Brassica* are susceptible to blackleg [50, 53, 60]. However, a recent study [61] evaluated three accessions of *B. oleracea* var. *virids*, collected from the USDA germplasm collection and found that the accession NSL6146 was moderately resistant to *L. maculans*.

Genetic resources for adult plant resistance are very limited and most of them are derived from the French cultivar Jet Neuf [62]. Efforts are currently being made to identify both qualitative and quantitative resistance in the Australian Brassica Germplasm Improvement Programs.

7. Inheritance of resistance to *L. maculans*

Genetic inheritance studies revealed that resistance to *L. maculans* is complex. Resistance is either described as qualitative (also referred as monogenic/seedling/race-specific resistance/ vertical resistance) or quantitative (also referred as polygenic/adult plant/race non-specific resistance/horizontal resistance) in *Brassica*.

7.1. Qualitative resistance

Monogenic inheritance was reported in several spring and winter cultivars of *B. napus* such as Cresor, Maluka, Dunkeld, Maluka, Skipton, and Major [32, 63-67]. Eighteen major genes for resistance to *L. maculans*; *Rlm1* to *Rlm11*, *RlmS*, *LepR1* to *LepR4*, *BLMR1* and *BLMR2*, have been identified in Brassica species; *B. rapa*, *B. napus*, *B. juncea* and *B. nigra* [31, 32, 40, 45, 68-73]. Six of them, *Rlm1*, *Rlm2*, *Rlm3*, *Rlm4*, *Rlm7* and *Rlm9* were identified in *B. napus*, all of them except *Rlm2* were clustered genetically on chromosome A07 [74]. *Rlm2* was mapped on chromosome A10 [45]. The *Rlm5* and *Rlm6* were identified in *B. juncea*; *Rlm8* and *Rlm11* in *B. rapa*, and *Rlm10* was identified in *B. nigra*. Four resistance genes; *LepR1*, *LepR2*, *LepR3*, and *LepR4* were introgressed into *B. napus* from *B. rapa* subsp. *sylvestris* (Table 1).

Species	Locus	*Population	Phenotyping stage	Marker type	Mapping strategy	chromosome	Linked markers/interval	Reference
B. napus	*Rlm1*	Maxol/S006 (140 DH)	Cotyledon inoculation	RAPD	Bulked segregant analysis	A7	T04.680 (14cM)	74
		Quinta/Score (110 F_2)	Cotyledon inoculation	RAPD	Bulked segregant analysis	A7	C02.1375/O15.1360 (19cM)	57, 74
		Maxol/Westar-10 (96 DH)	Cotyledon inoculation and stem canker	SSR, DArT	Whole genome mapping	A7	Xna12a-02a/Xra2-a05b	82
		Columbus/Westar-10	Cotyledon inoculation and stem canker	SSR	A7 chromosome specific mapping	A7	Xol12-e03a/Xna12-a02a	82
B. napus	*Rlm2*	Glacier/Score (110 F_2)	Cotyledon inoculation	RAPD	Bulked segregant analysis	A7	M08.1200, M08.600, P02.700	57, 74

Species	Locus	*Population	Phenotyping stage	Marker type	Mapping strategy	chromosome	Linked markers/interval	Reference
		Glacier/Yudal (BC189)	Cotyledon inoculation	RAPD	Bulked segregant analysis	A7	M08.1200, M08.600, P02.700	74
		Darmor/Samourai (133 DH)	Cotyledon, Field	RAPD	Bulked segregant analysis	A7	M08.1200 (10cM),	74
B. napus	*Rlm3*	Maxol/S006 (140DH)	Cotyledon inoculation	RAPD	Bulked segregant analysis	A7	Q12.750 (7cM)	74
B. napus	*Rlm4*	Quinta/Score (110F2)	Cotyledon inoculation	RAPD	Bulked segregant analysis	A7	C02.1375 (3.6 cM)/ O15.1360 (`33 cM)	74
		Skipton/Ag-Spectrum	Cotyledon and Stem canker	SSR	Whole genome mapping		BRMS075 (`0.7 cM)	32
B. juncea	*Rlm6*	Recombinant lines (*B. napus-B. juncea*)	Cotyledon and field test	RAPD/ RFLP	Bulked segregant analysis	B8	OPG02.800, OPT01	47
B. napus	*Rlm7*	2311.1/Darmor (221 F_2)	Cotyledon	RAPD	Bulked segregant analysis	A7	T12.650 (4cM)	74, 85
B. napus	*Rlm9*	Darmor-bzh/Yudal (132 DH)	Cotyledon	RAPD	Bulked segregant analysis	A7	T12.650/C02.1375	74
B. nigra	*Rlm10*	Addition lines (Darmor/Junius)	Cotyledon test	Isozyme RAPD	Whole genome mapping	B4	OPA11.1200, OPC19.3300	83, 84
B. rapa ssp. *sylvestris*	*LepR1*	6270/Springfield (DHP95)	Cotyledon inoculation and field resistance	RFLP	Whole genome analysis	A2 (N2)	pR4b, pO85h, pW180b, pN181a, pW207a	31
B. rapa ssp. *sylvestris*	*LepR2*	6279/3027 (DHP96)	Cotyledon inoculation and field resistance	RFLP	Whole genome analysis	A10 (N10)	pN21b, pR34b, pN53b	31
B. napus	*LepR3*	Surpass400/Westar (N-o-1)-BC	Cotyledon inoculation	SSR	A1 and A10 chromosome specific mapping		sR12281a (2.2 cM) sN2428Rb (0.7 cM)	69
		Topas (DH16516)/ Surpass400	Cotyledon inoculaton	SSR, SCAR	A10 chromosome specific mapping	A10 (N10)	Ind10-12	79
B. rapa ssp. *sylvestris*	*LepR4*	16S/PAS12//16S (BC_3S_2)	Cotyledon inoculation Disease nursery (field)	SSR	A genome specific marker analysis	A6	sN2189b (8.8cM) sR9571a (8.3 cM)	77
B. napus	*BLMR1*	Surpass400/Westar (1513 F_3BC_2)	Cotyledon inoculation	SRAP, SNP	Selective genotyping	A10 (N10)	80E24a (0.1 cM)	70
B. napus	*BLMR2*	Surpass400/Westar (1513 F_3BC_2)	Cotyledon inoculation	SRAP, SNP	Selective genotyping	A10 (N10)	R278 (1.2 cM)	70
B. napus	*LmFr1*	Cresor (resistant)/ Westar (susceptible)	Field/artificial inoculation	RFLP	Whole genome analysis	Linkage group 6 (A7)	cDNA011/cDNA110	64

Species	Locus	*Population	Phenotyping stage	Marker type	Mapping strategy	chromosome	Linked markers/interval	Reference
B. napus	*LEM1*	Major (resistant)/Stellar (susceptible)	Cotyledon Stem inoculation	RFLP	Whole genome analysis	A7	TG5D9b/WG5A1A	65
B. napus	*cLmR1*	Shiralee/90-3046 (153 DH lines)	Cotyledon incoulation	RFLP, RAPD	Bulked segregant analysis	A7	RAPD654 (~4.8cM)	66
B. napus	*cLmR1*	Shiralee/PSA12 (BC1 lines)	Cotyledon incoulation	RFLP, EST, SCAR	Bulked segregant analysis	A7	est126M9a/est149M9d	140
B. napus	*cLmR1*	DH12075/PSA12 (BC1 lines)	Cotyledon incoulation	RFLP, EST, SCAR	Bulked segregant analysis	A7	est126M9a/est149M9d	140
B. napus	*cLmR1*	Maluka/90-3046 (34 DH lines)	Cotyledon incoulation	RFLP, RAPD	Bulked segregant analysis	A7	RAPD654 (~4.8cM)	66
B. napus	*cRLM (cRLMm)*	Maluka/Westar	Cotyledon, Adult	RFLP, AFLP, RAPD	Bulked segregant analysis	A7	22-25	67
B. napus	*cRLM (cRLMrb)*	RB87-62/Westar	Cotyledon, adult plant	RFLP, AFLP, RAPD	Bulked segregant analysis	A7	22-25	67
B. napus	*cRLM (cRLMc)*	Cresor/Westar	Cotyledon, adult plant	RFLP, AFLP, RAPD	Bulked segregant analysis	A7	22-25	67
B. napus	*Rlm.wwai -A1*	Skipton/Ag-Spectrum (DH)	Cotyledon incoulation	SSR	Whole genome analysis	A1	Xpbcessrna16-Xbrms017b	32
B. napus	*QRlm.ww ai-A10a*	Skipton/Ag-Spectrum (DH)	Cotyledon inoculation	SSR	Whole genome analysis	A10	Xcb10079d-Xcb10079c	32
B. napus	*Rpg_3Dun*	Westar/Dunkeld (F_2)	Cotyledon inoculation	SRAP	Bulked segregant analysis	A7	$NA_{12}A_{02}$-200/$NA_{12}A_{02}$-190, $BG_{20}SA_{12}$-480/$BG_{20}SA_{12}$-475/ BN204	81
B. juncea	*#Rlm5*	150-2-1, 151-2-1, Aurea, Picra	Cotyledon inoculation	-	-	-	-	71
B. rapa	*#Rlm8*	156-2-1	Cotyledon inoculation	-	-	-	-	71
B. rapa	*#Rlm11*	02-159-4-1	Cotyledon inoculation	-	-	-	-	72
B. napus	*#RlmS*	Surpass400	Cotyledon inoculation	-	-	-	-	73
B. juncea	*LMJR1*	AC Vulcan/UM3132 (F_2)	Cotyledon test	RFLP, SSR	Whole genome mapping	J13 (B3)	PN199RV (22.1 cM), sBb31143F (8.7 $_c$M)	43
B. juncea	*LMJR2*	AC Vulcan/UM3132 (F2)	Cotyledon test	RFLP, SSR	Whole genome mapping	J18 (B8)	PN120cRI, sB1534	43
B. juncea	*rjlm2*	B genome introgression lines	cotyledon	RAPD, RGA & SCAR	B genome-specific	not defined	B5-1520, C5-1000, RGALm	80

Table 1. Molecular mapping of qualitative genes for resistance to *Leptosphaeria maculans* in *Brassica.** BC: Backcross population, DH: Doubled haploid population. # loci not mapped with molecular markers to date.

Recently, two genes *BLMR1* and *BLMR2* in Surpass 400; an Australian cultivar developed from an interspecific cross between wild *B. rapa* subsp. *sylvestris* (resistant) from Sicily and *B. oleracea* subsp. *alboglabra* were identified [70, 76]. However, *LepR1* to *LepR4* genes are thought not be related with *Rlm* genes on the basis of their map locations, except for *Rlm2* and *LepR3*, which are phenotypically different [31, 69, 77]. It appears that loci *LepR3*, *BLMR1* and *BLMR2* localised on chromosome A10 control resistance to *L. maculans* in Surpass 400. However, Van de Wouw et al. [73] demonstrated that two independently segregating *L. maculans* avirulence (Avr) genes, *AvrLm1* corresponding to *Rlm1* (on chromosome A7) and *AvrLmS*, are responsible for inducing resistance in this cultivar. Subsequently, Larkan *et al.* [78] investigated the interaction of *AvLm1* and *AvLmS* isolates with *B. napus* populations segregating for the resistance genes *Rlm1* (from the French cultivar Quinta) and *LepR3* (from Surpass 400). This study reported that (i) *AvrLm1* interacts in a gene-for-gene manner with both *Rlm1* and *LepR3*, (ii) *AvrLmS* is not responsible for triggering the *LepR3* mediated defence response, (iii) Surpass 400 does not contain *Rlm1*, and (iv) *Rlm1* and *LepR3* may be the same genes located in two distinct loci or may have evolved as two functional genes. Recently, *LepR3* has become the first functional *B. napus* resistance gene to be cloned and was shown to encode a receptor-like protein. Additionally, *LepR3*-transgenic *B. napus* and *AvrLm1*-transgenic *L. maculans* were used to demonstrate that *AvrLm1* conveys avirulence to *LepR3*. The shared genomic location of *LepR3* and *BLMR1* also suggested that these were the same gene [79]. Several other genes such as *LmR1, ClmR1, LmFr1, cRLMm, cRLMrb, aRLMrb,* and *LEM1* have also been identified using uncharacterised isolates, which are thought to be allelic to known *R*-genes [45, 68, 74]. Qualitative resistance conferred by single major genes is usually dominant and expressed at the seedling growth stage. Qualitative *R*-genes explain majority of phenotypic variation for blackleg resistance at adult plant stage [32, 74]. However, digenic mode of inheritance has also been reported in *B. napus and B. juncea* populations [40, 80].

7.2. Quantitative resistance

Quantitative inheritance for field resistance has been reported in segregating populations derived from *B. napus, B. juncea* and their hybrid derivatives [30, 32, 65, 80, 86]. Some of the QTLs identified are given in Table 2. Quantitative genetic analysis revealed that significant non-additive genetic variance for all measures of disease severity indicated the presence of strong dominance/epistasis at loci controlling blackleg resistance [36]. In the literature, the term 'QTL' as a quantitative locus has been used even when a large percent of genotypic variation is explained by the major locus. In classical genetics, QTL refers to genes that have, low heritability, non-Mendelian and quantitative accumulative effects. The majority of genetic analyses have utilised doubled-haploid (DH) populations, which are not suitable to infer modes of inheritance. Advanced intercross populations are required to interpret such phenomena, as used in [74].

Mapping Population	Stubble, Location	Flanking markers	Chromosome	LOD# score	%Genetic variance (R^2)#	Additive effect	Reference
Av-Sapphire/ Westar10	*B. napus,* Lake Bolac, Australia	E34M15_S190/ E35M53_S416	A1	2.5-5.6	14-16	Not known (-)	86*

Mapping Population	Stubble, Location	Flanking markers	Chromo-some	LOD# score	%Genetic variance (R^2)#	Additive effect	Reference
		E34M15_S218/ E35M53_S350	A2	1.3-3.8	4-26	-	
	Dahlen, Australia	CB10443_W258_ S269	C1	0.8-2.9	3-8	-	
	Lake Bolac	E36M47_W197/ E34M62_W127	LG1	1.0-3.6	4-10	-	
Caiman$_3$/Westar	*B. napus,* Lake Bolac	BRMS056/ E34M50_W140	A1	2.9-3.5	20-22.7	-	86*
	Dahlan	E35M53_C455/ E34M15_W271	A10	1.4-3.0	5-34	-	
		Not shown	C5	4.4-5.6	19-23	-	
Camberra$_4$/Westar	Lake Bolac	E36M55_C306/ E33M57_C306	A5	0.5-2.6	1.5-33	-	86*
	Dahlen	Na12D10_w203	A1/C1	2.9-5.1	17-18	-	
	Lake Bolac	E36M62_W414/0 1ju1fE07_cl_3b	A10	0.3-2.7	2-31	-	
		Not shown	C7-2	2.7-3.7	13-24	-	
		E33M59_W107/ E33M53_C75	LG2	2.1-2.8	14-28	-	
Darmor/Samourai	*B. napus*, Le Rheu	*BN483*	A1	2.3	6.7	Samourai	88
		BN239	A2	2.3-3.02	8.1-14.6	Darmor	
		BN182.1	A6	1.9-2.8	6.2-10.0	Samourai	
		At17	A10	2.7	11.0	Samourai	
		BN204	C2	2.0-2.2	8.0-8.4	Darmor	
		BN167	C4	2.4-3.2	6.7-12.2	Darmor	
		Vers6.9	C8	1.9	-	Samourai	
Darmor/Yudal	*B. napus*, Le Rheu, France	*OPE02.1200*	A2	2.4-5.5	3.8-8.5	Darmor	87
		OPW08.1620	A4	3.3	4.8	Darmor	Delourme et al, 2008; comm. pers.)
		OPW05.750-Bzh	A6	5-12.2	7.2-20	Darmor	
		Bras023	A7	4.5	6.9	Darmor	
		CB10026b	A8	7.2	13.0	Darmor	
		OPW15.1470	A9	3.3	4.8	Darmor	
		Fad8	C2	5.5-6.6	8.3-13.3	Yudal	
		OPD08.1310	C4	4.7-9.5	6.7-15.2	Darmor	
		OPH06.CD1	C8	4.2	6.2	Darmor	
Rainbow/Av-Sapphire	Lake Bolac	E33M57_R105	A9-2	3.7	13	-	
Skipton/Ag-Spectrum	*B. napus* Mixed stubble,	*Xbras123/Xem1-bg11-237*	A2	7.0	11.5	Ag-Spectrum	32

Mapping Population	Stubble, Location	Flanking markers	Chromo-some	LOD# score	%Genetic variance (R^2)#	Additive effect	Reference
	Wagga, Australia	*Xbrms319-Xbrms176*	A9	2.9	5.0	Skipton	
		Xcb10172-BnFLC10	A10b	2.2	6.2	Skipton	
		Xbrms287a-Xcb10034	C1	4.2	11.5	Ag-Spectrum	
		Xol10-c10/Xna12-c03	C2a	6.8	16.6	Skipton	
		Xpbcessrna13/ Xol13-d02a	C3	4.2	24.5	Skipton	
		Xem1-bg23-89/ Xol12-e03	C6	6.1	14.5	Ag-Spectrum	
	B. napus, ATR Beacon stubble, Wagga, Australia	*Xol12-f11/ Xpbcessrbr21*	A1a	6.1	26.1	Ag-Spectrum	

Table 2. Significant QTLs associated with blackleg resistance (scored as Internal infection due to canker development at adult plant stage) identified from mapping populations, * QTL with consistent effect, # range of LOD and R^2 varied with method of regression analysis (simple and composite interval mapping).* refers to predicted markers from supplementary figures ESM7-10 shown in Kaur et al [81]

8. Gene-for gene interactions

Host resistance genes (*R*-genes) interact in paired combination with pathogen avirulence (*Avr*) genes to condition resistance [89]. Two types of interactions may occur; compatible and incompatible. Compatible interaction occurs when there is an absence of an effective host defence response, due to a lack of a resistance allele in host (*r*) or an allele for virulence (*avr*) at the corresponding pathogen locus. An incompatible interaction occurs when there is no disease development due to the presence of both an effective host resistance allele (*R*) with an allele for *Avr* at the corresponding pathogen locus [90]. Biochemically, gene-for-gene interactions have been interpreted as the interaction of a race-specific pathogen elicitors with either cultivar-specific plant receptors or alternatively with a cultivar-specific signal transduction compounds [91]. Differential interaction between specific *R*-genes in the host (Brassica) and corresponding *Avr* genes of the pathogen *(L. maculans)* was first studied at the seedling stage using a cotyledon inoculation test in *B. napus* [92] and subsequently verified [57]. Qualitative and quantitative resistance differ with respect to host-pathogen interaction, as the latter does not appear to (but not proven) follow the gene-for gene hypothesis, being more effective against diverse pathogen populations (non-race specific). While quantitative resistance normally provides partial resistance to the pathogen and it is less likely to be rapidly overcome by shifting pathogen populations.

At least ten *Avr* genes have been identified in *L. maculans*, many of which map to two gene clusters; *AvrLm1-AvrLm2-AvrLm6* and *AvrLm3-AvrLm4-AvrLm7-AvrLepR1* ([71, 72, 86, 87]. Four of the *Avr* genes; *AvrLm1*, *AvrLm6*, *AvrLm4-7* and *AvrLm11* have been cloned. It has shown that although *AvrLm1* and *AvrLm6* are physically clustered together in the *L. maculans* genome, they are not allelic forms of a single gene [85, 96]. However, *AvrLm4* and *AvrLm7* are allelic variants of a single *Avr* gene that corresponds to the two resistance genes; *Rlm4* and *Rlm7* [71, 85]. It has also been demonstrated that *AvrLm1* interacts with two distinct resistance loci; *Rlm1* and *LepR3*, though these loci are located on different chromosomes (A7 and A10, respectively) [78]. The cloning and characterisation of additional Brassica *R*-genes and *L. maculans* Avr genes will lead to a better understanding of how these functional redundancies developed. In the recent years, understanding of *L. maculans/Brassica* interactions has increased our ability to deploy appropriate *R*-genes in new cultivars and manage blackleg disease with the increased knowledge of the distribution of *Avr* alleles in *L. maculans* populations [27, 94, 98]. Currently, it seems that the genes involved in race-specific resistance and polygenic non-specific resistance are distinct. A better understanding of the mechanisms underlying quantitative resistance would help our understanding of the relationships between quantitative and major resistance genes [99].

9. Alien gene introgression for blackleg resistance

Deployment of *R*-genes has been used as the most cost-effective and environmentally sound measure for disease control in various crops since a century ago when first *R*-genes were identified [100]. Conventional plant breeding methodologies have played an important role in gene introgression for disease resistance, especially in easily-crossed genetic backgrounds. As a result several cultivars rated for resistance to *L. maculans* now dominate commercial cultivation worldwide. There has been a continuous threat of 'breakdown' of resistance, especially when a resistant cultivar is grown extensively on large acreages over long period of time. For example, 'breakdown' of resistance in cultivar Surpass 400 occurred within three years of its release [101, 102] due to the evolution and spread of more virulent strain of *L. maculans*. 'Breakdown' of resistance implies that the resistance has not changed rather the pathogen population has shifted/been selected for virulence. The effectiveness of *Rlm1* in France was also greatly reduced from 1997 to 2000 following wide deployment of *Rlm1* varieties, effectively selecting for enrichment of the virulent *avrLm1* allele in *L. maculans* populations [34]. Interestingly, a similar enrichment for the virulent *avrLm1* allele was documented after the 'breakdown' of *LepR3* resistance in Australia [103]. Due to the threat of current resistance being rendered ineffective by shifting *L. maculans* populations, new effective sources of resistance are constantly in demand. In order to enlarge genetic variation for resistance to *L. maculans*, interspecific and intergeneric donor sources have been utilised. This has been achieved by conventional sexual crossing [44, 52, 75, 104] or via laboratory tools such as somatic hybridization [105], and embryo culture. Roy [52] crossed *B. juncea* and *B. napus* to introgress genes for blackleg resistance but none of the interspecific hybrids achieved the same level of *B. juncea* resistance as the donor parent. Wide hybrids (interspecific, intergeneric or intertribal) have also been produced either by sexual crossing followed by embryo culture or by somatic hybridisation as a result of protoplast fusion to transfer genes for blackleg resistance [106, 107]. Previous studies have reported hybrids between *B. napus* and *Arabidopsis thaliana*, belonging to different tribes; the Brassiceae and Sisymbrieae, respectively [108]. These hybrids were further utilized for identifying genetic regions associated with blackleg resistance [49]. Two regions localised on chromosome 3 of *A. thaliana* were shown to be linked with resistance to *L. maculans*.

Crouch *et al.* [75] transferred genes for resistance to *L. maculans* derived from *B. rapa* subsp. *sylvestris* into *B. napus*, using a resynthesised amphidiploid, as a result of hybridisation between *B. rapa* subsp. *sylvestris* and *B. oleracea* subsp. *alboglabra*. As a result, several cultivars derived from the re-synthesized *B. napus* lines were released for commercial cultivation in Australia such as Surpass 400, Surpass 404CL, Surpass 501TT, Surpass 603CL, Hyola 43, and Hyola 60. The *R*-genes *LepR1*, *LepR2* and *LepR4* have also been introgressed into *B. napus* via conventional interspecific crosses [75, 109]. Introgression of genes for resistance to *L. maculans* from *Sinapis arvensis*, *Coincya momensis* and *B. juncea* into *B. napus* was attempted [110]. Hybrid derivatives of *B. napus* and *S. arevensis*, and *B. napus* and *C. momensis* showed a high levels of resistance at the seedling (cotyledon) and/or adult plant stages. The offspring from asymmetric hybrids between *B. napus* and *B. nigra, B. juncea* and *B. carinata* were analysed for the presence of B genome markers and resistance to *L. maculans* [111]. This study revealed that resistance is conserved in one triplicate region in the B genome. Often, the majority of wide-hybrid derivatives exhibit unwanted traits and low frequencies of recombination between the different species which complicate the development of *B. napus* cultivars resistant to *L. maculans* by traditional breeding [43, 47]. Linkage drag due to suboptimal/undesired genes can be eliminated using the application of high density genome-wide molecular markers such as SNPs [112]. However, Rouxel and Balesdent [93] cautioned that before important breeding efforts are devoted to introgression of resistance genes from distant species into Brassica, there is a need thoroughly to evaluate their genetic control, putative redundancy and potential durability in the field.

Using transgenic technology, *R*-genes from other organisms can also be transferred irrespective of natural barriers to crossing. However, it is possible that transferred genes may not always contribute novel resistance specificities to the transgenic crop. Although several approaches have been used to induce host resistance in plants [113, 114] no major breakthrough has been made for an efficient management of blackleg disease. For example, Hennin *et al.* [115] demonstrated the expression of *Cf9* gene, which confers *Avr9*-dependant resistance to *Cladosporium fulvum* in tomato, along with co-expression of *Avr9* produced increased resistance to *L. maculans* in transgenic *B. napus* plants. Manipulation of plant defense responses is resource-expensive [116] and may be deleterious to the plant. Plants need to be selected for both appropriate expression of beneficial defense responses and avoidance of unnecessary ones [117], making artificially-induced constitutive expression of these responses an impractical solution to engineering resistance.

10. Durability of resistance to *L. maculans*

Durable disease resistance can be achieved by utilisation of one or more single dominant *R*-genes [118]. However, the effectiveness of the specific *R*-genes depends on the *L. maculans* population structure, i.e. on the frequency of the corresponding *Avr* allele, which is known to differ according to regions/countries [27, 94] and the rapid evolution of virulent pathotypes. For example, the mean number of virulence alleles per isolates was reported to be higher in Australia (5.11 virulence alleles) than in Europe (4.33) and Canada (3.46) [27]. It has been suggested that there is a fitness cost associated with pathogen evolution from avirulence to virulence to overcome host resistance [38, 119].

Previous research has shown that different qualitative gene sources for resistance vary in providing effective durable resistance over period of time. For example, Light *et al.* [120] reported that the adult plant survival of French winter lines such as Doublol (*Rlm1*), Capitol (*Rlm1, Rlm3*), Columbus*1 (*Rlm1, Rlm3*), Carolus (*Rlm1, Rlm2, Rlm3*) and Rlm_EX (*Rlm7*) was higher than the Australian cultivar, AV-Sapphire and concluded that French winter canola cultivars have effective resistance under Australian conditions.

Single resistance genes do not always provide a durable resistance as has been shown in a field experiment using the *Jlm1/Rlm6* gene introgressed into *B. napus* from *B. juncea* [121]. Several incidences on the breakdown/ineffectiveness of race-specific resistance genes in Surpass 400 (*(LepR3, RlmS)*), in Vivol and Capitol (*Rlm1),* and *Rlm6* genes in *Brassica* have been reported in literature particularly when they were grown extensively [34, 94, 122]. As a consequence, breeders have to develop new cultivars and replace 'old' cultivars in order to change pathogen specificity of *R-gene* even without the knowledge of comprehensive distribution of *Avr* genes. The latter is now feasible and being used in order to monitor the pathogen population [123]. In order to avoid selection pressure against a particular *Avr* gene in the pathogen population, pyramiding of several host *R*-genes and deployment of quantitative resistance is being practiced in several crops such as in wheat, and barley. However, this strategy has not resulted in greater durability of resistance [124, 125]. In contrast, a recent study [121] demonstrated that a major *R*-gene (*Rlm6*) is more durable when expressed in a genetic background that also has quantitative resistance, indicating the need to identify and combine both qualitative and quantitative loci for blackleg resistance. Although the proposed strategy may be useful for blackleg disease management in areas where 'less' disease pressure and low variability with *L. maculans* populations exists, in Australia polygenic resistance derived from the French cultivar Jet Neuf [87], was reported to become less effective over time [37]. Additionally, several Australian cultivars which are reported to harbour both qualitative and quantitative loci for blackleg resistance are susceptible to natural populations of *L. maculans* Delourme et al [99]. It is difficult to know whether this evolution results from a change in virulence, or in aggressiveness in the pathogen populations since these polygenic-resistance cultivars may also carry specific *R*-genes [99]. In order to keep the frequency of isolates virulent towards any race–specific gene under a 'threshold' level, an integrated approach based upon best farm practices such as crop rotation, stubble management, application of fungicides and deployment of resistance genes including rotation of race-specific genes [126] needs to be implemented for sustainable canola production, especially in areas where *L. maculans* populations are highly diverse and rapidly evolving.

11. Molecular dissection of qualitative and quantitative resistance loci

Molecular markers have been applied to identify loci associated with resistance to *L. maculans,* which relies on the availability of sequence variation among parental genotypes of mapping populations and diversity panels. Several genotyping methods based upon DNA hybridisation such as Restriction Fragment Length Polymorphism (RFLP) and Diversity Arrays Technology (DArT); PCR-based techniques such as Randomly Amplified Polymorphic DNA (RAPD), Simple Sequence Repeats (SSR) and Amplified Fragment Length Polymorphism (AFLP); Sequence-related amplified polymorphism (SRAP); and sequence-based analysis such as Single Nucleotide Polymorphism (SNP); Restriction site-associated DNA, (RAD) and Genotyping by Sequencing (GBS) have been developed for molecular analyses [81, 127 - 136]. RFLP, RAPD, SSR, SRAP and AFLP markers have all been used to map loci for resistance to *L. maculans* (Table 1). New marker technologies such as DArT, 60K SNP Infinium array, RAD and GBS are currently being developed and applied for mapping of blackleg resistance loci. These high-throughput approaches are expected to complement or replace low-throughput marker assays that were used previously to facilitate genetic and physical map-based cloning of resistance genes.

Loci for resistance to *L. maculans* have been mapped using linkage/QTL mapping and association mapping approaches [32, 74, 82, 86, 137] using structured (F_2, doubled-haploid (DH) and backcross) and unstructured (diversity sets/breeding lines) populations (Table 1). Bulked Segregant Analysis approach, used for the first time [138], is particularly useful when a limited number of traits are to be mapped and resources (money and time) required for extensive genotyping are limited [81]. Whole-genome analysis has been used to locate both qualitative and quantitative loci associated with resistance to *L. maculans* [32, 86]. Generally, it requires the framework linkage map of all 19 chromosomes (linkage groups) for linkage (QTL) analysis.

11.1. Qualitative resistance

The majority of genes for resistance to *L. maculans* have been genetically mapped with molecular markers (Table 1) on chromosomes A1, A2, A6, A7, A10, B3, B4 and B8 in *Brassica species: B. rapa, B. napus, B juncea* and *B. nigra* [31, 32, 45, 68-70, 99]. None of the race-specific genes have been mapped on the C genome yet. Previous linkage mapping studies revealed that at least five resistance genes (*Rlm1, Rlm3, Rlm4, Rlm7* and *Rlm9)* are localised in a cluster within a 35 cM genomic region on chromosome A7 [32, 45, 64-68, 74, 82]. This genomic region showed extensive inter- and intra-genomic duplications, as well as intra-chromosomal tandem duplications [140]. Whether some of these *R*-genes are allelic remains unknown. For example, it was concluded that at least four resistance genes *Rlm3*, *Rlm4*, *Rlm7*, and *Rlm9* could correspond to a cluster of tightly linked genes, to a unique gene with different alleles, or to a combination of these two hypotheses. However, *Rlm1* has been shown to be linked with *Rlm3* but is not allelic [74].

A major gene named *LmFr1* controlling adult plant resistance to blackleg was tagged in the DH population from French cultivar Cresor (resistant to *L. maculans*) and Westar (susceptible to *L. maculans*) with RFLP markers [64]. Similar study [65] mapped loci for blackleg resistance in a DH population from Major/Stellar and found that genetic control of resistance vary with inoculation techniques. A major gene designated as *LEM1* was mapped to linkage group 6 based on qualitative/quantitative scores of the interaction phenotype on inoculated cotyledons with a single ascospore-derived PG2 isolate, PHW1245. However, four other putative QTL for resistance were also identified on linkage groups LG8, LG17 and pair 4. This study further showed that none of the QTL that were associated with resistance at the seedling and stem stage had a significant effect in conferring resistance in the field. This may be attributed due to use of different pathogen population (PHW 1245 in cotyledon and stem experiments and natural *L. maculans* population in field experiment). The *Rpg3Dun* gene was mapped in an F_2 population from Westar/Dunkeld and identified a suite of SCAR markers that showed cosegregation with resistance to *L. maculans* [81]. Recently, the whole genome average interval mapping approach was applied to localise both qualitative and quantitative trait loci controlling blackleg resistance [32] in a DH population derived from the Australian *B. napus* vernalisation responsive cultivars, Skipton and Ag-Spectrum. Marker regression analyses revealed that at least fourteen genomic regions were associated with blackleg resistance, explaining 19.5% to 88.9% of genotypic variation. A major qualitative locus, designated *RlmSkipton (Rlm4),* was mapped on chromosome A7, within 0.8 cM of the SSR marker BRMS075 (Table 1).

Genomic regions of chromosome A10 harbours *Rlm2*, which has been shown to be the most common *R*-gene in winter *B. napus* varieties, such as Samourai, Eurol, Bristol, Symbol, Andol, Kintol, Akamar, Colvert, Synergy, and Tapidor, [41]. Chromosome A10 also harbours *LepR2*, *LepR3* and *BLMR2* genes derived from *B. rapa* subsp. *sylvestris* sources [31, 69, 70]. *LepR1* and *LepR2* were mapped on chromosomes A2 and A10, respectively with RFLP markers [31]. Genetic analysis revealed that both genes confer resistance independently and therefore are additive. *LepR1* was a dominant nuclear gene while *LepR2* was an incompletely dominant gene. This study further showed that *LepR1* generally conferred a higher level of resistance than *LepR2*. Both genes exhibited race-specific interactions with pathogen isolates.

The blackleg resistance gene *Rlm6* has been identified on B genome chromosome 8 [47]. *Rlm6* has been successfully introgressed to *B. napus* (AACC) from *B. juncea* (AABB) [47, 141] and provides excellent resistance to *L. maculans* isolates [58], though this gene has not yet been deployed in commercial cultivars [47, 58].

11.2. Quantitative resistance

The genetic basis of quantitative resistance has been investigated only in limited *B. napus* cultivars such as in Darmor; a derivative of Jet Neuf [119, 137, 142]. However, a number of DH populations have recently been utilised for identification of loci for quantitative resistance under field conditions [32, 86, 143], and are currently being validated (Raman *et al.*, unpublished, Larkan *et al.*, unpublished). Thirteen quantitative trait loci (QTL) on 10 linkage groups associated with quantitative field resistance to *L. maculans* were identified in a DH population from Darmor-*bzh*/Yudal [87]. Their detection was dependent upon phenotypic method used; seven QTL for mean disease index and six QTL for per cent survival (percentage of lost plants due to canker) and were also dependant on growing environment (year of evaluation). However, only four of the QTL were stable across experiments. These QTL accounted from 23% to 57% of the genotypic variation (Table 2). The unexplained variation was described due to non-detected additive QTL, G x E interaction and incomplete map coverage. This study further showed that resistance to *L. maculans* is influenced with growth habit. For example, one QTL, located close to a dwarf gene (*bzh*), was detected with a very strong effect, masking the detection of other QTL. This study further showed that these dwarfing genes also affect other traits such as earliness, and glucoinsolate content.

In order to validate the stability of QTL for field resistance to *L. maculans*, QTL were mapped and characterised in $F_{2:3}$ population from Darmor (resistant)/Samourai (susceptible) revealing only four QTL on LG3, LG11 and DY5 and DS6 that were consistent in Darmor/Yudal and Darmor/Samourai populations [143]. This study found that the genetic background and inoculum pressure are the major factors of the QTL instability and therefore suggested that QTL mapping must be carried out separately for each population. The genomic regions carrying the most consistent resistance QTL in Darmor do not correspond to the two regions on N7 (A7) and N10 (A10) identified as carrying race specific resistance genes to *L. maculans* [74]. The position of *Rlm2* on N10 (A10) corresponds to a QTL identified for adult plant resistance in the Darmor/Samourai DH population [88]. The cultivar Samourai carries both the resistance allele at this QTL and *Rlm2*. Since it has been reported that no French isolates of *L. maculans* carry *AvrLm2* [34], two hypotheses were proposed to explain this co-location; either the *Rlm2* gene has a residual effect at the adult plant stage, similar to that suggested in other pathosystems, or genes linked to *Rlm2* are responsible for part of variation for resistance at this QTL [99].

QTL for blackleg resistance were identified in four mapping populations derived from the crosses Caiman/Westar$_{10}$, Camberra/Westar$_{10}$, ^{AV}Sapphire/Westar$_{10}$ and Rainbow/^{AV}Sapphire [86]. Multiple QTLs were identified accounting for 13–33% of phenotypic variance. A recent study [32] identified seven significant QTL associated with blackleg resistance, scored on the basis of internal disease score, on chromosomes A2, A9, A10, C1, C2, C3 and C6 in a DH population derived from Skipton/Ag-Spectrum. The genotypic variation explained by the individual QTL ranged from 5% to 24.5%. Both parents contributed the alleles for blackleg resistance. This study showed poor correlation between canker lesion scores over the two years (2009, 2010). Some of the genomic regions for blackleg resistance may be the same as reported previously that have been identified using both classical QTL and association mapping approaches [31, 69, 87, 137, 144, 145]. The conservation of QTL between Australian and French studies is interesting and suggests the non-specificity of these QTL, irrespective of the environment, genetic background and G x E interactions [32]. However, it is possible that some of the original donor gene sources in French and Australian parental lines used for mapping resistance genes may be the same.

The majority of mapping populations used to map blackleg resistance genes in *B. napus* so far have been comparatively small (Table 1). The development of a high density map utilising larger populations, comprising several hundred to thousands lines, will allow for the precise mapping of resistance loci. Stability of QTL resistance needs to be tested in different environments. Although QTL mapping studies provide comprehensive information on the nature of inheritance, location, magnitude and allelic effects of QTL, much of the information tends to be 'population' specific. In biparental (structured) populations, generally two alleles at each locus are sampled and therefore trait-marker association may not be highly relevant to diverse genetic backgrounds. The validation of trait-marker association is necessary before their use for routine marker-assisted breeding (MAS). Association mapping can be utilised for investigating linkage disequilibrium close to loci of interest in a diverse germplasm [145-149] and therefore offers an alternative to linkage and QTL mapping. This approach has been applied in determining and confirming the markers located within the QTL associated with resistance to *L. maculans* previously identified in Darmor and established their usefulness in MAS [137]. A diverse set of an oilseed rape collection, comprised of 128 lines showing a large spectrum of responses to infection by *L. maculans*, was characterised using 72 SSR and other markers. At least 61 marker alleles were found to be associated with resistance to stem canker. Some of these markers were associated with previously identified QTL, which confirms their usefulness in MAS. Markers located in regions not harbouring previously identified QTL were also associated with resistance, suggesting that new QTL or allelic variants are present in the collection [137]. Genome-wide association based on 1513 markers enabled identification and validation of genomic loci associated with blackleg resistance. This study detected significant marker - race-specific blackleg resistance associations ($P<0.01$) at the seedling and adult plant stages. Loci for resistance were located on chromosomes A1, A2, A3, A5, A6, A7, A10, C1, and C2. Both studies suggested that association mapping is an efficient approach for identifying novel loci/alleles associated with blackleg resistance in diverse germplasm [137, 142]. Superior molecular marker allele(s) associated with resistance to *L. maculans* may be captured by canola breeding programs. Molecular markers associated with seedling and stem canker resistance will help identify accessions carrying desirable alleles and facilitate QTL introgression to develop elite germplasm having new gene/allele combinations for blackleg resistance [32].

12. Host *R*-gene cloning and candidate gene analysis

At least 20 *R*-genes and several allele variants and haplotypes of cloned *R*-genes have been identified in plants [151-158]. Molecular analyses revealed that these genes belong to large multiple gene families, which encode nucleotide binding site- leucine–rich repeats (NBS-LRRs), serine-threonine-kinases, leucine zipper and protein kinase domains, and toll/interleukin-1 receptor domains [159-164]. These genes are often clustered in many plant species including crops such as rice, maize and soybean and transduce the hypersensitive response to defend against pathogen attack [164-167]. At least 30 CC-NBS-LRR and TIR-NBS-LRR non-redundant genes have been identified in *B. rapa* [167]. Two major gene clusters for resistance to *L. maculans* exist on chromosomes A7 [74] and A10 [31, 69, 70], along with other genes dispersed on different chromosomes. It is possible that some of these *R*-genes may represent to multiple copies of the same functional gene. A recent study has shown that at least eight functional copies of *FLOWERING TIME LOCUS C* (*FLC*) exist within *B. napus* [6] which may modulate flowering time and other functions in different cultivars [168].

In *B. napus*, only few studies aimed at characterizing the genes underlying the resistance to *L. maculans* have been attempted. The recent cloning of the first functional *B. napus* resistance gene *LepR3* revealed a receptor-like protein responsible for conferring resistance to *AvrLm1 L. maculans* isolates [79]. Resistance genes effective against *L. maculans* have also been cloned in *A. thaliana* [169-171], which encode Toll interleukin-1 receptor-nucleotide binding (TIR-NB) or TIR-NB-LRR class proteins. Based on the synteny between *B. napus* and *A. thaliana*, it was deduced that several *B. napus* resistance genes are localised in a region of A7 (N7) that corresponds to the chromosome segment on *Arabidopsis* chromosome 1 which harbours *RLM1*Col [139, 167]. However, a recent report detailing the gene responses to *L. maculans* infections suggests very different responses in *B. napus* and *A. thaliana* [172]. Both salicylic acid and ethylene signaling was triggered in *B. napus*, possibly due to the hemibiotrophic nature of the infection. This stands in contrast to the JA signaling observed in *A. thaliana*, suggesting *L. maculans* is acting as a necrotroph during infection of susceptible *A. thaliana* lines. Since many *R*-genes are conserved and share sequence similarity, degenerated primers based on conserved motifs of *R*-genes have also been used to localise potential resistance gene loci in Brassica species such as *B. oleracea* (on chromosomes C1 (O1), C4 (O4), C8 (O8) and C9 (O9) and *B. napus* on linkage groups LG1a, LG1b, LG2, LG5, LG8, LG12, LG13, LG14, LG15 and LG18 [173, 174]. However their association with loci controlling resistance to *L. maculans* have not yet been established/validated.

In order to clone genes controlling blackleg resistance in *B. napus* population, high resolution mapping of *LmR1* and *ClmR1* loci was performed using 2500 backcross lines from two crosses between PSA12 and Shiralee, and PSA12 and Cresor, respectively [140], and reported that both resistance loci are located in a highly duplicated genomic region on chromosome A7. This region contained several genes encoding protein kinases or LRR domains. It is reported that the SCAR marker (BN204) that showed cosegregation with *RpgDun* locus for resistance to *L. maculans* is derived from a region showing 92% amino acid identity with the defense-related gene serine threonine 20 (ste-20) protein kinase of *Arabidopsis thaliana* [81]. A proteomic approach has also been utilised to understand gene expression in response to *L. maculans* infection [176]. However, candidacy of any of these genes has not yet been reported.

Recently an alternative approach for identifying candidate *R*-genes has been employed based on genomics [177]. Next-generation massively parallel sequencing platforms such as the Roche 454 genome sequencer FLX instrument, the Illumina Genome Analyser (HiSeq), and the ABI SOLiD System have revolutionized genome sequencing by providing high throughput and cost-effective high coverage sequencing [179-182] and has enabled much quicker identification of candidate genes [178]. Molecular markers associated with *RlmSkipton* (*Rlm4*) locus in the DH population from Skipton/Ag-Spectrum were aligned with the complete genome sequence *B. rapa* as reported in [32]. Eighteen candidate genes, designated as *BLR1-18* with disease resistance characteristics, several of which were clustered around a region syntenic to *Rlm4*.

Among candidates, *BLR2* and *BLR11* were the promising candidates for *Rlm4*-mediated resistance [178]. High resolution mapping and gene sequencing of different sources of *L. maculans* resistance will allow for a better understanding of the structural organisation and function of *R*-genes. Recently, the reference genome of *B. rapa* has been published [182] and genomes of *B. oleracea*, *B. nigra* and *B. napus* are expected to be published in coming years. Re-sequencing of whole genomes of known blackleg-resistant genotypes will allow identification of genetic variation between individuals, which can provide molecular genetic markers and insights into gene function [183]. Sequencing of different *R*-genes and understanding their function will also enable us to manipulate resistance to *L. maculans*, as genes with different specificities can be created.

13. Predictive breeding for resistance to *L. maculans* using molecular markers

Success of new disease resistance genes relies heavily on the successful transfer of target genomic regions from donor sources and the development of rigorous selection methods. Molecular markers have been used to improve the effectiveness and efficiency of selection strategies in predictive breeding in several agricultural crops. However, the development of molecular markers in *B. napus* and their application in breeding is a challenging exercise due to the large genome size, amphidipliod (4X) nature, open-pollination and lower research funding as compared to other key crops such as wheat, barley, maize and soybean. The *B. napus* genome is highly complex and homologous recombination plays a major role in chromosome rearrangements such as duplications and reciprocal translocations. These arrangements further add to the complexity of molecular analysis and interpretation. *B. napus* chromosomes C6 and A7, which harbours *Rlm1*, *Rlm3*, *Rlm4*, *Rlm7* and *Rlm9* genes for resistance, produced a reciprocal translocation in some cultivars such as in Westar, Marnoo, Monty and Maluka [185, 186] which makes analysis of resistance genes difficult [142].

In most of the breeding programs, selection for blackleg is conducted once a year during the growing season, hampering selection efficiency. Several studies suggest a significant correlation between cotyledon test and canker lesion scores. Therefore, cotyledon tests can be used for selection for resistance to *L. maculans*. However, in many developed countries, it is costly and laborious to perform, particularly as compared to molecular marker analysis, when several tests need to be carried to screen large populations. Furthermore, analysis of different blackleg resistance genes in a canola breeding program using a differential set of *L. maculans* isolates at various stages of the breeding cycle is a very slow process [39]. Interpretation of *R*-gene content using a differential set of control *B. napus* varieties, especially of Australian origin, is a challenging exercise, as majority of cultivars used are heterozygous and/or heterogeneous [32, 41]. In addition, phenotypic tests are dependent upon the growing environment (microclimate conditions and other factors such as powdery and downy mildew), which can complicate scoring of inoculated seedlings. Molecular markers generally out-perform conventional seedling assays, in both efficiency and reliability. It is also possible to identify haplotypes using molecular markers and then validate trait-marker associations, in conjunction with comprehensive phenotyping and conventional allelism tests.

The published literature suggests that little effort has been made to evaluate the allelic relationship among the known genes from different sources, to test stability of majority of QTL or qualitative genes identified over diverse growing environments, or to test their usefulness in achieving long term durable control of the disease. Table 1 also suggests that majority of markers are not very closely linked (<1cM) with resistance loci. Diagnostic or perfect markers for resistance genes are required for routine MAS and will assist allele enrichment strategies in breeding programs, although this is not always possible, even if the complete gene is cloned and characterised for its functionality [187]. The linkage between molecular markers and *Xbn204* flanking the *RlmSkipton* locus was verified in an F_2 population derived from Skipton/Ag-Spectrum [32]. The results showed that SSR markers linked to *RlmSkipton* are suitable for enrichment of favourable alleles for blackleg resistance in breeding programs. A separate study [82] validated the map location of *Rlm1* in the DH population derived from Maxol/Westar with SSR and DArT markers. Previously, *Rlm1* and *Rlm3* genes were mapped on chromosomes A7 in the Maxol (resistant to blackleg)/S006 (susceptible to blackleg) utilising RAPD markers and with single spore isolates with known *Avr* genotypes in the *B. napus* European cultivars, Columbus and Maxol [41, 71, 74]. RAPD markers are not amenable for high throughput marker analysis, as they are assayed on low-throughput agarose or polyacrylamide gel systems. Validation of a large array of genes for blackleg resistance in diverse segregating populations representing *B. napus* germplasm is a challenging exercise. However, an association mapping approach can be employed to test trait-marker associations in a large set of germplasm as demonstrated recently [137, 142].

14. Conclusions

It is now clear that major resistance genes will be overcome in time, as has been seen in many crop plants. Therefore, there is constant need to identify new sources of both qualitative and quantitative resistance loci and to properly utilise the resources available to us so that resistance can be deployed long term. Recent advances in molecular marker systems, such as the development of highly-parallel systems for genotyping and sequencing, have created new opportunities and strategies to select for qualitative and quantitative traits, including resistance to *L. maculans*. Strategies for deploying resistance in breeding programs will vary with individual breeding programs; monitoring introgression of specific loci, using whole-genome marker scans (genomic selection) or identifying individual plants that may offer the greatest opportunity for genetic gain. This is now becoming reality as several genome-wide signals associated with blackleg resistance have been identified (but need to be validated) and alleles at these loci can be selected efficiently and at a cheaper rate with new marker technologies. Development and validation of tightly-linked molecular markers amenable to high throughput marker screening with both qualitative and quantitative resistance and cost effective systems will enable the increased adoption in *B. napus* breeding programs. In addition to genetic resistance, deployment of agronomic practices such as use of rotation and stubble management will remain key management tools for reducing pathogen inoculum for subsequent crops.

Acknowledgements

Authors are thankful to Dr Regine Delourme, INRA, Le Rheu, Cedex France for providing critical comments and QTL information for quantitative resistance in the Darmor/Yudal population.

Author details

Harsh Raman[1*], Rosy Raman[1] and Nick Larkan[2]

*Address all correspondence to: harsh.raman@dpi.nsw.gov.au

1 Graham Centre for Agricultural Innovation (an alliance between NSW Department of Primary Industries and Charles Sturt University), Wagga Wagga Agricultural Institute, Wagga Wagga, Australia

2 Saskatoon Research Centre, Agriculture and Agri-Food Canada, Saskatoon, Canada

References

[1] Tode HI. *Fungi Mecklenburgenses Selecti*. Fasciculus. 1791;II(51, Plate XVI, Fig 126).

[2] Olsson G. Species Crosses within the Genus *Brassica*. I: Artificial *Brassica napus*. Hereditas. 1960;46:351-96.

[3] U N. Genomic Analysis in Brassica with Special Reference to the Experimental Formation of *B. napus* and Peculiar Mode of Fertilisation. Jpn J Bot. 1935;7:389-452.

[4] Gómez-Campo C, Prakash S. Origin and Domestication. In: C.Gómez-Campo (Ed.), Biology of Brassica Coenospecies. Elsevier, Netherlands, 33-58. 1999.

[5] Baranyk P, Fábry A. History of the Rapeseed (*Brassica Napus* L.) Growing and Breeding from Middle Age Europe to Canberra. Proceedings 10th International Rapeseed Congress, Canberra, Australia (http://regionalorgau/au/gcirc/4/374htm). 1999.

[6] Zou X, Suppanz I, Raman H, Hou J, Wang J, Long Y, et al. Comparative Analysis of *FLC* Homologues in Brassicaceae Provides Insight into Their Role in the Evolution of Oilseed Rape. PLoS One 2012 ; 7(9): e45751.

[7] FAO: Food and Agriculture Organisation (2012) http://faostat.fao.org/.

[8] Fitt B, Brun H, Barbetti M, Rimmer S. World-Wide Importance of Phoma Stem Canker (*Leptosphaeria maculans* and *L. biglobosa*) on Oilseed Rape (*Brassica napus*). European Journal of Plant Pathology. 2006;114(1):3-15.

[9] West JS, Kharbanda PD, Barbetti MJ, Fitt BDL. Epidemiology and Management of *Leptosphaeria maculans* (Phoma Stem Canker) on Oilseed Rape in Australia, Canada and Europe. Plant Pathol. 2001;50(1):10-27.

[10] Howlett BJ. Current Knowledge of the Interaction between *Brassica napus* and *Leptosphaeria maculans*. Canadian Journal of Plant Pathology. 2004;26(3):245-52.

[11] Marcroft S, Bluett C. Blackleg of Canola. Agriculture Notes, State of Victoria, Department of Primary Industries, May 2008, Ag1352, ISSN 1329-8062. 2008.

[12] Henderson MP. The Black-Leg Disease of Cabbage Caused by *Phoma lingam* (Tode) Desmaz. Phytopathology. 1918;8:379-431.

[13] Sosnowski MR, Scott ES, Ramsey MD. Infection of Australian canola cultivars (*Brassica napus*) by *Leptosphaeria maculans* is influenced by cultivar and environmental conditions. Australasian Plant Pathology. 2004;33(3):401-11

[14] Petrie GA. Variability in *Leptosphaeria maculans* (Desm.) Ces et de Not., the Cause of Blackleg of Rape. PhD Thesis, University of Saskatchwen, Canada. 1969.

[15] Hall R. Epidemiology of Blackleg of Oilseed Rape. Canadian Journal of Plant Pathology 1992;14:46-55.

[16] Alabouvette C, Brunin B. Recherches Sur La Maladie Du Colza Due a *Leptospharia maculans* (Desm.) Ces. Et De Not. 1. Role Des Restes De Culture Dans La Conservation Et La Dissemination Du Parasite. Ann Phytopathol 2(3): 463-475. 1970.

[17] Bokor A, Barbetti MJ, Brown AGP, MacNish GC, Poole ML, Wood P. Blackleg - Major Hazard to the Rapeseed Industry. Journal of Agriculture, Western Australia. 1975;16:7-10.

[18] Ghanbarnia K, Fernando WGD, Crow G. Developing Rainfall- and Temperature-Based Models to Describe Infection of Canola under Field Conditions Caused by Pycnidiospores of *Leptosphaeria maculans*. Phytopathology 2009;99(7):879-86.

[19] Ghanbarnia K, Fernando WGD, Crow G. Comparison of Disease Severity and Incidence at Different Growth Stages of Naturally Infected Canola Plants under Field Conditions by Pycnidiospores of *Phoma lingam* as a Main Source of Inoculum. Canadian Journal of Plant Pathology. 2011;33(3):355-63.

[20] Chen CY, Howlett BJ. Rapid Necrosis of Guard Cells Is Associated with the Arrest of Fungal Growth in Leaves of Indian Mustard (*Brassica juncea*) Inoculated with Avirulent Isolates of *Leptosphaeria maculans*. Physiological and Molecular Plant Pathology. 1996;48(2):73-81.

[21] Hua L, Sivasithamparam K, Barbetti MJ, Kuo J. Germination and Invasion by Ascospores and Pycnidiospores of *Leptosphaeria maculans* on Spring-Type *Brassica napus* Canola Varieties with Varying Susceptibility to Blackleg. Journal of General Plant Pathology 2004;70(5):261.

[22] Hammond KE, Lewis BG, Musa TM. A Systemic Pathway in the Infection of Oilseeed Rape Plants by *Leptosphaeria maculans*. Plant Pathology. 1985;34:557-65.

[23] Travadon R, Marquer B, Ribule A, Sache I, Masson JP, Brun H, et al. Systemic Growth of *Leptosphaeria maculans* from Cotyledons to Hypocotyls in Oilseed Rape: Influence of Number of Infection Sites, Competitive Growth and Host Polygenic Resistance. Plant Pathology. 2009;58:461-9.

[24] Sprague SJ, Watt M, Kirkegaard JA, Howlett BJ. Pathways of Infection of *Brassica napus* Roots by *Leptosphaeria maculans*. New Phytologyst. 2007;176: 211-222.

[25] Cunningham GH. Dry-Rot of Swedes and Turnips: Its Causes and Control. Wellington, New Zealand: New Zealand Department of Agriculture: Bulletin 133. 1927.

[26] Kutcher HR, van den Berg CGJ, Rimmer SR. Variation in Pathogenicity of *Leptosphaeria maculans* on *Brassica Spp.* Based on Cotyledon and Stem Reactions. Can J Plant Pathol 1993;15:253-8.

[27] Balesdent MH, Barbetti MJ, Li H, Sivasithamparam K, Gout L, Rouxel T. Analysis of *Leptosphaeria maculans* Race Structure in a Worldwide Collection of Isolates. Phytopathology. 2005 Sep;95(9):1061-71.

[28] Koch E, Song K, Osborn TC, Williams PH. Relationship between Pathogenicity Based on Restriction Fragment Length Polymorphism in *Leptosphaeria maculans*. Molecular Plant-Microbe Interactions. 1991;4:341-9.

[29] Aubertot J, West J, Bousset-Vaslin L, Salam M, Barbetti M, Diggle A. Improved Resistance Management for Durable Disease Control: A Case Study of Phoma Stem Canker of Oilseed Rape (*Brassica napus*). European Journal of Plant Pathology. 2006;114(1):91-106.

[30] Cargeeg LA, Thurling N. Contribution of Host-Pathogen Interactions to the Expression of the Blackleg Disease of Spring Rape (*Brassica napus* L.) Caused by *Leptosphaeria maculans* (Desm.) Ces. et de Not.. Euphytica. 1980;29:465-76.

[31] Yu F, Lydiate DJ, Rimmer SR. Identification of Two Novel Genes for Blackleg Resistance in *Brassica napus.* Theoretical and Applied Genetics. 2005;110:969-79.

[32] Raman R, Taylor B, Marcroft S, Stiller J, Eckermann P, Coombes N, et al. Molecular Mapping of Qualitative and Quantitative Loci for Resistance to *Leptosphaeria maculans*; Causing Blackleg Disease in Canola (*Brassica napus* L.). Theoretical and Applied Genetics. 2012;125(2):405-18.

[33] Bansal VK, Kharbanda PD, Stringam GR, Thiagarajah MR, Tewari J. A Comparison of Greenhouse and Field Screening Methods for Blackleg Resistance in Doubled Haploid Lines of *Brassica napus*. Plant Disease 1994;78:276-81.

[34] Rouxel T, Penaud A, Pinochet X, Brun H, Gout L, Delourme R, et al. A 10-Year Survey of Populations of *Leptosphaeria maculans* in France Indicates a Rapid Adaptation Towards the *Rlm1* Resistance Gene of Oilseed Rape. European Journal of Plant Pathology. 2003;109(8):871-81.

[35] McNabb WM, Van Den Berg CGJ, Rimmer SR. Comparison of Inoculation Methods for Selection of Plant Resistant to *Leptosphaeria Maculans* in *Brassica napus*. Can J Plant Sci 1993;73:1199-207.

[36] Pang ECK, Halloran GM. Genetics of Virulence in *Leptosphaeria maculans* (Desm.) Ces. et De Not., the Cause of Blackleg in Rapeseed (*Brassica napus* L.). Theoretical and Applied Genetics. 1996;93(3):301-6.

[37] Salisbury P, Ballinger DJ, Wratten N, Plummer K, Howlett BJ. Blackleg Disease on Oilseed Brassica in Australia: A Review. Australian Journal of Experimental Agricultural. 1995;35:665-72.

[38] Huang YJ, Li ZQ, Evans N, Rouxel T, Fitt BDL, Balesdent MH. Fitness Cost Associated with Loss of the *Avrlm4* Avirulence Function in *Leptosphaeria maculans* (Phoma Stem Canker of Oilseed Rape). European Journal of Plant Pathology. 2006;114(1): 77-89.

[39] Marcroft SJ, Elliott VL, Cozijnsen AJ, Salisbury PA, Howlett BJ, Van de Wouw AP. Identifying Resistance Genes to *Leptosphaeria maculans* in Australian *Brassica napus* Cultivars Based on Reactions to Isolates with Known Avirulence Genotypes. Crop and Pasture Science. 2012;63(4):338-50.

[40] Rimmer SR, van den Berg CGJ. Resistance to Oilseed Brassica Spp. To Blackleg Caused by *Leptosphaeria maculans*. Can J Plant Pathol. 1992;14: 56-66.

[41] Rouxel T, Willner E, Coudard L, Balesdent M-H. Screening and Identification of Resistance to *Leptosphaeria maculans* (Stem Canker) in *Brassica napus* Accessions. Euphytica. 2003;133(2):219-31.

[42] Marcroft SJ, Purwantara A, Salisbury P, Potter TD, Wratter N, Khangura R, et al. Reaction of a Range of *Brassica Species* under Australian Conditions to the Fungus, *Leptosphaeria maculans*, the Causal Agent of Blackleg. Australian Journal of Experimental Agriculture. 2002;42(5):587-94.

[43] Christianson JA, Rimmer SR, Good AG, Lydiate DJ. Mapping Genes for Resistance to *Leptosphaeria maculans* in *Brassica juncea*. Genome. 2006;49(1):30-41.

[44] Roy NN. Interspecific Transfer of *Brassica juncea*-Type High Blackleg Resistance to *Brassica napus*. Euphytica. 1984;33: 295-303.

[45] Delourme R, Chevre AM, Brun H, Rouxel T, Balesdent MH, Dias JS, et al. Major Gene and Polygenic Resistance to *Leptosphaeria maculans* in Oilseed Rape (*Brassica napus*). European Journal of Plant Pathology. 2006;114(1):41-52.

[46] Pang ECK, Halloran GM. The Genetics of Blackleg [*Leptosphaeria maculans* (Desm.) Ces. et de Not.] Resistance in Rapeseed (*Brassica napus* L.). II. Seedling and Adult-Plant Resistance as Quantitative Traits. Theoretical and Applied Genetics. 1996;93:941-9.

[47] Chèvre AM, Barret P, Eber F, Dupuy P, Brun H, Tanguy X, et al. Selection of Stable *Brassica napus-B. juncea* Recombinant Lines Resistant to Blackleg (*Leptosphaeria maculans*). 1. Identification of Molecular Markers, Chromosomal and Genomic Origin of the Introgression. Theoretical and Applied Genetics. 1997;95(7):1104-11.

[48] Snowden RJ, Winter H, Diestel A, Sacristan MD. Development and Characterisation of *Brassica napus-Sinapus arvensis* Addition Lines Exhibiting Resistance to *Leptosphaeria maculans*. Theoretical and Applied Genetics. 2000;101:1008-14.

[49] Bohman S, Wang M, Dixelius C. *Arabidopsis thaliana*-Derived Resistance against *Leptosphaeria maculans* in a *Brassica napus* Genomic Background. Theoretical and Applied Genetics. 2002;105(4):498-504.

[50] Sjödin C, Glimelius K. Screening for Resistance to Blackleg *Phoma lingam* (Tode Ex Fr.) Desm. Within Brassicaceae. Journal of Phytopathology. 1988;123(4):322-32.

[51] Leflon M, Brun H, Eber F, Delourme R, Lucas MO, Vallee P, et al. Detection, Introgression and Localization of Genes Conferring Specific Resistance to *Leptosphaeria maculans* from *Brassica rapa* into *B. napus*. Theoretical and Applied Genetics. 2007 Nov;115(7):897-906.

[52] Roy NN. A Study on Disease Variation in the Populations of an Interspecific Cross of *Brassica juncea* L. x *B. napus* L. Euphytica 27:145-149. 1978

[53] Mithen RF, Lewis BG, Heaney RK, Fenwick GR. Resistance of Leaves of Brassica Species to *Leptosphaeria maculans.* Trans Br Mycol Soc 88:525-531. 1987.

[54] Mitchell-Olds T, James RV, Palmer MJ, Williams PH. Genetics of *Brassica rapa* (Syn. *Campestris*). 2. Multiple Disease Resistance to Three Fungal Pathogens: *Peronospora parasitica, Albugo candida* and *Leptosphaeria maculans*. Heredity. 1995;75(4):362-9.

[55] Keri M, van den Berg CJG, McVetty PBE, Rimmer SR. Inheritance of Resistance to *Leptosphaeria maculans* in *Brassica juncea.* Phytopathology. 1997;87:594-8.

[56] Brun H, Levivier S, Somda I, Ruer D, Renard M, Chevre AM. A Field Method for Evaluating the Potential Durability of New Resistance Sources: Application to the *Leptosphaeria maculans-Brassica napus* Pathosystem. Phytopathology. 2000;90(9):961-6.

[57] Ansan-Melayah D, Balesdent MH, Delourme R, Pilet ML, Tanguy X, Renard M, et al. Genes for Race-Specific Resistance against Blackleg Disease in *Brassica napus* L. Plant Breeding. 1998;117(4):373-8.

[58] Plieske J, Struss D, Röbbelen G. Inheritance of Resistance Derived from the B-Genome of Brassica against *Phoma lingam* in Rapeseed and the Development of Molecular Markers. Theoretical and Applied Genetics. 1998;97(5):929-36.

[59] Barret P, Guérif J, Reynoird JP, Delourme R, Eber F, Renard M, et al. Selection of Stable *Brassica napus-Brassica juncea* Recombinant Lines Resistant to Blackleg (*Leptosphaeria maculans*). 2. A 'To and Fro' Strategy to Localise and Characterise Interspecific Introgressions on the *B. napus* Genome. Theoretical and Applied Genetics. 1998;96(8): 1097-103.

[60] Monteiro AA, Williams PH. The Exploration of Genetic Resources of Portuguese Cabbage and Kale for Resistance to Several Brassica Diseases. Euphytica. 989; 41:215-225. 1.

[61] Ananga AO, Cebert E, Soliman K, Kantety R, Pacumbaba RP, Konan K. Rapd Markers Associated with Resistance to Blackleg Disease in Brassica Species. African Journal of Biotechnology. 2006;5(22):2041-8.

[62] Wittern I. Wittern I (1984) Untersuchungen Zur Erfassung Der Resistenz Von Winterraps (*Brassica napus* L. Var. *oleifera* Metzger) Gegenüber *Phoma lingam* (Tode Ex Fr.) Desm. Und Zu Der Durch Den Erreger Verursachten Wurzelhals- Und Stengel- fäule. PhD Thesis, Universität Göttingen, Göttingen, Germany 1984.

[63] Stringam GR, Bansal VK, Thiagarajah MR, Tewari JP. Genetic Analysis of Blackleg (*Leptosphaeria maculans*) Resistance in *Brassica napus* L. Using the Doubled Haploid Method. XIII Eucarpia Congress, July 6-11, Angers, France. 1992.

[64] Dion Y, Gugel RK, Rakow GFW, Séguin-Swartz G, Landry BS. RFLP Mapping of Resistance to the Blackleg Disease [Causal Agent, *Leptosphaeria maculans* (Desm.) Ces. Et De Not.] in Canola (*Brassica napus* L.). Theoretical and Applied Genetics. 1995;91(8): 1190-1194.

[65] Ferreira ME, Rimmer SR, Williams PH, Osborn TC. Mapping Loci Controlling *Brassica napus* Resistance to *Leptosphaeria maculans* under Different Screening Conditions. Phytopathology. 1995; 85:213-217.

[66] Mayerhofer R, Bansal VK, Thiagarajah MR, Stringam GR, Good AG. Molecular Mapping of Resistance to *Leptosphaeria maculans* in Australian Cultivars of *Brassica napus*. Genome. 1997;40:294-301.

[67] Rimmer SR, Borhan MH, Zhu B, Somers D. Mapping Resistance Genes in *Brassica napus* to *Leptosphaeria maculans*. Proceeding 10th International Rapeseed Congress, Canberra, Australia. 1999. http://www.regional.org.au/au/gcirc/3/47.htm

[68] Rimmer SR. Resistance Genes to *Leptosphaeria maculans* in *Brassica napus*. Can J Plant Pathol-Rev Can Phytopathol. 2006;28:S288-S297.

[69] Yu F, Lydiate DJ, Rimmer SR. Identification and Mapping of a Third Blackleg Resistance Locus in *Brassica napus* Derived from *B. rapa* Subsp. *sylvestris*. Genome. 2008;51(1):64-72.

[70] Long Y, Wang Z, Sun Z, Fernando DW, McVetty PB, Li G. Identification of Two Blackleg Resistance Genes and Fine Mapping of One of These Two Genes in a *Brassica napus* Canola Cultivar 'Surpass 400'. Theoretical and Applied Genetics. 2011;122(6): 1223-31.

[71] Balesdent MH, Attard A, Kuhn ML, Rouxel T. New Avirulence Genes in the Phytopathogenic Fungus *Leptosphaeria maculans*. Phytopathology. 2002;92(10):1122-33.

[72] Balesdent MH, Fudal I, Ollivier B, Bally P, Grandaubert J, Eber F, et al. The dispensable chromosome of *Leptosphaeria maculans* shelters an effector gene conferring avirulence towards *Brassica rapa*. New Phytol. 2013;198(3):887-98.

[73] Van de Wouw AP, Marcroft SJ, Barbetti MJ, Hua L, Salisbury PA, Gout L, et al. Dual Control of Avirulence in *Leptosphaeria maculans* Towards a *Brassica napus* Cultivar with '*Sylvestris*-Derived' Resistance Suggests Involvement of Two Resistance Genes. Plant Pathology. 2008;58(2):305-13

[74] Delourme R, Pilet-Nayel ML, Archipiano M, Horvais R, Tanguy X, Rouxel T, et al. A Cluster of Major Specific Resistance Genes to *Leptosphaeria maculans* in *Brassica napus*. Phytopathology. 2004;94(6):578-83.

[75] Crouch JH, Lewis BG, Mithen RF. The Effect of a Genome Substitution on the Resistance of *Brassica napus* to Infection by *Leptosphaeria maculans*. Plant Breeding.1994; 112(4):265-278.

[76] Buzza G, Easton A. A New Source of Blackleg Resistance from *Brassica sylvestris*. In GCIRC Technical Meeting Poznan, Poland Bulletin No18. 2002.

[77] Yu F, Lydiate DJ, Hahn K, Kuzmisz Kuzmicz S, Hammond C, Rimmer SR. Identification and Mapping of a Novel Blackleg Resistance Locus *LepR4* in the Progenies from *Brassica napus* x *B. rapa* Subsp. *sylvestris*. Proc. 12th International Rapeseed Conference, Wuhan, China, March 2007.

[78] Larkan NJ, Kuzmicz S, Yu F, Lydiate D, Genetic Evidence for the Recognition of the *Leptosphaeria maculans* Avirulence Gene *AvrLm1* by Two *Brassica napus* Resistance Genes: *Rlm1* and *LepR3*. Proceedings 17th Crucifer-Genetics Workshop; 2010; Saskatoon, Canada.

[79] Larkan N.J., D.J. Lydiate, I.A.P. Parkin, M.N. Nelson, D.J. Epp, W.A. Cowling, et al. The *Brassica napus* blackleg resistance gene *LepR3* encodes a receptor-like protein triggered by the *Leptosphaeria maculans* effector *AvrLM1* New Phytologist. 2013, 197:595-605

[80] Saal B, Struss D, RGA- and RAPD-derived SCAR markers for a Brassica B-genome introgression conferring resistance to blackleg in oilseed rape. Theoretical and Applied Genetics, 2005; 111: 281-290

[81] Dusabenyagasani M, Fernando WGD. Development of a Scar Marker to Track Canola Resistance against Blackleg Caused by *Leptosphaeria maculans* Pathogenicity Group 3. Plant Disease. 2008;92(6):903-8.

[82] Raman R, Taylor B, Lindbeck K, Coombes N, Barbulescu D, Salisbury P, et al. Molecular mapping and validation of *Rlm1* genes for resistance to *Leptosphaeria maculans* in canola (*Brassica napus* L). Crop & Pasture Science. 2012;63:1007–1017.

[83] Delourme R, Piel N, Horvais R, Pouilly N, Domin C, Vallée P, et al. Molecular and Phenotypic Characterization of near Isogenic Lines at QTL for Quantitative Resistance to *Leptosphaeria maculans* in Oilseed Rape (*Brassica napus* L.). Theoretical and Applied Genetics. 2008(117):1055-67

[84] Eber F., Lourgant K., Brun H., Lode M., Huteau V., Coriton O., Alix K., Balesdent M., Chevre A.M. Analysis of *Brassica nigra* Chromosomes Allows Identification of a New Effective *Leptosphaeria maculans* resistance Gene Introgressed in *Brassica napus*. Proceeding of the 13th International rapeseed congress, Prague 5–9 June 2011.

[85] Parlange F, Daverdin G, Fudal I, Kuhn M-L, Balesdent M-H, ne, et al. *Leptosphaeria maculans* Avirulence Gene *Avrlm4-7* Confers a Dual Recognition Specificity by the *Rlm4* and *Rlm7* Resistance Genes of Oilseed Rape, and Circumvents *Rlm4*-Mediated Recognition through a Single Amino Acid Change. Molecular Microbiology. 2009;71:851-63.

[86] Kaur S, Cogan NOI, Ye G, Baillie RC, Hand ML, Ling AE, et al. Genetic Map Construction and QTL Mapping of Resistance to Blackleg (*Leptosphaeria maculans*) Disease in Australian Canola (*Brassica napus* L.) Cultivars. Theoretical and Applied Genetics. 2009 Dec;120(1):71-83.

[87] Pilet ML, Delourme R, Foisset N, Renard M. Identification of Loci Contributing to Quantitative Field Resistance to Blackleg Disease, Causal Agent *Leptosphaeria maculans* (Desm.) Ces. Et De Not., in Winter Rapeseed (*Brassica napus* L.). Theoretical and Applied Genetics. 1998;96:23-30.

[88] Delourme R, Piel N, Horvais R, Pouilly N, Domin C, Vallée P, et al. Molecular and Phenotypic Characterization of near Isogenic Lines at QTL for Quantitative Resistance to *Leptosphaeria maculans* in Oilseed Rape (*Brassica napus* L.). Theoretical and Applied Genetics. 2008;117(7):1055-67.

[89] Flor HH. The Current Status of the Gene-for-Gene Concept. Annu Rev Phytopathol. 1971;9:275-96.

[90] Keen NT. Gene-for-Gene Complementarity in Plant-Pathogen Interactions. Annu Rev Genet. 1990;24:447-63

[91] Flor HH. Inheritance of Pathogenicity in *Melampsora lini*. Phytopathology 1942;32:653-69.

[92] Williams PH, Delwiche PA, editors. Screening for Resistance to Blackleg of Crucifers in the Seedling Stage. Proceedings Eucarpia Conference, Breeding of Cruciferous Crops, Wageningen, Netherlands: 164-170; 1979.

[93] Rouxel T, Balesdent MH. The Stem Canker (Blackleg) Fungus, *Leptosphaeria maculans*, Enters the Genomic Era. Mol Plant Pathol. 2005;6(3):225-41.

[94] Balesdent MH, Louvard K, Pinochet X, Rouxel T. A Large-Scale Survey of Races of *Leptosphaeria maculans* Occurring on Oilseed Rape in France. European Journal of Plant Pathology. 2006;114(1):53-65.

[95] Ghanbarnia K, Lydiate D, Rimmer SR, Li G, Kutcher HR, Larkan N, et al. Genetic mapping of the *Leptosphaeria maculans* avirulence gene corresponding to the *LepR1* resistance gene of *Brassica napus*. Theoretical and Applied Genetics. 2012;124(3): 505-13.

[96] Gout L, Fudal I, Kuhn ML, Blaise F, Eckert M, Cattolico L, et al. Lost in the Middle of Nowhere: The *Avrlm1* Avirulence Gene of the Dothideomycete *Leptosphaeria maculans*. Mol Microbiol 2006;60:67-80.

[97] Fudal I, Ross S, Gout L, Blaise F, Kuhn ML, Eckert MR, et al. Heterochromatin-Like Regions as Ecological Niches for Avirulence Genes in the *Leptosphaeria maculans* Genome: Map-Based Cloning of *Avrlm6*. Mol Plant Microbe Interact 2007;20:459-70.

[98] Stachowiak A, Olechnowicz J, Jedryczka M, Rouxel T, Balesdent MH, Happstadius I, et al. Frequency of Avirulence Alleles in Field Populations of *Leptosphaeria maculans* in Europe. European Journal of Plant Pathology. 2006;114(1):67-75.

[99] Delourme R, Barbetti MJ, Snowdon R, Zhao J, Maria J. Manzanares-Dauleux. Genetics and Genomics of Disease Resistance Edwards D. Batley J, Parkin IAP, Kole C (Eds), USA: Science Publishers, CRC Press; 2011.

[100] Jackson AO, Taylor CB. Plant-Microbe Interaction:Life and Death at the Interface. The Plant Cell. 1996; 8:1651-68.

[101] Sprague S, Balesdent M-H, Brun H, Hayden H, Marcroft S, Pinochet X, et al. Major Gene Resistance in *Brassica napus* (Oilseed Rape) Is Overcome by Changes in Virulence of Populations of *Leptosphaeria maculans* in France and Australia. European Journal of Plant Pathology. 2006;114(1):33-40.

[102] Li H, Sivasithamparam K, Barbetti MJ. Breakdown of a *Brassica rapa* Subsp. *sylvestris* Single Dominant Blackleg Resistance Gene in *B. napus* Rapeseed by *Leptosphaeria maculans* Field Isolates in Australia. Plant Disease. 2003;87(6):752.

[103] Van de Wouw AP, Cozijnsen AJ, Hane JK, Brunner PC, McDonald BA, Oliver RP, et al. Evolution of linked avirulence effectors in *Leptosphaeria maculans* is affected by ge-

nomic environment and exposure to resistance genes in host plants.. PLoS Pathogens 2010;6: e1001180. doi:10.1371/journal.ppat.1001180. 2010.

[104] Howell PM, Sharpe AG, Lydiate DJ. Homoeologous Loci Control the Accumulation of Seed Glucosinolates in Oilseed Rape (*Brassica napus*). Genome. 2003;46:454-60.

[105] Sjödin C, Glimelius K. Transfer of Resistance against *Phoma lingam* to *Brassica napus* L. By Asymmetric Somatic Hybridisation Combined with Toxin Selection. Theoretical and Applied Genetics. 1989;78:513-20.

[106] Waara S, Glimelius K. The Potential of Somatic Hybridization in Crop Breeding Euphytica. 1995;85:217-33.

[107] Gerdemann-Kncörck M, Sacristan MD, Braatz C, Schieder O. Utilization of Asymmetric Somatic Hybridization for the Transfer of Disease Resistance from *Brassica nigra* to *Brassica napus*. Plant Breeding. 1994;113(2):106-13.

[108] Bauer-Weston B, Keller WA, Webb J. Production and Characterization of Asymmetric Somatic Hybrids between *Arabidopsis thaliana* and *Brassica napus*. Theoretical and Applied Genetics 1993;86:150-158

[109] Yu F, Lydiate DJ, Gugel RK, Sharpe AG, Rimmer SR. Introgression of *Brassica rapa* Subsp. *sylvestris* Blackleg Resistance into *B. napus.* Molecular Breeding 2012;30:1495-1506.

[110] Winter H, Gaertig S, Diestel A, Sacristan MD. Blackleg Resistance of Different Origin Transferred into *Brassica napus*. Proceeding 10th International Rapeseed Congress, Canberra, Australia. 1999. http://www.regional.org.au/au/gcirc/4/593.htm

[111] Dixelius C, Wahlberg S. Resistance to *Leptosphaeria maculans* Is Conserved in a Specific Region of the Brassica B Genome. Theoretical and Applied Genetics. 1999;99(1): 368-72.

[112] Michael TP, Alba R. The Tomato Genome Fleshed Out. Nature Biotechnology. 2012;30(8): 765-7.

[113] Strittmatter G, Janssens J, Opsomer C, Botterman J. Inhibition of Fungal Disease Development in Plants by Engineering Controlled Cell Death. Nature Biotechnology. 1995;13(10):1085-9.

[114] Keller H, Pamboukdjian N, Ponchet M, Poupet A, Delon R, Verrier J-L, et al. Pathogen-Induced Elicitin Production in Transgenic Tobacco Generates a Hypersensitive Response and Nonspecific Disease Resistance. The Plant Cell. 1999;11:223-35.

[115] Hennin C, Hofte M, Diederichsen E. Functional Expression of *Cf9* and *Avr9* Genes in *Brassica napus* Induces Enhanced Resistance to *Leptosphaeria maculans*. Molecular Plant-Microbe Interactions. 2001;14(9):1075-85.

[116] Bolton MD. Primary Metabolism and Plant Defense-Fuel for the Fire. Mol Plant-Microbe Interact. 2009;22:487-97.

[117] Katagiri F, Tsuda K. Understanding the Plant Immune System. Molecular Plant-Microbe Interactions. 2010;23(12): 1531-1536.

[118] Johnson R, Law CN. Cytogenetic Studies of the Resistance of the Wheat Variety Bersée to *Puccinia Striformis*. Cereal Rusts Bulletin 1973;1:38-43.

[119] Vera Cruz C, Bai J, On˜ a I, Leung H, Nelson R, Mew T-W, et al. Predicting Durability of a Disease Resistance Gene Based on an Assessment of the Fitness Loss and Epidemiological Consequences of Avirulence Gene Mutation. Proceedings of the National Academy of Sciences USA 2000;97: 13500-13505.

[120] Light KA, Gororo NN, Salisbury PA. Usefulness of Winter Canola (*Brassica napus*) Race-Specific Resistance Genes against Blackleg (Causal Agent *Leptosphaeria maculans*) in Southern Australian Growing Conditions. Crop and Pasture Science. 2011;62 162-8.

[121] Brun H, Chevre AM, Fitt BDL, Powers S, Besnard AL, Ermel M, et al. Quantitative Resistance Increases the Durability of Qualitative Resistance to *Leptosphaeria maculans* in *Brassica napus*. New Phytol. 2010;185(1):285-99.

[122] Sprague SJ, Marcroft SJ, Hayden HL, Howlett BJ. Major Gene Resistance to Blackleg in *Brassica napus* Overcome within Three Years of Commercial Production in Southeastern Australia. Plant Disease. 2006;90(2):190-8.

[123] Van de Wouw AP, Stonard JF, Howlett BJ, West JS, Fitt BDL, Atkins SD. Determining Frequencies of Avirulent Alleles in Airborne *Leptosphaeria maculans* Inoculum Using Quantitative PCR. Plant Pathol. 2010;59(5):809-18.

[124] Kolmer JA, Dyck PL, Roelfs AP. An Appraisal of Stem and Leaf Rust Resistance in North American Hard Red Spring Wheats and the Probability of Multiple Mutations to Virulence in Populations of Cereal Rust Fungi. Phytopathology 1991;81:237-9.

[125] Crute R, Pink D. Genetics and Utilization of Pathogen Resistance in Plants. Plant Cell. 1996;8:1747-55.

[126] Marcroft S, van De Wouw A, Salisbury P, Potter T, Howlett BJ. Rotation of Canola (*Brassica napus*) Cultivars with Differential Complements of Blackleg Resistance Genes Decreases Disease Severity. Plant Pathol. 2012;DOI: 10.1111/j.1365-3059.2011.02580.x.

[127] Raman H, Raman R, Kilian A, Detering F, Long Y, Edwards D, et al. A Consensus Map of Rapeseed (*Brassica napus* L) Based on Diversity Array Technology Markers: Applications in Genetic Dissection of Qualitative and Quantitative Traits. BMC Genomics 2013; 14:277.

[128] Li G, Quiros CF. Sequence-Related Amplified Polymorphism (SRAP), a New Marker System Based on a Simple PCR Reaction: Its Application to Mapping and Gene Tagging in Brassica. Theoretical and Applied Genetics. 2001;103(2):455-61.

[129] Sun Z, Wang Z, Tu J, Zhang J, Yu F, McVetty P, et al. An Ultradense Genetic Recombination Map for *Brassica napus* Consisting of 13551 SRAP Markers. Theoretical and Applied Genetics. 2007;114(8):1305-17.

[130] Durstewitz G, Polley A, Plieske J, Luerssen H, Graner EM, Wieseke R, et al. SNP Discovery by Amplicon Sequencing and Multiplex SNP Genotyping in the Allopolyploid Species *Brassica napus*. Genome. 2010;53(11):948-56.

[131] Trick M, Long Y, Meng J, Bancroft I. Single Nucleotide Polymorphism (SNP) Discovery in the Polyploid *Brassica napus* Using Solexa Transcriptome Sequencing. Plant Biotechnology Journal. 2009;7:334-46.

[132] Suwabe K, Iketani H, Nunome T, Kage T, Hirai M. Isolation and Characterization of Microsatellites in *Brassica rapa* L. Theoretical and Applied Genetics 2002;104:1092-8.

[133] Suwabe K, Tsukazaki H, Iketani H, Hatakeyama K, Kondo M, Fujimura M, et al. Simple Sequence Repeat-Based Comparative Genomics between *Brassica rapa* and *Arabidopsis thaliana*: The Genetic Origin of Clubroot Resistance. Genetics. 2006;173(1): 309-19.

[134] Lombard V, Delourme R. A Consensus Linkage Map for Rapeseed (*Brassica napus* L.): Construction and Integration of Three Individual Maps from DH Populations. Theoretical and Applied Genetics. 2001;103(4):491-507.

[135] Baird NA, Etter PD, Atwood TS, Currey MC, Shiver AL, Lewis ZA, et al. Rapid Snp Discovery and Genetic Mapping Using Sequenced RAD Markers. PLoS ONE. 2008;3(10):e3376.

[136] Miller MR, Dunham JP, Amores A, Cresko WA, Johnson GA. Rapid and Cost-Effective Polymorphism Identification and Genotyping Using Restriction Site Associated DNA (RAD) Markers. Genome Research. 2007;17:240-8.

[137] Jestin C, Lodé M, Vallée P, Domin C, Falentin C, Horvais R, et al. Association Mapping of Quantitative Resistance for *Leptosphaeria maculans* in Oilseed Rape (*Brassica napus* L.). Mol Breed. 2011;27:271-87.

[138] Michelmore RW, Paran I, Kesseli RV. Identification of Markers Linked to Disease-Resistance Genes by Bulked Segregant Analysis: A Rapid Method to Detect Markers in Specific Genomic Regions by Using Segregating Populations (Random Amplified Polymorphic DNA/Restriction Fragment Length Polymorphism). Proc Natl Acad Sci USA. 1991;88:9828-32,.

[139] Raman H, Milgate A. Molecular Breeding for Resistance to Septoria Tritici Blotch. Cereal Res Commun. 2012; 40:451-466

[140] Mayerhofer R, Wilde K, Mayerhofer M, Lydiate D, Bansal VK, Good AG, et al. Complexities of Chromosome Landing in a Highly Duplicated Genome: Toward Map-Based Cloning of a Gene Controlling Blackleg Resistance in *Brassica napus*. Genetics. 2005;171(4):1977-88.

[141] Chèvre AM, Brun H, Eber F, Letanneur JC, Vallee P, Ermel M, Glais I, Li H, Sivasithamparam K, Barbetti MJ. Stabilization of Resistance to *Leptosphaeria maculans* in *Brassica napus - B. juncea* Recombinant Lines and Its Introgression into Spring-Type *Brassica napus*. Plant Disease. 2008;92(8):1208-14.

[142] Raman H, Raman R, Taylor B, Lindbeck K, Coombes N, Eckermann P, et al. Blackleg Resistance in Rapeseed: Phenotypic Screen, Molecular Markers, and Genome-Wide Linkage and Association Mapping. Proceedings of the 17th Australian Research Assembly on Brassicas, 15-17 August, 2011, Wagga Wagga, pp 61-64.

[143] Pilet ML, Duplan G, Archipiano M, Barret P, Baron C, Horvais R, et al. Stability of QTL for Field Resistance to Blackleg across Two Genetic Backgrounds in Oilseed Rape. Crop Sci 2001;41:197-205.

[144] Piquemal J, Cinquin E, Couton F, Rondeau C, Seignoret E, Doucet I, et al. Construction of an Oilseed Rape (*Brassica napus* L.) Genetic Map with SSR Markers. Theoretical and Applied Genetics. 2005;111(8):1514-23.

[145] Breseghello F, Sorrells ME. Association Analysis as a Strategy for Improvement of Quantitative Traits in Plants. Crop Sci. 2006;46:1323-30.

[146] Breseghello F, Sorrells ME. Association Mapping of Kernel Size and Milling Quality in Wheat (*Triticum aestivum* L.) Cultivars. Genetics. 2006;172(2):1165-77.

[147] Buckler ES, Holland JB, Bradbury PJ, Acharya CB, Brown PJ, Browne C, et al. The Genetic Architecture of Maize Flowering Time. Science. 2009;325(5941):714-8.

[148] Flint-Garcia SA, Thornsberry JM, Buckler ES. Structure of Linkage Disequilibrium in Plants. Annu Rev Plant Biol 2003 54:357-74

[149] Hirschhorn JN, Daly MJ. Genome-Wide Association Studies for Common Diseases and Complex Traits. Nat Rev Genet. 2005;6:95-108.

[150] Raman H, Stodart B, Ryan P, Delhaize E, Emberi L, Raman R, et al. Genome Wide Association Analyses of Common Wheat (*Triticum aestivum* L) Germplasm Identifies Multiple Loci for Aluminium Resistance. Genome. 2010;53(11):957-66.

[151] Cloutier S, McCallum BD, Loutre C, Banks TW, Wicker T, Feuillet C, et al. Leaf Rust Resistance Gene *Lr1*, Isolated from Bread Wheat (*Triticum aestivum* L.) Is a Member of the Large *Psr567* Gene Family. Plant Mol Biol. 2007;65:93-106.

[152] Feuillet C, Travella S, Stein N, Albar L, Nublat A, Keller B. Map-Based Isolation of the Leaf Rust Disease Resistance Gene *Lr10* from the Hexaploid Wheat (*Triticum aestivum* L.) Genome. Proc Natl Acad Sci U S A. 2003;100(25):15253-8.

[153] Krattinger SG, Lagudah ES, Spielmeyer W, Singh RP, Huerta-Espino J, McFadden H, et al. A Putative ABC Transporter Confers Durable Resistance to Multiple Fungal Pathogens in Wheat. Science. 2009;323:1360-3.

[154] Michelmore RW, Meyers BC. Clusters of Resistance Genes in Plants Evolve by Divergent Selection and a Birth-and-Death Process. Genome Res 1998;8:1113-30.

[155] Srichumpa P, Brunner, S., Keller, B. & Yahiaoui, N. Allelic Series of Four Powdery Mildew Resistance Genes at the *Pm3* Locus in Hexaploid Bread Wheat. Plant Physiology 139, 885-895. 2005.

[156] Martin G, Brommonschenkel S, Chunwongse J, Frary A, Ganal M, Spivey R, et al. Map-Based Cloning of a Protein Kinase Gene Conferring Disease Resistance in Tomato. Science. 1993;262(5138):1432-6.

[157] Fu D, Uauy C, Distelfeld A, Blechl A, Epstein L, Chen X, et al. A Kinase-Start Gene Confers Temperature-Dependent Resistance to Wheat Stripe Rust. Science. 2009;323(5919):1357-60.

[158] Baumgarten A, Cannon S, Spangler R, May G. Genome-Level Evolution of Resistance Genes in *Arabidopsis thaliana*. Genetics. 2003;165 309-19.

[159] Persson M, Staal J, Oid S, Dixelius C. Layers of Defense Responses to *Leptosphaeria Maculans* Below the *Rlm1* - and Camelexin - Dependent Resistances. New Phytologist. 182, 470-482. 2009.

[160] Dangl JL, Jones JDG. Plant Pathogens and Integrated Defence Responses to Infection. Nature 2001;411:826-33.

[161] Dixon MS, Hatzixanthis K, Jones DA, Harrison K, Jones JDG. The Tomato *Cf-5* Disease Resistance Gene and Six Homologs Show Pronounced Allelic Variation in Leucine-Rich Repeat Copy Number. Plant Cell 10: 1915-1926. 1998.

[162] Dixon MS, Jones D, Keddie JS, Thomas CM, Harrison K, Jones JD. The Tomato *Cf-2* Disease Resistance Locus Comprises Two Functional Genes Encoding Leucine-Rich Repeat Proteins. Cell 84: 451-459. 1996.

[163] Song WY, Pi LY, Wang GL, Gardner J, Holsten T, Ronald PC. Evolution of the Rice *Xa21* Disease Resistance Gene Family. Plant Cell 9: 1279–1287. 1997.

[164] Ellis J, Jones D. Structure and Function of Proteins Controlling Strain-Specific Pathogen Resistance in Plants. Current Opinion in Plant Biology. 1998;1:288-93.

[165] Meyer JDF, Silva DCG, Yang C, Pedley KF, Zhang C, Mortel Mvd, et al. Identification and Analyses of Candidate Genes for *Rpp4*-Mediated Resistance to Asian Soybean Rust in Soybean. Plant Physiology. 2009;150:1 295-307

[166] Hulbert SH, Bennetzen JL. Recombination at the *Rp1* Locus of Maize. Mol Gen Genet 226: 377-382. 1991.

[167] Mun JH, Yu HJ, Park S, Park BS. Genome-Wide Identification of NBS-Encoding Resistance Genes in *Brassica rapa*. Molecular and General Genetics. 2009;282:617-31.

[168] Deng W, Ying H, Helliwell CA, Taylor JM, Peacock WJ, Dennis ES. Flowering Locus C (*FLC*) Regulates Development Pathways Throughout the Life Cycle of *Arabidopsis*. Proceedings of the National Academy of Sciences. 2011;108 (16):6680-5

[169] Staal J, Kaliff M, Bohman S, Dixelius C. Transgressive Segregation Reveals Two Arabidopsis TIR-NB-LRR Resistance Genes Effective against *Leptosphaeria maculans*, Causal Agent of Blackleg Disease. Plant J. 2006;46(2):218-30.

[170] Staal J, Dixelius C. *Rlm3*, a Potential Adaptor between Specific *TIR*-NB-LRR Receptors and DZC Proteins. Communicative & Integrative Biology 2008;1(1):59-61.

[171] Staal J, Kaliff M, Dewaele E, Persson M, Dixelius C. *Rlm3*, a TIR Domain Encoding Gene Involved in Broad-Range Immunity of Arabidopsis to Necrotrophic Fungal Pathogens. Plant Journal 2008;55(2):188-200.

[172] Šašek V, Nováková M, Jindřichová B, Bóka K, Valentová O, BurketováLenka. Recognition of Avirulence gene *AvrLm1* from hemibiotrophic ascomycete *Leptosphaeria maculans* triggers salicylic acid and ethylene signaling in *Brassica napus*. Molecular Plant-Microbe Interactions 25:9, 1238-1250. 2012.

[173] Vincente JG, King GJ. Characterisation of Disease Resistance Gene-Like Sequences in *Brassica oleracea* L. Theoretical and Applied Genetics. 2001;102:555-63.

[174] Fourmann M, Charlot F, Froger N, Delourme R, Brunel D. Expression, Mapping, and Genetic Variability of *Brassica napus* Disease Resistance Gene Analogues. Genome. 2001;44(6):1083.

[175] Sharma N, N. Hotte, M.H. Rahman, M. Mahammadi, M.K. Deyholos, N.N.V. Kav. Towards Identifying Brassica Proteins Involved in Mediating Resistance to *Leptosphaeria maculans*: A Proteomics-Based Approach. Proteomics. 2008;8:3516-35.

[176] Marra R, Li H, Barbetti MJ, Sivasithamparam K, Vinale F, Cavallo P, et al. Proteomic Analysis of the Interaction between *Brassica napus* Cv. Surpass 400 and Virulent or Avirulent Isolates of *Leptosphaeria maculans*. Journal of Plant Pathology. 2010;92:89-101.

[177] Tollenaere R, Hayward A, Dalton-Morgan J, Campbell E, Lee JRM, Lorenc M, et al. Identification and Characterization of Candidate *Rlm4* Blackleg Resistance Genes in *Brassica napus* Using Next-Generation Sequencing. Plant Biotechnology Journal. 2012;10(6):709-15.

[178] Wheeler DA, Srinivasan M, Egholm M, Shen Y, Chen L, McGuire A, et al. The Complete Genome of an Individual by Massively Parallel DNA Sequencing. Nature. 2008;452(7189):872-6.

[179] Metzker ML. Sequencing Technologies- the Next Generation. Nat Rev Genet. 2010;11(1):31-46.

[180] Ju YS, Kim J-I, Kim S, Hong D, Park H, Shin J-Y, et al. Extensive Genomic and Transcriptional Diversity Identified through Massively Parallel DNA and Rna Sequencing of Eighteen Korean Individuals. Nat Genet. 2011;43(8):745-52.

[181] Consortium TPGS. Genome Sequence and Analysis of the Tuber Crop Potato. Nature. 2011;475(7355):189-95.

[182] Wang X, Wang H, Wang J, Sun R, Jian Wu, Shengyi Liu, et al. The Genome of the Mesopolyploid Crop Species *Brassica rapa*. Nature Genetics. 2011;43:1035-9.

[183] Imelfort M, Edwards D. Next Generation Sequencing of Plant Genomes. Briefings in Bioinformatics. 2009;10:609-18.

[184] Osborn TC, Butrulle DV, Sharpe AG, Pickering KJ, Parkin IAP, Parker JS, et al. Detection and Effects of a Homeologous Reciprocal Transposition in *Brassica napus*. Genetics. 2003;165(3):1569-77.

[185] Kelly AL. The Genetic Basis of Petal Number and Pod Orientation in Oilseed Rape (*Brassica napus*). PhD Thesis, University of New Castle, UK. 1996.

[186] Wang J, Kaur S, Cogan N, Dobrowolski M, Salisbury P, Burton W, et al. Assessment of Genetic Diversity in Australian Canola (*Brassica napus* L.) Cultivars Using SSR Markers. Crop & Pasture Sci. 2009;60:1193-201.

[187] Raman H, Ryan PR, Raman R, Stodart BJ, Zhang K, Martin P, et al. Analysis of *TALMT1* Traces the Transmission of Aluminum Resistance in Cultivated Common Wheat (*Triticum aestivum* L.). Theoretical and Applied Genetics. 2008;116:343–54.

Chapter 5

Marker Assisted Selection for Common Bean Diseases Improvements in Tanzania: Prospects and Future Needs

George Muhamba Tryphone,
Luseko Amos Chilagane, Deogracious Protas,
Paul Mbogo Kusolwa and Susan Nchimbi-Msolla

Additional information is available at the end of the chapter

http://dx.doi.org/10.5772/52823

1. Introduction

Common bean (*Phaseolus vulgaris* L.) is an important grain legume for direct human consumption [1]. It is an important source of dietary protein, calories, dietary fibres, and minerals especially iron and zinc in Africa and a primary staple in parts of the Great Lake Regions (GLR) [2, 3]. Beans consuming have medicinal benefits [4]. It is estimated that over 75% of rural households in Tanzania depend on it for daily dietary requirements [5]. Bean production also provides farm households with both income and food for nutrition [1]. Bean is a cash income earner crop where the dry seeds and fresh pods attract a higher market price [6].

Despite the importance of common bean in Tanzania and other developing countries, its production mostly relies on local cultivars [7- 9]. The local cultivars however, are commonly known to produce notoriously low yields as they are highly constrained by several biotic and abiotic factors, including diseases, insect pests, poor seed quality, drought, low soil fertility and poor crop management [1, 10-12]. Yield losses caused by bean diseases are very significant and devastating in the bean industry [11, 13-15]. The economic losses caused by diseases results from reduction of seed quality and yield [16]. Since most of landraces and improved cultivars grown in Tanzania are susceptible to the diseases, there is a need therefore to incorporate resistance against them in adapted cultivars. Currently, none of the commercial genotypes has multiple resistances to common bean diseases. However, using classical breeding, significant strides have been made in crop improvement through phenotypic selections for agronomical important traits. Considerable difficulties however, are often encountered during this process, due to genotype-environment interactions [17]. Furthermore, resistance to some diseases is complex as they are quantitatively inherited making it difficult to achieve rapid progress through classical breeding [13]. In addition, breeding is complicated by the pathogens variability and different genes conditioning resistances [1, 13]. The identification of plants carrying two or more resistance alleles of different genes using standard inoculation test is impractical because several races would be needed to screen for specific alleles [16]. Thus classical breeding is limited by the length of screening procedures and reliance on the environmental factors. Hence, deployment of the molecular markers linked to resistance genes could be an alternative, more reliable screening procedure to increase the efficiency of breeding for disease resistance using marker assisted selection (MAS) [13]. Molecular marker available include 23 RAPD and five SCAR markers linked to 15 different resistance genes in addition to QTL conditioning resistance to seven major pathogens of common bean [13, 66]. The use of DNA molecular markers will improve understanding of the genetic factors conditioning these traits and is expected to assist in the selection of superior genotypes [17, 18]. Molecular marker assisted selection can be used to simultaneously screen for resistance to diseases without affecting the growth of the plants [13, 19]. Selection for genetic markers linked with resistance genes and QTL can accelerate development of multiple resistant varieties and increase efficacy [14, 20, 21]. The use of disease resistant cultivars in combination with appropriate cultural practices is essential for the management of bean diseases [14, 22, 23]. This chapter discusses the importance of MAS and how it can be integrated into breeding programs for enhancing selection efficiency in developing disease resistant bean varieties in Tanzania.

2. Economic important of common bean

Common bean (*Phaseolus vulgaris* L.) is an important grain legume for the direct human consumption in the World [1]. It is a staple food for more than 100 million people in Africa with per capita consumption of 60 kg/person/year in the Great Lakes Regions (GLR) [24]. Beans represent one of the principal crops in East Africa in terms of total area planted and number of farmers involved in production [25]. Bean production also provides farm households with both a source of income and food for nutrition through sales and consumption of part of the produce. Tanzania ranks 6th among top 10 bean producers worldwide [26] and is the largest producer in Africa with 850,000 MT produced per year which is equivalent to a commercial value of US$ 246,583,000. Production of common beans in Tanzania is higher than any other pulses estimated at 300 000 tonnes annually, representing 82% of the total pulse production [5, 27]. The dry bean is the major product although green beans are also widely consumed. It complements cereals and other carbohydrate rich foods by providing near perfect nutrition to people of all ages. Common bean has the nutritional benefits such as high source of proteins and high mineral contents especially Fe and Zn which combat high prevalence related micronutrient deficiencies [3, 6]. Consuming beans also have medicinal benefits as it is recognized that they contribute to treating human aliments like cancer, diabetes, and heart diseases [2, 4].

3. Constraints in bean production

The average yields of common bean has remained low (>500 kg/ha) [11] while the potential of current promising released varieties are at 1500 kg/ha [11, 28]). Across farming systems, biotic and abiotic stresses continue to present the major constraints for increased bean production and high yields with bean diseases representing the major constraints to production by reducing yields and seed quality. In Tanzania and other parts of the world, large yield losses of common bean are due to a great number of diseases affecting the crop. The major diseases affecting bean production in Tanzania include Bean Common Mosaic Necrosis Virus, common bacterial blight (*Xanthomonas axonopodis pv. phaseoli*), halo bacterial blight (*Pseudomonas syringae pv phaseolicola*), angular leaf spot (*Phaeoisariopsis griseola*), anthracnose (*Colletotricum lindemuthianum*) and rust (*Uromyces phaseoli*) [11]. On sandy soils the root-knot nematodes (*Meloidogyne incognita* and *M. javanica*) are the main problems [11]. The angular leaf spot (ALS), the common bacterial blight (CBB), the bean common mosaic virus (BCMV) and the bean common mosaic necrosis virus (BCMNV) are diseases which are endemic in Tanzania occurring across all production ecologies [1]. They can cause yield loss up to 100% of the expected yield, depending on the environment and the cultivars used [29]. There is thus a need to breed for high resistance levels and one option is to introgress resistance genes in adapted cultivars grown locally or into one line.

4. Breeding for disease resistance

The low bean yields in developing countries among others are due to a lack of effective diseases management practices including the lack of disease resistant cultivars and when such cultivars are available, they are not integrated in the disease management packages. The development of cultivars with improved resistance to biotic and abiotic stresses has long been a primary goal for many bean breeding programs [8]. It is considered that the use of resistant cultivars is an efficient, safe and inexpensive technique accessible for bean growers [14]. In fact, this strategy is the most effective and sustainable method for controlling bean diseases [29]. Resistant varieties therefore provide distinct channels for achieving high productivity through productivity maintenance, where benefits are not derived from the avoidance of yield losses associated with disease pressure and the yield gains the resistant varieties can give under disease pressure [30]. The use of resistant varieties leads to a reduction in both production costs especially pesticide cost and lower the quantity of pesticides or their residues released into the environment [14, 16]. Thus, varieties with improved disease resistance can reduce reliance on pesticides in high input systems, avert the risk of yield loss from diseases in low- and high-input systems, and enable more stable bean production across diverse and adverse environments [30]. However, the development of resistant variety is an obstacle for breeders as most pathogen exhibits a great variability for pathogenicity which mostly overcomes the resistance in the released cultivars. Breeders are thus continuously forced to look for new sources of resistances. The screening procedures to ascertain resistance is another setback as pathogenicity tests need to be reliable by exhibiting comparable and reproducible results [13]. The other constraint is whatever resistances detected with those tests should be efficient in controlling the target diseases in the field. Finally, methods usable by breeders for speeding up the breeding work should be developed. Genomics of *P. vulgaris* appear to be promising in discovering and tagging novel alleles [19, 31]. If closely linked to resistant genes, molecular markers such as Sequence Characterized Amplified Region (SCAR), Simple Sequence Repeats (SSR), Restriction fragment length polymorphism (RFLP), Amplified fragment length polymorphism (AFLP) can enhance the efficiency of breeding programs especially in the so-called marker assisted selection (MAS) and can be used in initial and intermediate stages of the breeding process. The target traits can be achieved indirectly using molecular markers closely linked to underlying genes or that have been developed from the actual gene sequences [32]. MAS can be used to simultaneously screen for resistance to diseases without affecting the growth of the plants. Selection for genetic markers linked with resistance genes and QTL can accelerate development of multiple resistant varieties and increase efficacy [20, 21]. The uses of MAS enable the introgression of resistance genes into a cultivar, decreases population size and ultimately reduce the time required to develop a new variety.

5. Molecular markers

Genetic markers represent genetic differences between individual organisms or species. Generally, they do not represent the target genes themselves but act as signs or flags and they are used as chromosome landmarks to facilitate the introgression of chromosome regions with genes associated with economically important traits [19]. However, such markers themselves do not affect the phenotype of that trait of interest because they are located only near or are linked to genes controlling the target traits [31]. Various types of molecular markers are utilized to evaluate DNA polymorphism and are generally classified as either hybridization-based or polymerase chain reaction (PCR)-based markers [19]. DNA markers are useful particularly if they can reveal difference between individuals of the same species or different species [32, 33].

There are three types of genetic markers: morphological (or classical or visible) markers, which themselves are phenotypic traits or characters, biochemical markers which include allelic variants of enzymes called isozymes and DNA (or molecular) markers, which reveal sites of variation in DNA [19]. Morphological markers are usually visually characterized and include phenotypic characters such as flower colour, seed shape, growth habits or pigmentation [34]. However, these markers are limited in number so only small portion of the genome can be assayed for contribution towards complex characters. Also, the genes controlling morphological markers have pleiotropic effects on the characters under investigation; this eludes the actual location of genes due to distortion of segregation ratio. Isozyme markers are differences in enzymes that are detected by electrophoresis and specific staining. The number of useful protein markers is very small. Both morphological and biochemical markers are influenced by environmental factors and/or developmental stages of the plants [20, 16, 19, 34].

However, the properties to be considered desirable for ideal DNA markers for their use as DNA markers in MAS as suggested by authors in reference [32, 33] as: highly polymorphic nature, codominant inheritance (distinguishing homozygous and heterozygous states of diploid organisms), quality and quantity of DNA required, frequent occurrence in genome (reliability), selective neutral behaviour (the DNA sequences of any organism are neutral to environmental conditions or management practices), easy access (availability), easy and fast assay, high reproducibility and easy exchange of data between laboratories. However, it is not easy to find a molecular marker which meets all these criteria. Depending on the type of study undertaken, a marker system can be identified that would fulfill at least a few of these criteria.

5.1. Restricted Fragment Length Polymorphism (RFLP)

RFLPs are simply inherited naturally and are Mendelian characters. They have their origin in the DNA rearrangements that occur due to evolutionary processes, point mutations within the restriction enzyme recognition site sequences, insertions or deletions within the fragments, and unequal crossing over. The usefulness of these markers in improvement of common bean have been the assessment of genetic diversity as they are useful in detecting polymorphism among different lines and hence being used to determine how diverse the genome being assessed [35] and they have been found superior over isozymes for their better coverage of the genome and higher level of polymophiosm. These markers are useful in breeding for disease resistance when they are linked to disease resistant genes. For example, four RFLPs were found to be linked to *Are* gene for resistance to Anthracnose of common bean [36] and in this matter then the RFLPs can be used to breed for resistance.

5.2. Microsatellite markers (SSR-Simple Sequence Repeats)

They essentially belong to the repetitive DNA family. Fingerprints generated by these probes are also known as oligonucleotide fingerprints. The methodology has been derived from RFLP and specific fragments are visualized by hybridization with a labelled microsatellite probe. Microsatellites or short tandem repeats/simple sequence repeats consist of 1 to 6 bp long monomer sequence that is repeated several times. These loci contain tandem repeats that vary in the number of repeated units between genotypes and are referred to as variable number of tandem repeats. Microsatellites thus form an ideal marker system creating complex banding patterns by simultaneously detecting multiple DNA loci. Some of the prominent features of these markers are that they are dominant fingerprinting markers and codominant sequence tagged microsatellites markers. If many alleles exist in a population, the level of heterozygosity is high and they follow Mendelian inheritance.

These markers have been utilized in a variety of ways in bean improvement since they are linked to disease resistance genes and in diversity analysis [37]. The SSR markers have been used in diversity assessment in common bean because of their utilities like low costs, high efficiency, whole genome coverage, robustness and minimum DNA requirements [20, 37]. In addition these markers are preferred for use because of being highly polymorphic, co-dominant, being PCR based and easily detected [19, 37]. The SSR markers have been utilized in assessing the genetic structure and diversity among common beans [38]. In MAS some SSR markers have been identified to be linked to disease resistance genes as the case for Angular leaf spot genes where the primer *PV-atct001* was found to be linked to resistant allele to ALS [16, 39] and some markers have been used in Marker assisted backcrossing [29].

5.3. Random Amplified Polymorphic DNA (RAPD)

This procedure detects nucleotide sequence polymorphisms in DNA by using a single primer of arbitrary nucleotide sequences. In this reaction, a single species of primer anneals to the genomic DNA at two different sites on complementary strands of DNA template. If these priming sites are within an amplifiable range of each other, a discrete DNA product is formed through thermocyclic amplification. On an average, each primer directs amplification of several discrete loci in the genome, making the assay useful for efficient screening of nucleotide sequence polymorphism between individuals.

These markers have been used in a variety of ways in genetic analysis. They have been used in gene pyramiding especially where conventional procedures couldn't solve the problem when there is epistasis between resistance genes to be pyramided [40, 41]. Some of the RAPD markers have been used to pyramid three rust resistance alleles *Up2, Ur-3* and *B-190* [42] with other epistatic resistance alleles from plant introduction collection [40, 43]. Similarly, pyramiding was also suggested in reference [44] where the two genes linked to *I* and *bc-3* genes for resistance to bean common mosaic virus disease and bean common mosaic necrosis virus disease respectively were incorporated in elite cultivar/line.

These markers have also been used in the assessment of genetic diversity of common bean. In reference [45] reported the potential of using RAPD markers as compared to RFLP, DAMD-PCR, ISSR and AFLP for assessing diversity of common bean and in this finding it shows that these markers were able to produce higher percentage of polymorphism than the others used hence being very useful in detecting polymorphism.

5.4. Sequence Characterized Amplified Region (SCAR) markers

In SCAR markers, the RAPD marker termini are sequenced and longer primers are designed (22–24 nucleotide bases long) for specific amplification of a particular locus [16]. The presence or absence of the band indicates variation in sequence. These are better reproducible than RAPDs. SCARs are usually dominant markers, however, some of them can be converted into codominant markers by digesting them with tetra cutting restriction enzymes and polymorphism can be deduced by using simple non denaturing gels to detect whether the products has different restriction sites for the different alleles. Compared to arbitrary primers, SCARs exhibit several advantages in mapping studies (codominant SCARs are informative for genetic mapping than dominant RAPDs), map-based cloning as they can be used to screen pooled genomic libraries by PCR, physical mapping, locus specificity, etc. SCARs also allow comparative mapping or homology studies among related species, thus making it an extremely adaptable concept in the near future [16, 19]. These markers have been widely used in breeding for disease resistance especially where the disease is controlled by dominant gene since these markers are dominant in nature. Different SCAR markers have been identified linked to resistance genes to many common bean diseases [46].

5.5. Sequence Tagged Sites (STS)

RFLP probes specifically linked to a desired trait can be converted into polymerase chain reaction (PCR)-based Sequence-Tagged Sites (STS) markers based on nucleotide sequence of the probe giving polymorphic band pattern, to obtain specific amplicon. Using this technique, tedious hybridization procedures involved in RFLP analysis can be overcome. This approach is extremely useful for studying the relationship between various species. When these markers are linked to some specific traits, for example the powdery mildew or stem rust resistance genes in barley, they can be easily integrated into plant breeding programmes for MAS of the trait of interest [47].

5.6. Amplified Fragment Length Polymorphism (AFLP)

The technique based on the detection of genomic restriction fragments by PCR amplification and can be used for DNAs of any origin or complexity. The fingerprints are produced, without any prior knowledge of sequence, using a limited set of generic primers. The number of fragments detected in a single reaction can be 'tuned' by selection of specific primer sets. AFLP technique is reliable since stringent reaction conditions are used for primer annealing. This technique thus shows an ingenious combination of RFLP and PCR techniques and is extremely useful in detection of polymorphism between closely related genotypes. Due to their characteristics, these markers are useful in assessing diversity of common bean and in case the marker is linked to a trait of importance in common bean then it can be useful for MAS in selecting or screening genotypes for that particular trait [48, 49]. For example, AFLP studies conducted to determine genetic relatedness of two near-isogenic Teebus lines and Teebus of common bean to CBB resistance [44, 50]. These markers despite being useful, their analysis is too difficult and troublesome, for this they can be converted to other types of markers like SCAR or STS which is also a difficult thing to achieve.

6. Molecular Marker Assisted Selection (MAS)

By using DNA markers to assist in plant breeding, efficiency and precision could be greatly increased. Use of markers in plant breeding is called marker-assisted selection (MAS) and is a complement of the new discipline of molecular breeding [33]. MAS is the novel approach in which individuals for intercrossing are selected using selection index based on genotypic data controlled by few or several genes (Quantitative linked traits or QTL). The gain from selection using such index is expected to be higher than phenotypic selection used in conventional recurrent methods [21]. Significant progress has been made through phenotypic selections for agronomic traits. However, difficulties are often encountered due to the genotype x environment interactions [17]. For example, significant progress has been achieved in selecting BCMV and BCMNV resistant lines [13]. However, some of the traits are controlled by multiple genetic loci (Quantitative Trait Loci) and display a strong interaction with the environment. Molecular markers linked to such traits are available and have increased the efficiency of breeding for diseases in MAS programmes [13, 19]. The use of DNA molecular markers will improve understanding of the genetic factors conditioning these traits and is expected to assist in the selection of superior genotypes [18]. The use of disease resistant cultivars in combination with appropriate cultural practices is essential for the management of these bean diseases [2].

MAS is an approach designed to avert problems encountered with conventional/classical plant breeding by increased precision of selection, selecting phenotypes through the selection of genes that control the traits of interest [19, 51]. This is because molecular markers are clearly not influenced by environment and are detectable at all stages of plant growth [20, 28]. With the availability of an array of molecular markers and genetic maps, MAS has become possible for traits governed by single gene or QTLs. MAS is a good approach for bean breeders who also work to improve bean for disease resistance. For MAS to be highly successful, a high correlation and/or tight linkage must exist between the genes for resistance to diseases and molecular markers, and the markers must be stable, reproducible and easy to assay [52].

MAS provide an effective and efficient breeding tool for detecting, tracking, retaining, combining, and pyramiding disease resistance genes [31]. DNA based markers can be effectively utilized for the following basic purposes (i) tracing favorable alleles (dominant or recessive) across generations and (ii) identifying the most suitable individual (s) among the segregating progeny, based on allelic composition across a part or the entire genome [20, 32].

7. Why MAS in plant breeding

Justifications for the application of MAS in plant breeding fall into four broad areas that are relevant to almost all target crops [53, 54, 55] (i) traits that are difficult to manage through conventional phenotypic selection because they are expensive or time-consuming to measure, or have low penetrance or complex inheritance; (ii) traits whose selection depends on specific environments or developmental stages that influence the expression of the target phenotypes; (iii) maintenance of recessive alleles during backcrossing or for speeding up backcross breeding in general; and (iv) pyramiding multiple monogenic traits (such as pest and disease resistances or qualitative traits) or several QTL for a single target trait with complex inheritance (such as drought tolerance or other adaptive traits). Introgression and pyramiding of multiple genes affecting the same trait is a great challenge to breeding programs.

The target cropping environments of many breeding programs require a combination of diverse biotic stress resistances, agronomic and quality trait profiles, plus abiotic stress tolerances to improve performance, yield stability, and farmers' acceptance. The greatest impact from MAS will only be realized when breeding systems are adapted to make best use of large-scale genotyping for both multiple target traits and the genetic background. The greatest benefits from this type of integrated molecular breeding approach will be to achieve the same breeding progress in a much shorter time than through conventional breeding, and from pyramiding combinations of genes that could not be readily combined through other means.

8. MAS' requirements

Success of marker based breeding system depends on several factors as described by [20, 19], a genetic map with an adequate number of uniformly-spaced polymorphic markers to accurately locate desired QTLs or major gene (s); close linkage between the QTL or a major gene of interest and adjacent markers; adequate recombination between the markers and rest of the genome; an ability to analyze a large number of plants in a time and cost effective manner.

9. Applications of MAS

The key success of integrating MAS into breeding programmes lies in identifying applications in which markers offer real advantages over conventional/classical breeding methods or complement them in a novel way. MAS offer significant advantages in cases where phenotypic screening is expensive, difficult or impossible or traits are of low heritability and/or the selected trait is expressed late in plant development. Also, for incorporating genes for resistance to diseases or pests that cannot be easily screened due to special requirements for the genes to be expressed; the expression of the target gene is recessive; there is a need to accumulate multiple genes for one or more traits within the same cultivar, or improving perennial/biennial crops with long life cycle using a process called gene pyramiding [13, 20, 32, 33]. The success of MAS depend upon the distance between the markers and the target gene, the number of target genes to be transferred, the genetic basis of the trait, the number of individuals that can be analyzed and the genetic background in which the target gene has to be transferred, the type of molecular marker (s) used and the availability of specific technical facilities [20, 21].

Conventional breeding has been successfully applied in several crops' breeding programmes and a large number of varieties or lines possessing multiple attributes have been produced. However, the difficulties associated with this method are due to the dominance and epistasis effects of genes governing the target disease resistances, for example, the CBB resistance in case common bean. Therefore, MAS has been especially suggested for increasing the selection efficiency and timely delivery of cultivars in the particular case of breeding for resistant cultivars. The benefits from the use of genomics tools include (i) more effectively identify, quantify and characterize genetic variation from all available germplasm resources; (ii) tag, clone and introgress genes and/or QTLs that are useful for enhancing the target trait using either genetic transformation, facilitating pyramiding or recurrent selection, by differentiating and selecting particular genotypes in breeding populations [20, 32].

10. Molecular markers assisted selection for bean diseases

Breeders used to rely on visual screening of genotypes to select for traits of economic importance. However, successful application of this method depends on its reproducibility and heritability of the trait. Therefore, the use of molecular markers in the bean breeding programmes has improved the accuracy of crosses to carry out and allowed breeders to produce germplasm with combined traits that were hazardous and difficult before the advent of DNA technology [13].

10.1. Angular leaf spot

Resistance genes against *Phaeoisariopsis griseola* the causal agent of ALS are controlled by major genes, that are either dominant or recessive, acting singly or duplicated and which may interact in an additive manner with or without epistasis [56]. Inheritance of resistance is controlled by a single recessive gene [57], but in an earlier study, resistance to ALS was reported to be controlled by a single dominant gene. This shows that inheritance of ALS resistance is complex, involving both dominant and recessive genes that may be or may not be independent. Major and minor genes mediate angular leaf spot (ALS) resistance in beans (*P. vulgaris)* and a number of sources for these resistance genes have been identified [56]. Diverse sources of resistance to angular leaf spot in bean genotypes have been reported [58]. Examples of resistant cultivars include A 75, A 140, A 152, A 175, A 229, BAT 76, BAT 431, BAT 1432, BAT 1458 and G5686, MAR 1, MAR 2 [59]. In reference [60] found the ALS resistance in AND 277 to race 63:23 to be conferred by a single dominant gene (*Pgh-1*). Cornell 49-242 has *Pgh-2* which confers resistance to *P. griseola* pathotype 31:17 [61] while [41] found that resistance to ALS in Mexico 54 is due to a single dominant gene that confers resistance to pathotype 63:63 and G06727 has resistance to *P. griseola* pathotype 63:59. In reference [120] reported that 'Ouro Negro' had resistance to 8 pathotypes, including *P. griseola* race 63:63 from Brazil. G5686 and Mexico 54 display fairly good levels of resistance to nearly all races [59]. These cultivars are not only good sources of resistance to *P. griseola* but could also serve as reliable indicators of new races of the pathogen in the future [62]. Mexico 54 has shown to be resistant to all *P. griseola* isolates characterized in Africa [63]. Resistance in G5686 is conditioned by two dominant epistatic genes and Amendoim by two recessive genes [64]. Resistance to specific isolates of *P. griseola* has been reported to be simply inherited and molecular markers have been identified for some of these resistance genes [14, 41, 65, 66]. Sources of resistance reported from Africa include GLP 24, GLP X-92, GLP - 806 and GLP 77 [59]. Resistance to various diseases is monogenically determined, but cases of duplicate,

http://dx.doi.org/10.5772/52823

complementary and other interactions have been reported [67]. The breed for ALS resistance, molecular markers linked to angular leaf spot resistance genes have been identified in beans. SCAR markers for selecting for genes for resistance to ALS include SH13 for *phg-1* gene in linkage group *6 [68]* and SNO2 for phg-2 gene in linkage group 8 [69, 61]. Others include, SAA19 [68], SBA16 [68] and SMO2 [68] which is ouro negro dominant gene.

10.2. Common bacterial blight

The control of common bacterial blight (CBB) disease caused by *Xanthomonas axonopodis pv phaseoli (Xap)* is challenging due to its complexity and seed borne nature [67]. The number of genes involved in resistance to *Xap* range from one to several genes with varying degrees of action and interactions [70, 71]. Breeding for CBB resistance is complicated pathogen genetic diversity and coevolution [72, 73] different genes conditioning resistance in leaves, pods and seeds [16, 73, 74, 76] and linkage of resistance with undesirable traits [16, 76]. Resistance of CBB is quantitatively and qualitatively controlled depending on the source of germplasm with pod and leaf resistance being controlled by different genes [9, 67, 77]. Quantitative inheritance was observed after making original interspecific crosses between resistant *P. acutifolius* 'tepary 4' and susceptible *P. Vulgaris* [67]. Sources of resistance to *Xap* in common bean have been reported [66, 78]. Other sources of resistance have been identified in tepary bean (*P. acutifolius*) [79, 80], and runner bean, (*P. coccineus*) [81]. Resistance to common bacterial blight has been reported in *Phaseolus acutifolius* [77], *P. coccineus* and lines of *P. vulgaris* [82]. CIAT lines VAX 3, VAX 4, VAX 6, and XAN 159 have also been reported to have good level of resistance to common bacterial blight [67]. Increased resistance can be developed by selecting for horizontal resistance [83].

Albeit, genetic studies have shown that resistance to CBB is quantitatively inherited, it involves a few major genes [13]. The identification of QTL influencing resistance to CBB combined with phenotypic data implying the involvement of few genes, suggests that MAS may be useful in combining resistance sources to CBB in common bean. To date, SCAR markers used in selecting resistance to CBB are dominant and are scored as presence or absence of a single band on an agarose gel. SCAR markers available in screening are SU91, BC420, SAP 6, BAC 6, R7313 and R4865. SU91 is linked to a QTL for CBB resistance in bean in the linkage group B8 [16, 84]. BC420 is linked to a QTL for CBB resistance on bean linkage group B6. SAP 6 is for a major QTL in the linkage group B10 [84], BAC 6 for a major QTL in linkage group B10 [85] R7313 for a major QTL in linkage group B8 [86] and R4865 for another major QTL [86]. Thus, molecular markers allow distinct QTLs to be screened and consequently provide an opportunity to pyramid multiple QTL for CBB resistance into a single genotype.

10.3. Bean common mosaic virus and bean common mosaic necrosis virus

Genetic resistance to both potyviruses is conditioned by a series of independent multi-allelic loci in common bean is affected by four different loci: bc-1, bc-2, bc-3 and bc-u [87]. Resistance controlled by alleles at these loci is inherited as recessive characters [88]. In addition to the recessive bc genes, the dominant I gene in *P. vulgaris* confers resistance to BCMV and other potyviruses through a hypersensitive response [88, 89] and has also been the focus of positional gene cloning activities [90]. The *I* gene located on B2 [91], is independent of recessive resistance conditioned by three different *bc* genes. The *bc-3* gene is located on B6 [84, 92, 93], whereas the *bc-12* allele was mapped to B3 [84]. The non-specific *bc-u* allele, needed for expression of *bc-22* resistance, also resides on B3 based on the loose linkage with the *bc-1* locus [94].

The independence of the BCMV resistance genes provides opportunities to use gene pyramiding as a strategy in breeding for durable resistance. Bean breeders recognize that the combination of the dominant *I* gene with recessive *bc* resistance genes offers durability over single gene resistance to BCMV and BCMNV, since the two types of genes have distinctly different mechanisms of resistance [95]. The dominant *I* gene is defeated by all necrotic strains, whereas the three most effective recessive genes (*bc-1, bc-2 and bc-3*) act constitutively by restricting virus movement within the plant, probably through the virus movement proteins. The action of the dominant *I* gene is masked by the recessive *bc-3* gene, so as efforts to incorporate the *bc-3* gene into new germplasm proceed, the risk of losing the *I* gene in improved germplasm increases, since direct selection for the *I* gene is not possible. Linked markers offer the only realistic opportunity to maintain and continue to utilize the *I* gene as a pyramided resistance gene in future bean cultivars.

A marker tightly linked to the *I* gene [96] has been demonstrated in many laboratories to be effective across a wide range of germplasm from both gene pools. Breeders have used markers linked to the *I* gene to develop enhanced germplasm with the *I +bc-3* gene combination. In addition, [92] developed SCAR markers from the OC11350/420 (ROC11) and OC20460 RAPD markers linked to the *bc-3* gene to improve their utilization. The use of these markers in MAS, however, has been limited due to a lack of polymorphism and reproducibility across diverse genetic backgrounds and gene pools of common bean [91].

Direct screening with strains of BCMV and BCMNV is still required to confirm the presence of the *bc-3* gene. To efficiently introgression the *bc-3* gene for resistance to BCMV and BCMNV into susceptible bean cultivars, there is a need to identify more robust DNA markers tightly linked to the *bc-3* gene that will demonstrate reproducibility across laboratories and be functional in different genetic backgrounds. Similarly, the hypostatic *I* gene is retained in the presence of the *bc-3* gene by MAS for the SW13 SCAR [69, 96]. This combination of a dominant and a recessive gene, likely possessing different resistance mechanisms, should provide more durable resistance to bean common mosaic virus.

At CIAT, bean cultivars have been bred which combine *I* gene and recessive resistance genes. These have been evaluated in areas of East Africa where BCMNV is known to occur [96]. Several commercial varieties combining the *I* gene and recessive resistance genes are now available [97, 99].

10.4. Anthracnose

Two new sources of anthracnose resistance within the Andean gene pool were identified in germplasm from Brazil [10, 100; 101]. The two independent genes were identified as Co-12 in Jalo Vermelho and Co-13 in Jalo Listras Pretas and represent unique resistance patterns.

These are significant findings as the multiallelic Co-1 locus with five alleles was the only resistance sources previously known in Andean germplasm. This is particularly important given the recent breakdown of the Co-12 gene by race 105 in Manitoba. The rapid evolution of this new race underscores the need to monitor the pathogenic variability in different production areas. The availability of new resistance genes of Andean origin offers breeders more choices for pyramiding genes with the more common Middle American resistance sources.

10.5. Root rots

Root rot of dry bean is a yield-limiting disease problem for growers in the North-Central region of the U.S. [102]. In North Dakota and Minnesota, *Fusarium solani* was considered to be the most common causal agent of root rot followed by *Rhizoctonia solani* [103]. However, recent findings have highlighted the ability of other Fusarium species to cause root rot in dry beans [104, 105]. Little is known about the prevalence and virulence of the four subspecies of *Rhizoctonia solani* that are found on common bean. Crops grown in rotation with beans, such as sugar beets, are also hosts for *R. solani*. [106]) found low genetic diversity among 166 isolates of the Fusarium wilt pathogen from the U.S. Central High Plains using RAPD markers. Resistance to Fusarium wilt in race Durango dry beans CO 33142 and Fisher were controlled by a single dominant gene, whereas polygenic control (h^2 ranged from 0.25 to 0.60) was found for resistance in race Mesoamerica cultivars Rio Tibagi and Jamapa [107, 108]. In addition, limited research has been conducted on *Aphanomyces euteiches f.sp. phaseoli*, but this fungus occurs frequently in the sandy soils in the Upper Midwest.

10.6. Rust

Two new races of rust have been recently reported in Michigan and North Dakota. The new races have reoccurred in Michigan since 2007 and in North Dakota since 2008. Preliminary results are showing that both races are similar, but not identical [109]. Resistance to both races is conditioned by the Ur-5, Ur-11, and CNC genes. A new source of resistance was mapped to LG 4 near the Ur-5 and Ur-Dorado108 loci in black bean populations derived from Tacana [110]. Several new cultivars with different combinations of rust resistance genes have been released [111]. Salient among these are six unique great northern bean germplasm lines named BelDakMi-RMR-8, to -13. These are the first great northern beans that combine four genes for rust resistance and two genes for resistance to the two bean common mosaic potyviruses. These beans combine two Andean (Ur-4 and Ur-6) and two Middle American (Ur-3 and Ur-11) rust resistance genes [111]. Other rust resistant cultivars include great northern bean cultivars ABC-Weihing (Ur-3 and Ur-6) [112], and Coyne (Ur-3 and Ur-6) [113], and Pinto CO46348 (Ur-4 and Ur-11) [114]. In the case of soybean rust, the common bean lines Compuesto Negro Chimaltenengo (CNC) and PI 181996 were among the most resistant to all six isolates. Inheritance of SBR resistance in CNC was studied by crossing Mx309/CNC. Based on severity, the segregation for SBR resistance in the F_2 population fit a 9 resistant to 7 susceptible ratio.

11. Other case studies of MAS

MAS has been proposed as the most practical and realistic approach to provide efficient long term control of bean anthracnose, ashly stem, bean common mosaic virus, common mosaic necrosis virus, bean golden mosaic virus [69], bean rust [115] and common bacterial blight [16, 64]. It has been or is being used to assist the simultaneous transfer of resistance genes for rust, anthracnose and angular leaf spot into Brazilian commercial cultivars [29]. Several lines resistant to rust [115, 116]; bean golden mosaic virus [69] and anthracnose [117] are being obtained using MAS.

12. Cost effectiveness of MAS to conventional screening method

As conventional breeding systems attempt to combine more and more target traits, there are tends to lose overall of breeding gains and an increase in the number of breeding cycles required to generate a finished product. In contrast, MAS offers the potential to assemble target traits in single genotypes more precisely, with less unintentional losses and in fewer selection cycles [20]. By means of MAS, breeding programmes have reported twice the rate of genetic gain over phenotypic selection for multiple traits such as yield, biotic and abiotic stress resistance and quality attributes [29, 32].

It has been described that the time, precision, number of traits and efficiency for traits with low heritability has increased with MAS. The cost-effectiveness of MAS depends on four parameters which are: the relative cost of phenotypic versus marker screening; the time saved by MAS; the time and temporal distribution of benefits associated with accelerated release of improved germplasm; the availability in the breeding program of operating budgets [20]. For example, in [16] estimated the cost for using SCAR and RAPD markers to analyse 100 bean samples (lines) would be $4.24 and 4.59 per data point, respectively after the markers were developed. This included the costs of labour to plant seeds, watering the plants daily for eight days, extract genomic DNA and conduct PCR and electrophoresis as well as the costs for chemicals and greenhouse space, but not the initial costs of developing the markers. Conversely, conventional greenhouse screening was estimated to cost approximately $6.99 per data point. This included the costs of labour to prepare inoculums, inoculate the plants, take care of plants for 32 days (fertilizer application, daily plant watering, insect control, growth room cleaning) and rate disease symptoms as well as the cost of greenhouse rental.

13. Historical background of common bean improvement in Tanzania

Bean production in Tanzania is affected by many problems that range from diseases to poor soil fertility as well as drought as the production is heavily rain-fed [11]. Some of the major bean production areas have acid soils with pH <5.5 which limit crop productivity [1].

Effort has been put on developing varieties that are resistant to biotic and abiotic stresses. This came in when breeding programs that set up across the country. Since the initiation of the breeding programme in Tanzania in 1959 [11], the white haricot beans was produced for the canning industry though it is susceptible to bean rust disease and has a poor seed quality. The objectives were to i) determine the reasons for poor bean yields among smallholders in the Southern Highlands and ii) to select high-yielding cultivars. It was established that diseases were the major yield-limiting factor and disease resistance became the main thrust of the programme. Therefore, its first step was to identify resistance sources among the available lines. The first line adapted in East Africa as being resistant to rust with good quality was Mexico 142 [11].

Since 1984, CIAT has introduced a number of varieties with different attributes into its breeding programmes for the mid- and high altitude areas of central, eastern and southern Africa. Twenty three bean varieties have been released in Tanzania since 1970 and several of these have been CIAT lines or were selections made in Tanzania from CIAT crosses [11, 118, 119].

Classical breeding methods were also used by CIAT in East Africa to develop a population from multi-parent crosses among genetically diverse lines from Andean and Mesoamerican gene pools. Several new lines were selected with combined resistance to ALS, root rot, low soil N, low soil P and low soil pH. These lines are being evaluated in seven countries in the region including Tanzania [121]. The plant breeders in the national and regional breeding programmes have been able to release a number of varieties in Tanzania as shown in Table 1 [119]. However, none of those varieties have been developed through marker assisted selection technique.

SN	Name of varieties	Year of release	Institutions involved	Yield (t/ha)	Reaction to diseases
1	Canadian wonder	1977	ARI Selian	1.1-2.4	Moderately resistant to halo blight and bean common mosaic virus
2	Kabanima	1980	ARI Uyole	1.5-1.8	Resistant to anthracnose and rust
3	Uyole 84	1984	ARI Uyole	1.5-2.0 (non staked) 2.5-4.0 (staked)	Resistant to anthracnose and halo blight
4	Uyole 90	1990	ARI Uyole	1.5-2.0	It is tolerant to halo blight and angular leaf spot
5	Uyole 94	1994	ARI Uyole	1.0-1.8	Resistant to *ascochyta* and rust, tolerant to Bean Common Mosaic Virus and Angular Leaf Spot
6	Uyole 96	1996	ARI Uyole	1.0-1.8	Tolerant to rust, ascochyta and Bean Common Mosaic Virus

SN	Name of varieties	Year of release	Institutions involved	Yield (t/ha)	Reaction to diseases
7	Uyole 98	1998	ARI Uyole	1.2-2.0	Resistant to anthracnose, angular leaf spot and rust. Tolerant to halo blight and *ascochyta*
8	Ilomba	1990	ARI Uyole	1.5-2.5	Resistant to anthracnose, halo blight and rust, Tolerant to *ascochyta*
9	Lyamungu 85	1985	ARI Selian	1.2-1.5	Resistant to anthracnose, angular leaf spot, Bean Common Mosaic Virus and intermediate to common bacteria blight.
10	Lyamungu 90	1990	ARI Selian	1.2-1.6	Resistant to leaf rust and anthracnose
11	Selian 94	1994	ARI Selian	2.5-3.5	Moderately susceptible to anthracnose and angular leaf spot
12	Jesca	1997	ARI Selian	2.0-3.4	Resistant to anthracnose, Bean Common Mosaic Virus and halo blight, moderately resistant to bean rust, angular leaf spot, common bacterial blight
13	Selian 97	1997	ARI Selian	2.0-2.8	Resistant to anthracnose, Bean Common Mosaic Virus and halo blight, moderately resistant to bean rust, angular leaf spot, common bacterial blight
14	Rojo	1997	SUA	2.2	Resistant to Bean Common Mosaic Virus, moderately resistant to common bacterial blight and nematodes.
15	Wanja	2002	ARI Uyole	1.5	Drought tolerant.
16	Bilfa	2004	ARI Uyole	1.5-2.5	Tolerant to Halo blight, Drought resistant Resistant to Anthracnose and bean rust
17	Uyole 04	2004	ARI Uyole	2.0 – 2.5	Resistant to Bean rust, Anthracnose and Tolerant to Halo blight and drought
18	Pesa	2006	SUA	0.9-1.5	Moderate resistant and Angular Leaf Spot. Resistant to Bean Common Mosaic Virus
19	Mshindi	2006	SUA	0.9-1.5	Moderate resistant to Angular Leaf Spot and Resistant to Bean Common Mosaic Virus
20	Selian 05	2005	ARI Selian	1.0-1.6	Resistant to Bean rust, Anthracnose, Mosaic Virus, and Halo blight
21	Selian 06	2007	ARI Selian	2.5-3.0	Resistant to Bean rust, Anthracnose, Mosaic Virus, and Halo blight

http://dx.doi.org/10.5772/52823

SN	Name of varieties	Year of release	Institutions involved	Yield (t/ha)	Reaction to diseases
22	Cheupe	2007	ARI Selian	2.5-3.0	Resistant to Bean rust, Anthracnose, Mosaic Virus, and Halo blight
23	Njano Uyole	2008	ARI Uyole	2.5 – 3.0	Resistant to Anthracnose

Source: MAFSC, 2008 [119]

Table 1. Common bean varieties released in Tanzania since 1970s and their characteristics

14. Conclusion

Plant breeders have traditionally and routinely used various recurrent selection methods to cumulate favourable alleles for yield and other polygenic traits. This selection will provide the population or breeding lines with diverse genetic recombination. The selection methods using classical breeding should be compared with that of MAS. To make it successful to the breeder, gains made from MAS must be more cost effective as compared to gains through classical breeding. It is anticipated that the applications and technology improvements will result in a reduction in the cost of markers, which will subsequently lead to a greater adoption of using molecular markers in plant breeding. The obstacles in using MAS are equipment, infrastructure, skilled man power and supplies or consumables. The available projects in Tanzania which involves the use MAS are time based and focuses on few bean pathogen. The available projects are facing several problems such as timely purchase and acquisition of consumables for molecular biology laboratories is frustrating even when funds are available. The main reasons include the reduced number of commercial flights between the supplier countries and Tanzania, the lack of proper cold chains in the supply chain and inappropriate policies hampering imports. The benefits of using MAS need to be critically compared to those achieved or expected from any existing classical breeding programmes. This is because; although classical breeding programme have their limitations, they have also shown over time that they can be highly successful. The use of molecular tools should not be a substitute for classical breeding methods but these two approaches should complement one another so as to archieve the benefits of both in crop breeding programmes. Development of comprehensive crop improvement programmes that will deploy the available sources of resistance to diseases and make proper use of MAS in selection is very important and this can in a proper way leap the benefits associated with these new tools and technologies as MAS in breeding for disease resistance. That can be true if government, donors and private sectors can join efforts to invest on facilities which can be shared for cost effective and efficiency delivery of services using MAS in breeding for disease resistance.

Author details

George Muhamba Tryphone, Luseko Amos Chilagane, Deogracious Protas,
Paul Mbogo Kusolwa and Susan Nchimbi-Msolla

Department of Crop Science and Production, Faculty of Agriculture, Sokoine University of Agriculture, Chuo Kikuu, Morogoro, Tanzania

References

[1] Wortmann, C. S., R. A. Kiluby, C. A. Eledu, D. J. Arron *Atlas of Common Bean (Phaseolus vulgaris L.) Production in Africa*. CIAT. Cali. Columbia, 1998, p. 133.

[2] Singh, S. P. Broadening the genetic base of common bean cultivars: A Review. Crop Science 2000; 41: 1659 - 1675.

[3] Tryphone, G.M. and S. Nchimbi-Msolla. Diversity of common bean (Phaseolus vulgaris L.) genotypes in iron and zinc contents under screenhouse conditions. African Journal of Agricultural Research 2010; 5(8):738-747

[4] Hangen, L. A. and M.R. Bennink, Consuption of black beans and navy beans (*Phaseolus* Tanzania, 1959-2005. Euphytica 2006, 150: 215 - 231.

[5] CIAT, The impact of improved bean production technologies in Northern Tanzania. http//www.ciat.cgiar.org/work/Africa/Documents/highlights no. 42.pdf. 2008; 2pp.

[6] Broughton, W. J.; Hernandez, G.; Blair, M.; Beebe, S.; Gepts, P and Vanderleyden, J. Beans (*Phaseolus spp.*) – model food legumes. Plant Soil 2003; 252: 55 – 128.

[7] Gepts, P. and Debouck, D. Origin, domestication and evolution of the common bean (*Phaseolus vulgaris*). In: *Common beans: Research for crop improvement (Edited by Van Schoonhoven, A. and Voysest, O.)* CABI/CIAT, Wallingford, UK. 1991; 7-53.

[8] Miklas P. N, Kelly J. D, Beebe S. E, Blair M. W. Common bean breeding for resistance against biotic and abiotic stresses: from classical to MAS breeding. Euphytica 2006; 147:105-131

[9] Chataika, B.Y.E., J. M. Bokosi, M. B. Kwapata, R. M. Chirwa, V. M. Mwale,P. Mnyenyembe, J. R. Myers, Performance of parental genotypes and inheritance of Angular Leaf Spot (*Phaeosariopsis griseola*) resistance in the common bean (*Phaseolus vulgaris*). African Journal of Biotechnology 2010; 9(28): 4398-4406.

[10] Mkandawire, A. B. C., Mabagala, R. B., Guzman, P., Gepts, P and Gilbertson, R. L. Genetic and Pathogenic variation of common blight bacteria (Xanthomonas axonopodis pv. Phaseoli and X. axonopodis pv. phaseoli var. fuscans). Phytopathology 2004; 94: 593-603.

[11] Hillocks, R. J., Madata, C. S., Chirwa, R., Minja, E. M., and Msolla, S. Phaseolus bean improvement in Tanzania 1959-F2005. Euphytica 2006; 150: 225-231.

[12] Mwang'ombe, A.W., Wagara, I.N., Kimenju, J.W. and Buruchara, R. Occurance and severity of Angular leaf spot of common bean in Kenya as influenced by geographical location, altitude and agroecological zones. Plant Pathology Journal 2007; 6 (3): 235-241.

[13] Kelly, J. D. and Miklas, P. N. The role of RAPD markers in breeding for disease resistance in common bean. Kluwer Academic Publishers. Molecular Breeding 1998; 4: 1-11.

[14] Ferreira, C.F., Borém, A., Caravalho, G.A., Neitsche, S., Paula, T. J., De Barros, E.G. and Moreira. M. A. Inheritance of angular leaf spot resistance in common bean and identification of a RAPD marker linked to a resistance gene. Crop Science 2000; 40: 1130-1133.

[15] Coyne D.R, Steadman J.R, Godoy-Lutz G, Gilbertson R, Arnaud- Santana E, Beaver J.S, Myers J.R. Contribution of the bean/cowpea CRSP to management of bean disease. Field Crops Research 2003; 82:155-168.

[16] Yu, K., Park, S.J. and Poysa, V. Marker-assisted selection of common beans for resistance to common bacterial blight: efficacy and economics. Plant Breeding 2000; 119: 411-415

[17] Tar`an, B., Michaels. T. E. and Pauls, K. P. Genetic mapping of agronomic traits in common bean. Crop Science 2002; 42: 544 - 556.

[18] Bezawada, C., Saha, S., Jenkins, J.N., Creech, R.G. and McCarty, J.C. SSR Marker(s) associated with root knot nematode resistance gene(s) in cotton. Journal of Cotton Science 2003; 7: 179-184

[19] Collards, B.C.Y, Jahufer, M.Z.Z., Brouwer, J.B., Pang, E.C. K. An introduction to markers, quantitative trait loci (QTL) mapping and marker assisted selection for crop improvement: the basic concept. Euphytica 2005; 169-196.

[20] Babu, R., Nair, S.K., Prasanna, B.M and Gupta H.S. Integrating marker-assisted selection in crop breeding-Prospects and challenges. Crop Science 2004; 87 (5): 606-619.

[21] Semagn, K., Bjornstad, A. and Ndjiondjop, M.N. Progress and prospects of marker assisted backcrossing as a tool in crop breeding programs. African Journal of Biotechnology 2006; 5(25): 2588-2603.

[22] Singh, S. P., Munoz, C. G. and Teran, H. Registration of common bacterial blight resistant dry bean germplasm VAX 1, VAX 3, and VAX 4. Crop Science 2001; 41: 275-276.

[23] Gomez, O. Evaluation of Nicaragua common bean (Phaseolus vulgaris L.) landraces. Doctors Dissertation. National agrarian university, Managua, Nicaragua. 2004; 30

[24] CTA (2010): Techinical Center for Agricultural and Rural Cooperation (Dry Beans: Grains of Hope), Spore 146/April, 2010.

[25] Kelly, J.D. Advances in common bean improvement: some case histories with broader applications. Acta horticulture 2004; 637: 99-121

[26] Food and Agriculture Organization of the United Nations (FAO), (April 2005). FAOSTAT DATABASE. [http://www.appsl.fao.org.serlet] site visited on 10/06/2005.

[27] NBS (bureau of statistics). United Republic of Tanzania: Socio-economic profile. National Bureau of Statistics 2006; 245p

[28] Miklas. P.N; Stone, V; Urrea, C. A, Johnson, E., Beaver, J. S. Inheritance and QTL analysis of field resistance to ashy stem blight. Crop Science 1998; 38:916–921

[29] Oliveira, L.K., Melo, L.C., Brondani, C., Peloso, M.J.D and Brondani, R.P.V. Backcross assisted by microsatellite markers in common bean. Genetics and Molecular Research 2008; 7 (4): 1000-1010

[30] Mooney, Daniel F. The Economic Impact of Disease-Resistant Bean Breeding Research in Northern Ecuador. M.S. thesis, Michigan State University, December 2007. 153pp

[31] O'Boyle, P. D., James D. Kelly, J. D. and Kirk, W.W. Use of Marker-assisted Selection to Breed for Resistance to Common Bacterial Blight in Common Bean. Journal of American Society of Horticultural Science 2007; 132(3): 381–386.

[32] Xu, Y. and Crouch, J. H. Marker assisted selection in plant breeding: from publication to practices: Review and interpretation. Crop science 2008; 48: 391-407.

[33] Collard BCY; Mackill DJ. 2008. Marker-assisted selection: an approach for precision plant breeding in the twenty-first century. Philosophical Transactions of the Royal Society B 363(1491):577–572.

[34] Winter, P. and Kahl, G. Molecular markers technologies for plant improvements. World Journal of Microbiology and Biotechnology 1995; 11:438-448.

[35] Velasquez, V. L and Gepts, P. RFLP diversity of common bean (*Phaseolus vulgaris*) in its centres of origin. Genome 1994; 37(2): 256-63.

[36] Adam-Blondon, A.; Sevignac M.; Bannerot, H. and Dron, M. SCAR, RAPD and RFLP markers linked to ARE, a simple dominant gene conferring resistance to C. lindemuthianum, the causal agent of antracnose in french bean. Theoretical and Applied Genetics 1994; 88: 865-870

[37] Blair, M. W., Buendía, H. F., Giraldo, M. C.,Métais, I., Peltier, D. Characterization of AT-rich microsatellite markers for common bean (*Phaseolus vulgaris* L.) based on screening of non-enriched small insert genomic libraries. Genome 2008; 52: 772–782.

[38] Burle, M.L., Fonseca, J.R., Kami, J.A., Gepts, P. Microsatellite diversity and genetic structure among common bean (*Phaseolus vulgaris* L.) landraces in Brazil, a secondary center of diversity. Theoretical and Applied Genetics 2010 121: 801-813.

[39] Ferreira da Silva, G. dos Santos, J. B. and Ramalho, M. A. P. Identification of SSR and RAPD markers linked to a resistance allele for angular leaf spot in the common bean (*Phaseolus vulgaris*) line ESAL 550. *Genetics and Molecular Biol*ogy 2003; 26 (4): 459-463

[40] Young, R. and Kelly, J.D. RAPD Markers flanking the Are gene for anthracnose resistance in common bean. Journal of American Society of Horticultural Science 1996; 121: 37-41.

[41] Mahuku,G. Montoya, C., Henríquez, M.A. Jara, C. Teran, H. Beebe, S. Inheritance and characterization of angular leaf spot resistance gene presence in common bean accession G 10474 and identification of an AFLP marker linked to the resistance gene, Crop Sci. 44 (2004) 1817-1824.

[42] Kelly, J. D. Use of random-amplified polymorphic DNA markers in breeding for major resistance to plant pathogens. Horticulture Science 1995; 30:461- 465.

[43] Johnson, E., Miklas, P.N., Stavely, J. R and Martinez-Cruzado, J. C. Coupling- and repulsion-phase RAPDs for marker-assisted selection of the PI 181996 rust resistance in common bean. *Theoretical Applied Genetics* 1995; 90:659–664.

[44] Haley, S. D., Afanador, L. K and Kelly, J. D. Selection for monogenic resistance traits with coupling and repulsion-phase RAPD markers. Crop Science 1994; 34: *1061–1066*.

[45] Métais, I., Aubry, C., Hamon, B., Jalouzot, R. and Peltier, D. assessing common bean genetic diversity using RFLP, DAMD-PCR, ISSR, RAPD and AFLP markers. *Acta Horticturae* (ISHS) 2001; 546:459-461

[46] Miklas, P.N., D. Fourie, J. Wagner, R.C. Larsen, and C.M.S. Mienie. Tagging and mapping Pse-1 gene for resistance to halo blight in common bean host differential cultivar UI-3. Crop Science 2009; 49:41-48

[47] Joshi, B. K., Bimb, H .P., Parajuli, G., and Chaudhary , B. Molecular Tagging , Allele Mining and Marker Aided Breeding for Blast Resistance in Rice. BSN E-Bulletin 2009; 1: 1-23.

[48] Šustar-Vozlič, J., Maras, M., Javornik, B and Meglič, V. Genetic Diversity and Origin of Slovene Common Bean (*Phaseolus vulgaris* L.) Germplasm as Revealed by AFLP Markers and Phaseolin Analysis. American society of Horticultural Science 2006; 131(2): 242 – 249.

[49] Hernández-Delgado, S., Reyes-Valdés, M. H., Rosales-Serna, R and Mayek-Pérez, N. Molecular markers associated with resistance to *Macrophomina phaseolina* (Tassi) goid. in common bean. Journal of Plant Pathology 2009; 91 (1): 163 – 170

[50] Fourie, D. Herselman, L. and Mienie , C. Improvement of common bacterial blight resistance in South African dry bean cultivar teebus. African Crop Science Journal 2011; 19 (4): 377-386

[51] Ribaut, J. M. and Betran, J. Single large scale marker assisted selection (SLC-MAS). Molecular Breeding 1999; 531-541

[52] Yu, K., Park, S.J., Zhang, B., Haffner, M., & Poysa, V. An SSR marker in the nitrate reductase gene of common bean is tightly linked to a major gene conferring resistance to common bacterial blight. Euphytica, 2004; 138: 89–95.

[53] Ribaut, J. M and Hoisington, D. Marker assisted selection: New tools and strategies. Trends Plant Sciences 1998; 236-239.

[54] Xu, Y. B., McCouch, S. R. and Zhang, Q. F. How can we use genomics to improve cereals with rice as a reference Genome. Plant Molecular Biology 2005; 59:7–26

[55] Kasha, K. J. Biotechnology and world food supply. Genome 1999; 42: 642-645

[56] Mahuku, G.S., Jara, C., Cajiao, C. and Beebe, S. Sources of resistance to angular leaf spot (*Phaeoisariopsis griseola*) in common bean core collection, wild *Phaseolus vulgaris* and secondary gene pool. Euphytica 2003; 130:303-313.

[57] Santos-Filho HP, Ferraz S and Sediyama CS (1976) Isolamento e esporulac ˜ ¸ao ''in vitro'' de Isariopsis griseola Sacc. Experientiae 7: 175–193

[58] Beebe, S.E. and Pastor-Corrales, M.A. 1991. Breeding for disease resistance. In: van Schoonhoven, A. and Voysest, O. (Eds.). Common beans: Research for crop improvement. C.A.B. Intl., Wallingford, UK and CIAT, Cali, Colombia. 1991, 561-617pp.

[59] Ferreira, C. F., Borém, A., Caravalho, G. A., Neitsche, S., Paula, T. J. de Barros, E. G. Inheritance of angular leaf spot resistance in common bean and identification of a RAPD marker linked to a resistance gene, Crop Science 2000; 40: 1130-1133.

[60] Ragagnin, V., Sanglard, D., de Souza, T. L., Costa, M., Moreira, M. and Barros, E. A new inoculation procedure to evaluate angular leaf spot disease in bean plants (*Phaseolus vulgaris* L.) for breeding purposes. Bean Improvement Cooperative 2005; 48: 90-91.

[61] Nietsche, S., A. Borém, G. A. Carvalho, R. C. Rocha, T. J. Paula, E. G. de Barros, M. A. Moreira, RAPD and SCAR markers linked to a gene conferring resistance to angular leaf spot in common bean, Phytopathology 2000; 148: 117-121

[62] Ngulu, F. S. Final Report on Pathogenic Variation in *Phaeoisariopsis griseola* in Tanzania. Selian Agricultural Research Institute, Arusha, Tanzania.1999;13pp

[63] Mahuku, G. S., M.A. Henriquez, J. Munoz, R.A. Buruchara, Molecular markers dispute the existence of the Afro-Andean Group of the bean angular leaf spot pathogen, *Phaeoisariopsis griseola*, Phytopathology 2002; 92 580–589.

[64] CIAT. (2001). Solutions that cross-frontiers. [http://www.ciat.cgiar.org/beans] site visited on 27/04/2006

[65] Carvalho, G. A., T. J. Paular, A. L. Alzate-Marin, S. Nietsche, E. G. Barros, M. A. Moreira. Inheritance of line resistance AND277 of common bean plants of the race 63-23 of *Phaeoisariopsis griseola* and identification of RAPD markers linked to the resistant gene). Fitopatologia Brasia 1998; 23: 482-485.

[66] Miklas, P. N. List of DNA SCAR markers linked with disease resistance traits in bean. [http://www.usda.prosser.wsu.edu/miklas/Scartable3.pdf] site visited on 13/04/2012. (2005).

[67] Singh, S.P. and Munoz, C.G. Resistance to common bacterial blight among Phaseolus species and common bean improvement. Crop Science 1996; 39: 80–89.

[68] Queiroz V.T., C.S. Sousa, M.R. Costa, D.A. Sanglad, K.M.A. Arruda, T.L.P.O. Souza, V.A. Regagnin, E.G. Barros, M.A. Moreira. Development of SCAR markers linked to common bean anthracnose resistance genes *Co-4* and *Co-6*. Annual Report of the Bean Improvement Cooperative 2004; 47:249-250

[69] Miklas, P. N., Pastor-Corrales, M. A, Jung, G., Coyne, D. P., Kelly, J. D., McClean, P. E., and Gepts, P. Comprehensive linkage map of bean rust resistance genes. Bean Improvement Cooperative 2002; 45: 125-129.

[70] Pastor-Corrales M.A. Estandarización de variedades diferenciales y designación de razas de Colletotrichum lindemuthianum. Phytopathology 1991; 81:694

[71] Zapata, M., Beaver, J.S. and Porch, T.G. Dominant gene for common bean resistance to common bacterial blight caused by Xanthomonas axonopodis pv. phaseoli. Euphytica 2010; 179:373-382

[72] Hanounik, S.B., Jelly, G. J., Hussein, M. M. Screening for disease resistance in faba bean. In Breeding for stress tolerance in cool-season food legumes, K. B. Singh and M. C. Saxena (Eds). Chichister, John Wiley. 1993; 97-106 pp.

[73] Allen, D.J. and Lenne, J.M. Diseases as constraints to production of legumes in agriculture. In Pathology of Food and Pasture Legumes. Allen, D. J. and Lenne, J.M. (Eds.). CAB International, Wallingford, UK. 1998; p1-61.

[74] Arnaud-Santana, E., Coyne, D.P., Steadman, J.R., Eskridge, K.M. and Beaver, J.S. Heritabilities of seed transmission, leaf and pod reactions to common blight, leaf reaction to web blight and plant architecture and their associations in dry beans. Annual Report of the Bean Improvement Cooperative 1994; 37: 46-47.

[75] Zapata, M. Pathogen variability of *Xanthomonas campestris pv. phaseoli*. Annual Report of Bean Improvement cooperative 1996; 39:166 – 167.

[76] Crous PW, Slippers B, Wingfield MJ, Rheeder J, Marasas WFO. Phylogenetic lineages in the Botryosphaeriaceae. Studies in Mycology 2006; 55: 235–253

[77] Park, S.O., Coyne, D.P. and Jung, G. Gene estimation, associations of traits, and confirmation of QTL for common bacterial blight resistance in common bean. Annual Report of the Bean Improvement Cooperative 1998; 41:145-146.

[78] Zapata, M., G.F. Freytag and R.E. Wilkinson. Registration of five common bean germplasm lines resistant to common bacterial blight: W-BB-11, W-BB-20-1, W-BB-35, W-BB-52, and W-BB-11-56. Annual Report of the Bean Improvement Cooperative 2004; 47:333-337.

[79] Schuster, M.D., Coyne, D.P., Behre, T. and Leyna, H. Sources of *Phaseolus* species resistance and leaf and pod differential reactions to common blight. *Horticulture Science 1983;*18:901-903.

[80] Drijfhout, E. and Blok, M.J. Inheritance to *Xanthomonas axonopodis pv. phaseoli* in tepary bean (*Phaseolus acutifolius*). Euphytica 1987; 36: 803-808.

[81] Mohan, S.T. (1982). Evaluation of *Phaseolus coccineus* Lam. Germplasm for resistance to common bacterial blight of bean. Turrialba 1982; 32: 489–490.

[82] Miklas, P.N., R. Delorme, W.C. Johnson, and P. Gepts. 1999. Dry bean G122 contributes a major QTL for white mold resistance in the straw test. Annu. Rpt.Bean Improvement Coop. 42:43–44.

[83] Garcia-Espinosa, R. Breeding for horizontal resistance in bean: an example from Mexico. Biotechnology and Development Monitor 1997; 33:5

[84] Miklas, P.N., Smith, J.R., Riley, R., Grafton, K.F., Singh, S.P., Jung, G. and Coyne, D.P. Marker-assisted breeding for pyramided resistance to common bacterial blight in common bean. Annual Report of the Bean Improvement Cooperative 2000; 43: 39-40.

[85] Jung, G., Coyne, D.P., Scroch, P.W., Nienhuis, J., Arnaud-Santana, E., Bokosi, J., Ariyarathne, H.M., Steadman, Beaver, J.S. and Kaeppler, S.M. Molecular markers associated with plant architecture and resistance to common blight, web blight, and rust in common beans. Journal of the American Society for Horticultural Science 1996; 121:794-803.

[86] Bai, Y., Michaels, T.E., & Pauls, K.P. Identification of RAPD markers linked to common bacterial blight resistance genes in *Phaseolus vulgaris* L. Genome, 1997; 40: 544–551.

[87] Drijfhout, E. Genetic interaction between *Phaseolus vulgaris* and BCMV with implication for strain identification and breeding for resistance. Centre for Agricultural Publication and Documentation, Wageningen. 1978; 33 – 50pp.

[88] Naderpour, M., Søgaard Lund, O., Larsen, R. and Johansen, E. Potyviral resistance derived from cultivars of *Phaseolus vulgaris* carrying *bc-3* co-segregates with homozygotic presence of a mutated *eIF4E* allele. 2008

[89] Collimer, C. W., Marston, M. F., Taylor, J. C. and John, M. Dominant *I* gene of bean a dose dependent allele conferring extreme resistance, hypersensitive resistance, or

spreading vascular necrosis in response to Bean common mosaic virus. Molecular Plant-Microbe Interaction 2000; 13: 1266 - 1270.

[90] Vallejos, C. E., Malandro, J. J., Sheehy, K. and Zimmermann, M. J. Detection and cloning of expressed sequences linked to a target gene. Theoretical and Applied Genetics 2000; 101: 1109–1113.

[91] Kelly, J. D., Gepts, P., Miklas, P. N., and Coyne, D. P. Tagging and mapping of genes and QTL and molecular marker-assisted selection for traits of economic importance in bean and cowpea. Field Crops Research *2003;* 82: 135–154.

[92] Johnson, W.C., Guzman, P., Mandala, D., Mkandawire, A. B. C., Temple, C., Gilbertson, R. L. and Gepts, P. Molecular tagging of the bc-3 gene for introgression into Andean common bean. Crop Science 1997; 37:248–254

[93] Mukeshimana, G., Pa˜neda, A., Rodriguez, C., Ferreira, J. J. Giraldez, R. and Kelly, J. D. Markers linked to the bc-3 gene conditioning resistance to bean common mosaic potyviruses in common bean. Euphytica 2005; 144: 291–299

[94] Strausbaugh C.A., Overturt K., Koehn A.C. Pathogenicity and real-time PCR detection of Fusarium spp. in wheat and barley roots. Canadian Journal of Plant Pathology 2005; 27: 430–438.

[95] Kelly, J. D. A review of varietal response to bean common mosaic potyvirus in *Phaseolus vulgaris*. Plant Varieties and Seeds 1997; 10: 1- 6.

[96] Melotto, M., L. Afanador, and J.D. Kelly. Development of a SCAR marker linked to the I gene in common bean. Genome 1996; 39:1216-1219.

[97] Kelly, J.D., Hosfield, G. L., Varner, G. V., Uebersax, M. A. and J. Taylor, J. 1999. Registration of 'Matterhorn' great northern bean. Crop Science 1999; 39: 589–590.

[98] Miklas, P.N., Beaver, J.S., Steadman, J.R., Silbernagel, M.J.,Freytag, G.F., 1997. Registration of three bean common mosaic virus-resistant navy bean germplasms. Crop Science 1997; 37: 1025.

[99] Park, S.J. and Tu, J. C. Association between BCMV resistant *I* gene and eye color of cv. Steubean. Annual Report of the Bean Improvement Cooperative 1989; 29:4–5

[100] Gonçalves-Vidigal, M.C., P.S. Vidigal Filho, A.F. Medeiros, and M.A. Pastor-Corrales. 2009. Common bean landrace Jalo Listras Pretas is the source of a new Andean anthracnose resistance gene. Crop Science 2009; 49:133-138.

[101] Vidigal Filho, P.S., M.C. Gonçalves-Vidigal, J.D. Kelly, and W.W. Kirk. 2007. Sources of resistance to anthracnose in traditional common bean cultivars from Paraná, Brazil. J. Phytopathology 155:108-113.

[102] Bradley, C.A., and J.L. Luecke. 2004. 2002 dry bean grower survey of pest problems and pesticide use in Minnesota and North Dakota. Ext. Rep. 1265. North Dakota State Univ. Fargo.

[103] Vennette, J.R., and Lamey, H.A. Dry Edible Bean Diseases. NDSU Extension Service Publication 1998;576pp

[104] Bilgi, V.N., C.A.Bradley, S. Ali, S.D. Khot, and J.B. Rasmussen. 2007. Reaction of dry bean genotypes to root rot caused by Fusarium graminearum. Phytopathology 2007; 97:S10.

[105] Gambhir, A., R.S. Lamppa, J.B. Rasmussen, and R.S. Goswami. 2008. Fusarium and Rhizoctonia species associated with root rots of dry beans in North Dakota and Minnesota. Phytopathology 2008; 98:S57.

[106] Cramer, R.A., P.F. Byrne, M.A. Brick, L. Panella, E. Wickliffe, and H.F. Schwartz. 2003. Characterization of Fusarium oxysporum isolates from common bean and sugar beet using pathogenicity assays and random-amplified polymorphic DNA markers. J. Phytopathology 2003; 151:352-306.

[107] Cross, H., M.A. Brick, H.F. Schwartz, L.W. Panella, and P.F. Byrne. 2000. Inheritance of resistance to Fusarium wilt in two common bean races. Crop Science 2000; 40:954-958.

[108] Velasquez, V.R. and Schwartz, H. F. Resistance of two bean lines to wilt by Fusarium oxysporum f. sp. phaseoli under different soil temperatures. Agro-Ciencia 2000; 16:81-86

[109] Markell, S.M., M.A. Pastor-Corrales, J.G. Jordahl, R.S. Lampa, F.B. Mathew, J.M. Osorno, and R.S. Goswami. Virulence of Uromyces appendiculatus to the resistance gene Ur-3 identified in North Dakota in 2008. Annual Report of the Bean Improvement Cooperative 2009; 52: 82-83.

[110] Wright, E.M., Awale, H.E., M.A. Pastor-Corrales, and J. D. Kelly. Persistence of a new race of the common bean rust pathogen in Michigan. Annual Report of the Bean Improvement Cooperative 2009; 52: 84-85.

[111] Pastor-Corrales, M.A., A. Sartorato, M.M. Liebenberg, M.J. del Peloso, P.A. Arraes-Pereira, J. Nunes-Junior, and H. Dinis-Campo. 2007. Evaluation of common bean cultivars from the United States for their reaction to soybean rust under field conditions in Brazil and South Africa. Annual Report of the Bean Improvement Cooperative 2007; 50: 123-124.

[112] Mutlu, N., Vidaver, A. K., Coyne, D. P., Steadman, J. R., Lambrecht, P. A., and Reiser, J. 2008. Differential pathogenicity of Xanthomonas campestris pv. phaseoli and X. fuscans subsp. Fuscans strains on bean genotypes with common blight resistance. Plant Disease 2008; 92:546-554.

[113] Urrea, C.A., Steadman, J. R. Pastor-Corrales, M.A. Lindgren, D.T. and Venegas J.P. Registration of great northern common bean cultivar Coyne with enhanced disease resistance to Common bacterial blight and bean rust. Journal of Plant Registrations 2009; 3: 219-222

[114] Brick, M. A., Ogg, J.B., Singh, S.P., Schwartz, H.F., Johnson, J.J., and Pastor-Corrales, M.A. 2008. Registration of drought tolerant, rust resistant, high yielding pinto bean germplasm line CO46348. Journal of Plant Registration 2008; 2: 120-124

[115] Stavely, J.R. Pyramiding rust and viral resistance genes using traditional and marker techniques in ommon bean. Annual Report of the Bean Improvement Cooperative 2000; 43:1–4.

[116] Feleiro, F.G., Vinhadelli, W. S., Ragagnin, V.A., Stavely, J. R., Moreira, A. M. and Barros, E. G. Resistance of bean lines to four races of *Uromyces appenduculata* isolated in the state of Minas Gerais. Fitopatologia Brasileiara 2001; 26: 77-80

[117] Alzate-Marin AL, Menarim H, Carvalho GA, Paula Jr TJ, Barros EG, Moreira MA. Improved selection with newly identified RAPD markers linked to resistance gene to four pathotypes of *Colletotrichum lindemuthianum* in common bean. Phytopathology 1999; 89:281–285

[118] CIAT (Centro Internacional de Agricultura Tropical). Pathology in Africa. CIAT Annual Report 2005. CIAT Bean Programme, Cali, Colombi. 2005. Pp 232.

[119] MAFSC (Ministry of Agriculture, food security and cooperative). Tanzania Variety List Updated to 2008. 2008; 64p

[120] Sartorato, A. Resistance of Andean and Mesoamerican common bean genotypes to *Phaeoisariopsis griseola.* Annual Report of the Bean Improvement Cooperative 2005; 48:88-89.

[121] Kimani, P.M., Burachara, R., Muthamia, J., Mbikayi, N., Namayanja, A., Otsyula, R. and Blair, M. Selection of marketable bean lines with improved resistance to angular leaf spot, root rot and yield potential for smallholder farmers in eastern and central Africa. Paper presented at the 2nd General Meeting on Biotechnology, Breeding and Seed Systems, Nairobi, Kenya, 24–27 January 2005.

Section 2

Crop Breeding for Complex Phenotypes

Chapter 6

Breeding for Drought Resistance Using Whole Plant Architecture — Conventional and Molecular Approach

H.E. Shashidhar, Adnan Kanbar, Mahmoud Toorchi,
G.M. Raveendra, Pavan Kundur, H.S. Vimarsha,
Rakhi Soman, Naveen G. Kumar,
Berhanu Dagnaw Bekele and P. Bhavani

Additional information is available at the end of the chapter

http://dx.doi.org/10.5772/54983

1. Introduction

Drought, also referred to as low-moisture stress, is a form of abiotic stress. It is a challenge posed by the environment to the survival and productivity of a plant/crop that occupies a large area. This directly translates to economic loss to the farmer(s) who depend on the harvest. The plant has a wide range of genetic and phenological adaptations innate or triggered to cope with the stress. The extent of loss to productivity depends on the periodicity (over years), timing within the season when it occurs, rate of onset of the stress, severity, duration and a few other minor factors. At certain geographical locations, drought occurs at periodical intervals over years in a cycle. Should it occur, all the stages of the crop are likely to be affected. Vulnerability of crops to drought is likely to be intensified due to climate change [1].

When challenged by drought, a plant struggles to survive. If it succeeds to survive, it tries to complete the life cycle, which in annual crops means production of grains. When challenged by stress the phenology of the plant is severely altered. Altered phenology is often reflected as advancing flowering and maturity or by delaying flowering so that the critical stages of the crop do not get severely affected. Either way, it tries to circumvent the stressful period. This is a form of drought escape. The pattern of response will depend on the time of onset, intensity and nature of stress. Alternatively, it triggers a series of biological processes that helps the plant take the challenge 'head on' and complete the lifecycle with high grain yields. It is this pattern of responses that are a subject matter of systematic plant breeding endeavor. Collectively the latter strategy is referred to as drought resistance and scientists seek to study, understand and use it to enable farmers to get as good a harvest as possible.

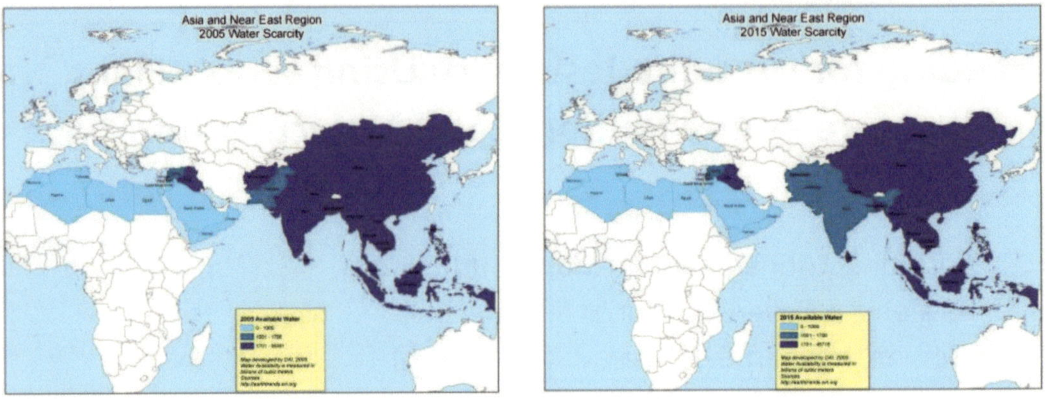

Daek blue – countries with plentiful water (>1,700 m^3/person/day)
Medium blue – countries with water stress (<1,700 m^3/person/day)
Light blue countries with water scarcity (<1,000 m^3/person/day)

Figure 1. Water scarcity map of the most vulnerable parts of the world. Left 2005, Right 2015. Borrowed from "Blue revolution initiative Strategic framework for Asia and the Near East, Bureau for Asia and the Near East, USAID, May 2006. P 37 [2]"

Breeding for drought tolerance in any given crop, has immense value to the farmers as their livelihood depends on the harvest(s). It bears a positive effect on the farmers' economic health, family well-being and harmony in the society. It affects poor farmers more than the rich ones. Complete or partial loss of harvest in drought years is known to trigger panic reaction, migration and decrease or extinction of flora and fauna of the particular habitat. There have been scores of farmer suicides due to losses caused by drought and associated problems in different States of India [3, 4]. A link between drought and suicides has been established in Australia [5], Africa, and in the South America. Thus as a trait, drought resistance has immense value to the individual farmer and the society. According to [6] the "future imperative is clear —Asia cannot continue to depend on the quantity and quality of freshwater for rice cultivation in the traditional manner".

2. What is drought resistance?

The ability of a plant to maintain favorable water balance in its tissues (turgidity/turgor) when exposed to drought stress is a manifestation of drought resistance. Turgidity refers to the condition of the leaf when it is wide open and fully facing the sky. When a leaf loses turgor it rolls (in crops like rice) wilts (in crops like legumes) and ultimately dries up. Loss of turgor is an indication that the transpiration demand is more than the water being supplied from the soil through the plant. Sometimes, the loss of turgor can be a temporary phase during high temperatures prevalent during midday.

Maintenance of turgor under low-moisture conditions is crucial. It implies continued transpiration. This requires the stomata to be open thus facilitating gas exchange, a prerequisite for photosynthesis. The transpiration pull thus generated provides the suction force (one of the requirements) for water uptake by roots. This also keeps the leaf cool and prevents drying and subsequent dying. Thus, a favorable water balance under drought condition is a key to a plant's survival and productivity.

While continued transpiration has many advantages to the plant/crop survival, the final and economically useful manifestation of drought resistance is the magnitude of grain yield that is obtained at the end of the season, when the crop has been challenged by drought. Maintenance of turgor, transpiration, biomass or greenness is of little use to the farmer who wishes grain yield. While maintenance of turgor and survival under stress are of academic interest, grain yield is of practical value. Thus, ultimately, in grain crops the grain yield is the manifestation of drought resistance. Even under non-stress conditions, it is the grain yield (or the economic product in non-grain crops) that is a measure of a plants' performance [7]. Any trait that contributes to this would be a useful selection criteria in a breeding program.

The pattern of responses that a plant choses to trigger has been collectively referred to as drought resistance. Further classifications of responses fall into three categories namely, drought escape, dehydration avoidance and dehydration tolerance [8]. Dehydration avoidance is a reaction when the plant maintains a high level of water status or turgor under conditions of increasing soil-moisture deficit. Finally, drought resistance is referred to as a plants' ability to sustain the least injury to life functions at decreasing levels of tissue water status or turgor. Drought escape refers to the ability of the plant to complete its lifecycle before the onset of drought or adjust its phenology so that the crucial developmental stages escape the adverse impacts of drought [9]. Delayed flowering, is one such phenological adjustment.

Broadly, plants adopt two strategies, which involve reducing their water expenditure called "water savers" or "pessimistic plants" or accelerating water uptake sufficiently so as to replenish the lost water called as "water spenders" or "optimistic plants". A plant can maintain turgor by adopting one or both of the following strategies depending on genotype and environmental factors.

1. The mechanism of conserving water: includes stomatal mechanism, increased photosynthetic efficiency, low rate of cuticular transpiration, reduced leaf area, effect of awns, stomatal frequency and location.

2. Improving the water uptake: the mechanisms are efficient root system, high root to shoot ratio (R/S), difference in the osmotic potential of the plants and conservation of water.

The drought resistant variety or hybrid that is developed is also expected to possess the ability to contend with excess moisture. Many times low-moisture and excess moisture can also cause stress to the crop within the particular season. The variety or hybrid must also possess certain degree of resistance to common diseases or pests that are prevalent in the area that is targeted.

3. What characters are associated with drought resistance?

All parts of the plant are affected by drought stress. Conversely, all parts of the plant can potentially contribute to augment/enhance stress resistance. Among the plant species that inhabit the earth a wide range of traits enable plants to either tolerate excess water (submergence) or very low-water (drought). Each species has a wide range of characters accumulated during the course of evolution to adapt to the habitat. Crops have evolved over centuries in a particular habitat and have, over time, adapted to the adverse conditions. All the crops occupying a habitat share the same/similar set of adaptive traits as per the law of homologous series of variation [10]. For example, in rice there are accessions, which tolerate short span to long periods of submergence. They outgrow the water level and produce panicles above (like lotus flowers) or kneel down when water recedes, all the time keeping panicles facing upwards. On the other hand, there are accessions of rice, which tolerate prolonged periods of drought. Referred to as upland rice, these accessions grow like other arable crops with no need for standing water, ever. In the middle of this wide range are genotypes, which grow under submerged soils (irrigated rice).

Extensive studies of gross morphology and hard pan penetration ability of roots among traditional and improved accessions of rice had brought out the fact that the most deep-rooted accessions were traditional accessions and improved varieties had relatively shallow roots. The traditional accessions had greater hard pan penetration ability compared to improved accessions [11]. Most likely, this was due to the natural selection over decades/centuries or crop improvement efforts in well-endowed habitats. Most traditional accessions manifested low grain yield, but had high degree of tolerance to drought [12] but improved varieties were susceptible to drought, shallow rooted and were high yielders. Based on the germplasm study, it almost appeared that the drought resistance and grain yield were under such a genetic control that bringing them together was impossible. This would have been the case if the two sets of traits were pleiotropic. Extensive QTL mapping studies for root traits and grain yield in the same mapping population in similar habitats contradicted this [13].

Considerable amount of investment has been made by the scientific community in studies associated with drought resistance. Several crops have been studied. A wide range of traits is found to be associated with drought resistance (Table 1). Ironically, the only trait that the farmer is interested in is that which fetches him/her an income from what constitutes a marketable produce [6]. Thus, finally, for practical breeding purposes, manifestation of drought resistance can be summarized as increase in the economic product(s). In food crops, it would be the grain, in fruit crops it would be fruit and in vegetable crops it would be the edible part, whatever it is root, leaves or stem. Thus, yield is one single trait that could be considered as a manifestation of drought resistance. As yield is a result of a well-grown plant, biomass could be the cause or a prerequisite to high yield. Further, good biomass is a result of adequate quantity of water and nutrients made available at appropriate growth of the plant. This implies a well-endowed root system. As a breeding objective, the plant traits that could be selected among segregants are robust and efficient root systems, well-endowed shoot system and finally grain yield. This means selection for the entire plant characters and not only for shoots that are easy to see, measure and select. Every part of the plant, above-ground or below-ground should be subjected to selection pressure.

Traits associated with drought tolerance	
Morphological & Anatomical:	Grain Yield; Maximum Root length, Root Volume, Root Dry Weight, Root Thickness; Root surface area, above-ground Biomass; Harvest index; Leaf drying; Leaf tip firing; Delay in flowering. Aerenchyma, Leaf Pubescence.
Phenological:	Earliness; Delay in Flowering; Anthesis-Silking Interval; Seedling vigor; Weed competitiveness; Photosensitivity; perennially.
Physiological & Biochemical	Osmotic Adjustment; Carbon Isotope Discrimination; Stomatal conductance; Remobilization of stem reserves; Specific leaf weight; ABA; Electrolyte leakage; leaf rolling, tip firing, Stay-green; Epicuticular wax; Feed forward response to stress
Oxygen scavenging;	Heat shock proteins; Cell Wall proteins; Leaf water potential; Water use efficiency; Aquaporins; Nitrogen use efficiency; Dehydrins;

Table 1. Development of drought tolerant quality rice varieties

All the traits fit well in the well-known formulae given below

Grain Yield – Transpiration x Water Use Efficiency

Finally, for a trait(s) to be of use, it should be correlated with or causally related to yield, easy to select for and should not be a drain on the energy reserves of the plant. For a breeder to use such a trait there should be ample genetic variability for the trait in the germplasm accessions. The heritability of the trait must be greater than heritability of the grain yield per se.

4. Genetic elements associated with drought resistance

Drought resistance is a complex trait/phenomenon [14]. Some people think that it is not an individual trait and refers to the response of a plant/crop to an environmental condition. Purported complexity of the trait deterred many scientists to work on the trait in several crops. Most of the investment in the green revolution era was focused on favorable habitats. The research investment in terms of time, effort and funds on unfavorable habitats was significantly less compared to the favorable ones and this was due to the high rate of returns on the investment (in the private sector). One of the favorite arguments extolling the difficulty in breeding for drought resistance was that the genetic basis of the trait was not discerned and that it was controlled by many traits. In fact literature is replete with many reasons to almost dissuading a not so determined breeder/researcher.

As an avocation, breeding for any trait can be done irrespective of the complexity of the trait. Neither is it necessary to fully understand the trait's inheritance. Crop improvement can be accomplished in spite of this. The argument is amply exemplified by the rapid strides and break-through accomplished in the 1. Semi-dwarfism, 2. Heterosis 3. Development of synthetic varieties of *Triticum aestivum*,L. and 4. Continuous improvements in grain yield and quality parameters across crops over years Table 2. In all cases listed above, one common issue is that the genetic basis is still not 'clear'. While concerted efforts are underway in several crops to discern the mode of action, number of genes governing the trait, the promoters, QTLs, etc., plant breeders have gone ahead and improved each one of the traits.

No.	Trait	Crop
1	Grain yield	Rice, Wheat, Finger millet, Bajra
2	Heterosis	Maize, Sorghum, Cotton, Tomato,
3	Semi-dwarfism	Wheat and Rice
4	Synthetics (reconstituted allo-hexaploid genome)	Synthetic wheat
5	Genome diplodization	Triticale, Synthetic wheat

Table 2. Traits for which genetics has not been discerned but have been subject of continued improvement over decades.

5. Breeding for drought resistance — Selection environment

Breeding for drought must be conducted with adequate concern for the selection environment. Adequate care and appropriate consideration must be given to the genotype X environmental interaction during selection of parents and segregants at each filial generation. Ideally, the selection environment(s) must adequately represent the target environment(s) for which the variety/hybrid is being developed. Usually the target environment is highly variable in edaphic, climatic and hydrological status. Every cubic centimeter of soil is different from the other. Aboveground also, the plant faces differences in climatic condition during the day/night, across the season and over year(s). Thus, every cubic centimeter aboveground and below-ground is likely to be different and the plant has to adapt to this. If the habitat covers a large geographic area, so as to explain the variability that exists, it is usually referred to as a 'population of habitats'.

Any significant deviation between the selection environment (where the parents and the segregants chosen are evaluated/advanced) and the target population of habitats would make the final selected variety/hybrid inadequately adapted contributing to failure of the crop improvement program. An alternative to having the selection environment geographically isolated or distant from the target environment is to perform selection in the target environment itself. The farmers of the target habitat(s) could be involved in the selection process. Such a breeding program, conducted on the farmers' fields (target environments) involving target farmers is referred to as 'participatory plant breeding'.

Unjustifiably it is perceived that breeding for drought resistance is difficult because

a. It is a complex trait,

b. There are too many secondary traits associated with it and heritabilities are low,

c. There is inadequate knowledge about the inheritance mechanism involved,

d. Predicting the magnitude of drought that might occur, if at all it occurs, is difficult and

e. No single trait manifests direct correlation with grain yield under stress.

This argument is invalid because breeders, over years, have been improving traits and crop plants without adequate knowledge about the genetics of the trait they are breeding for. Four classic examples are given in Table 2. Thus, complexity of a trait or lack of information on the inheritance mechanism of a trait has not bothered breeders much. The innovative selection strategies applied in a well understood environment has yielded results year after year in crop after crop. Thus, while breeding for drought resistance too, not having 'complete' knowledge of inheritance of traits, will not be a deterrent.

With reference to the inability to predict the occurrence of drought and the stage at which it would occur within the cropping duration, it is prudent to build drought resistance to a genotype irrespective of the crops' developmental stage. A plant should be able to face the challenge, posed by low-moisture regime, whenever, should it occur [13].

Genetic variability for traits is harnessed by the breeders in a breeding program. There is ample variation for all traits in the germplasm accessions within a given species and across species that are amenable for use. Selection strategies need to be designed to be able to select for traits especially if it involves destructive sampling (example, root traits). Studying roots in segregating populations is not as easy as studying shoot traits and grain yield. A plant has to be uprooted to expose roots for analysis. This would kill the plant if it is not already mature. The root traits are ideally studied at peak vegetative stage. At maturity there would be decline in the root traits. Thus innovative selection strategies need to be adapted depending on the mode of propagation, reproduction etc. Traits associated with drought resistance valuated under the stress-full environment manifest lower heritability values making selection an unattractive proposition. This is because of the high G x E interactions. This is manifested by 'crossover interactions' typical of improved and traditional accessions when evaluated in the same study [15, 16]. Any effort to improve the Environment (E) in the experimental site might contribute to improve heritability (H) values. But increase the risk of misrepresenting the target population of environment. Crossover effects are not universal and it is possible to break the trend and select for high productivity under stress and relatively high yields under non-stress habitats too [14, 17].

Two examples where selection for root traits was seamlessly incorporated into the breeding program are discussed below in detail.

6. Breeding for drought resistance — Marker-assisted selection

Marker-assisted selection is expected to boost the pace of crop improvement especially for complex traits. This was the feeling of molecular biologists who want about discovering DNA markers in large numbers. Overtime, the markers have evolved. There is always a search for ideal markers which can be used by breeders. Characteristics of ideal markers are as follows

1. Tightly linked to gene that controls the trait either individually (monogenic trait) or in groups (polygenic trait)

2. Co-dominant in inheritance. It will help identify heterozygotes and homozygotes with ease. Dominant markers are also useful but they identify only one of the homozygous allelic combination

3. PCR based so that it can be analyzed faster. It would be better if the amplified bands could be resolved on agarose gels or data acquired as quickly as possible.

4. The marker should account for a large proportion of the genetic variability for the trait of interest.

5. The marker must be able to identify all other allelic forms associated with the trait.

The first QTL tagging work, for root traits was done by IRRI, Philippines in 1995 [18]. Ever since a very large number of QTLs have been discovered for every component trait expected to contribute to drought in several crops. Each one of them, proposed that the QTLs discovered would help MAS for drought. A large number of QTLs associated with traits related to drought have been tagged to different kinds of molecular markers [13, 19]

So far, the only documented success stress with MAS for root traits has been the work of [20] in rice. In this paper too, out of the five loci selected for MAS, only one locus of chromosome 9 had a significant and positive effect on root traits. Phenotyping done among the transgressants aided in the selection process.

A novel upland rice variety, BirsaVikasDhan 111 (PY 84), has recently been released in the Indian state of Jharkhand. It was bred using marker-assisted backcrossing with selection for multiple quantitative trait loci (QTL) for improved root growth to improve its performance under drought conditions. It is an early maturing, drought tolerant and high yielding variety with good grain quality suitable for the direct seeded uplands and transplanted medium lands of Eastern India. PY84 is the first example of a rice variety bred through the combined use of marker-assisted selection and client-oriented breeding, and a rare success story for the use of marker-assisted selection to improve a quantitative trait. It out-yields the recurrent parent by 10% under rain fed conditions. The variety was developed in a collaborative partnership between CAZS-NR; GraminVikas Trust, Ranchi, Jharkhand, India and Birsa Agricultural University (BAU), Ranchi, Jharkhand, India. The target QTL was first identified by Adam Price (Aberdeen University, UK) and Brigitte Courtois (CIRAD, France/IRRI, Philippines) [20].

In this marker assisted backcrossing program (MABC) was used. The strategy was to pyramid different QTLs situated on different chromosomes. All these QTLs were related to root traits.

http://dx.doi.org/10.5772/54983

An Indian *indica* rice variety was used as the recurrent parent. The donor for deep-rooting and grain aroma was Azucena, a *japonica* from Philippines. Five segments on different chromosomes were targeted for introgression; four segments carried QTLs for improved root morphological traits (root length and thickness) and the fifth carried a recessive QTL for aroma. Twenty-two near-isogenic lines (NILs) were evaluated for root traits in five field experiments in Bangalore, India by Dr. H.E. Shashidhar. The target segment on chromosome 9 (RM242-RM201) significantly increased root length under both irrigated and drought stress treatments, confirming that this root length QTL from Azucena functions in a novel genetic background. No significant effects on root length were found at the other four targets. Azucena alleles at the locus RM248 (below the target root QTL on chromosome 7) delayed flowering. Selection for the recurrent parent allele at this locus produced early-flowering NILs that were suited for upland environments in eastern India (Figure 2).

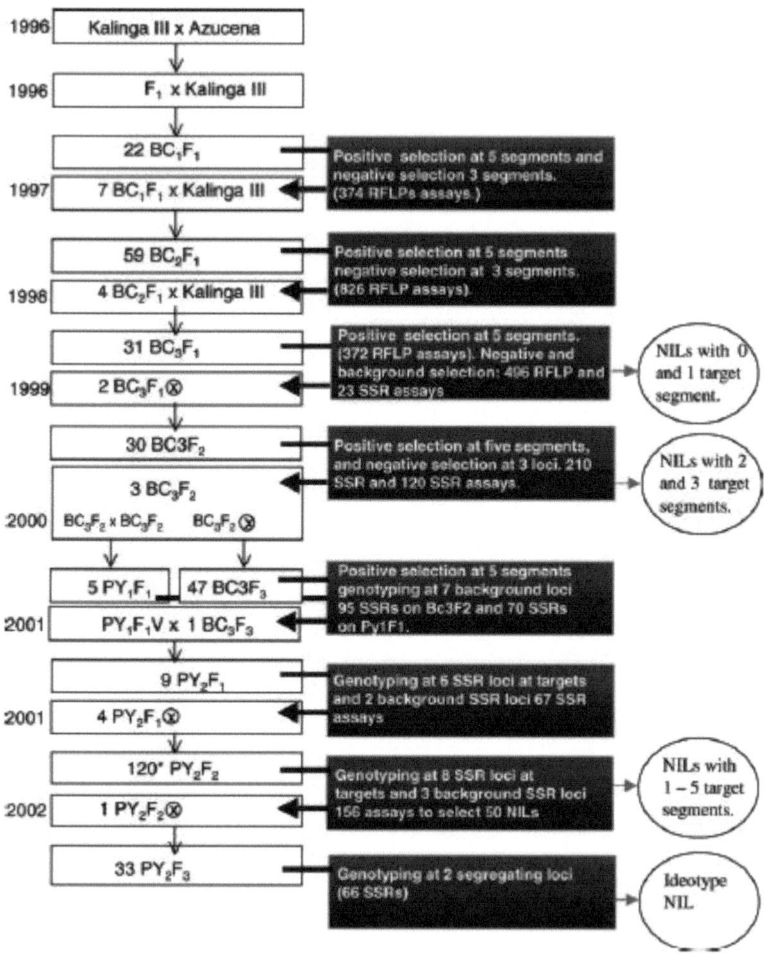

Figure 2. A flow chart for MAS for drought resistance.

7. Breeding for drought resistance — Conventional approach

Selection in the target habitat has been the standard way of breeding for drought resistance across crops. Over the past decade several OPVs and Hybrids have been developed with the active participation of the national programs across the target countries (Table. 3). Grain yield and other shoot traits has been the focus in most of their projects. This is a typical case of plant breeding. Selection for a plant's performance would have been better understood and most effective selection would have resulted probably by using root characters in the parental selection and breeding program.

In rice, an innovative strategy was adapted to breed for drought resistance. The donor for characteristic deep root was a local variety Budda. The donor for grain yield was IR-64. The generations were advanced by raising the families derived from F3 onwards in farmers' fields and involving farmers in the selection process. Each of the F3 families was divided into two parts with one being directly sown and maintained under well-watered conditions, while the other one was maintained under drought stress. Water was provided to each one (WW and LMS) by precise measurements. While WW set received 80 % of the water lost due to evaporation, the other one (Stress) received 60 % of water evaporated (Evaporation was measured by in installing and maintaining a pan-evaporimeter in the field). Data was recorded on grain yield and biomass at harvest. Selection at each generation was based only on biomass. High biomass types under both conditions were forwarded to next generation. In the next generation, one tiller from each plant was grown in PVC pipes to study root traits (Figure 3). All subsequent generations were forwarded in three places. Two in field (WW and drought) and one in PVC tubes. The selection was based on all three traits: Good Roots + Shoots + Grain yield [21].

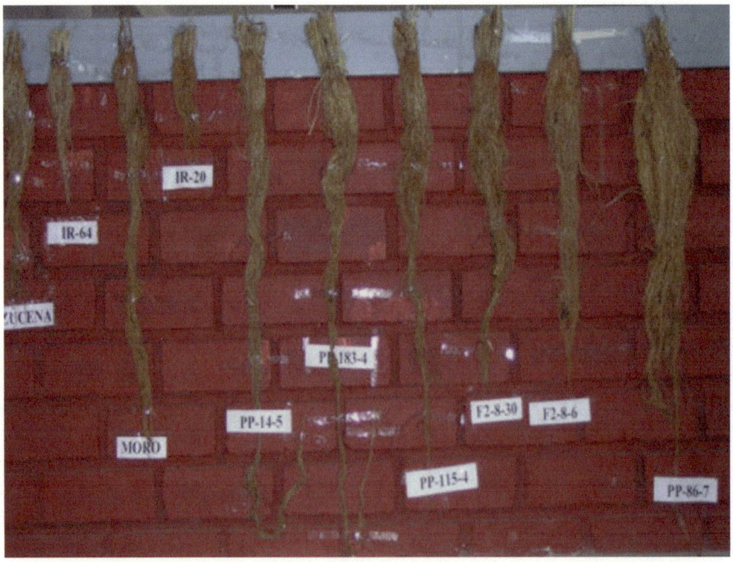

Figure 3. Manifestation of transgressive segregation for root traits in rice.

Several varieties have been developed in different countries adopting conventional plant breeding principles (Table 3). Some of these have been accomplished using markers and some without.

No.	Variety	Trait + Selection Strategy	Crop	Developing Institute, Country
1	Ashoka 228 (BVD 109)	MAS+ PPB, Root+Shoot+Yield	Rice	GrameneVikas Trust, BAU, Jharkhand, India
2	Ashoka 220 (BVD 110)	MAS + PPB, Root+Shoot+Yield	Rice	GrameneVikas Trust, BAU, Jharkhand, India
3	PY 84	MAS + PPB, Root+Shoot+Yield	Rice	GrameneVikas Trust, BAU, Jharkhand, India and UAS, Bangalore
4	ARB6	Conventional Pedigree PPB + Root + Shoot + grain yield	Rice	UAS, Bangalore, India
5	MAS946-1	Conventional breeding Pedigree	Rice	UAS, Bangalore, India
	MAS26	Conventional breeding Pedigree	Rice	UAS, Bangalore, India
6	Poornima	Conventional breeding Pedigree	Rice	IGKV, Raipur, India
7	Danteshwari	Conventional breeding Pedigree	Rice	IGKV, Raipur, India
8	Indira BharaniDhan 1	Conventional breeding & selection for roots	Rice	IGKV, Raipur, India
9	Kamaleshwari	Conventional breeding Pedigree	Rice	IGKV, Raipur, India
10	Han Dao 502	Conventional Pedigree	Rice	China Agril. University, India
11	Han Dao 297	Conventional Pedigree	Rice	China Agril. University, India
12	Jin Dao 305	Conventional Pedigree	Rice	China Agril. University, India
13	ZM 309, 401, 423, 523, 623, 625, and 721	Conventional	Maize	South Saharan Africa
14	KDV1, 4, and 6	Conventional	Maize	South Saharan Africa
15	WS103	Conventional	Maize	South Saharan Africa
16	Melkassa 4	Conventional	Maize	South Saharan Africa
17	WH 403, 502 and 504, ZMS402 and 737	Conventional	Maize	South Saharan Africa
18	Rd 12, and 33	Conventional	Rice	Thailand
19	Hanyou 2 and 3 (Hybrids)	Conventional and MAS	Rice	Zhejiang Yuhul Agro-technology Company Zhejiang

MAS= Marker-assisted selection, PPB= Participatory plant breeding, ARB = Aerobic rice Bangalore

Table 3. Drought resistant lines/ list of varieties developed

In conclusion, breeding for drought resistance can do only as much as develop a genotype that can tolerate to moisture stress and respond to incremental water inputs should that be possible in the given habitat. The final answer to maximizing productivity comes from an integrated approach where genotype, agronomy, management, economics and policy come together to maximize the water productivity, the key limiting natural resource. Water is not equitably distributed in the world and the scarcity of water is assuming ominous dimensions (Figure 3).

8. Time tested tips for breeding for drought across crops

A deluge of information and knowledge has been generated over time. Considerable investment has been made by the international community and funding agencies. The collective intelligence can be summarized as under.

1. Screen parents and segregants in a habit that most closely represent/ resemble the target population of habitats.

2. Repeat phenotyping over years and seasons so that maximum possible variations in the environmental conditions are represented.

3. Impose selection starting from early generation (not F2) in well-watered and stress conditions. This will ensure selection for potential productivity (should stress not occur in the farmers' fields) and still maximize productivity under stress (should it occur). This will ensure that the farmer is likely to harness the full potential of every incremental drop of water above the threshold called drought.

4. Quantify the water that is received by the field during the experimental period. Input of water could come in the form of rainfall or surface irrigation. It would be ideal to also document the evapotranspiration from the field. This will help budget water at the level of each genotype/segregant/plot. With such data, water productivity could be computed for each segregant, genotype.

5. While stability of the drought variety is highly desirable, local adaptability is also very important. A genotype may manifest low stability and may be use-full for the particular habitat.

6. High yield under favorable conditions (moisture regimes) can be combined with the high degree of drought resistance. Thus, traits associated with drought need not be a penalty to the plant under well-watered condition.

7. Selection for root and shoot morphology can be judiciously combined in ongoing breeding program while selecting for resistance to diseases and pests.

8. Instead of incorporating growth stage specific drought resistance (vegetative stage drought resistance, reproductive stage drought resistance etc.) it is more appropriate to make any and every growth stage of the crop drought resistant as the timing of occurrence of drought, if at all in the farmers' field is unpredictable. It would be counterproductive

if stage specific drought resistance is built into a variety and should drought occur at some other stage. Breeding effort would be futile.

9. Need to select for combination of stresses that challenge the crop in the farmers' field rather than only drought resistance. This will ensure longer survival of the variety in the farmers' field [22].

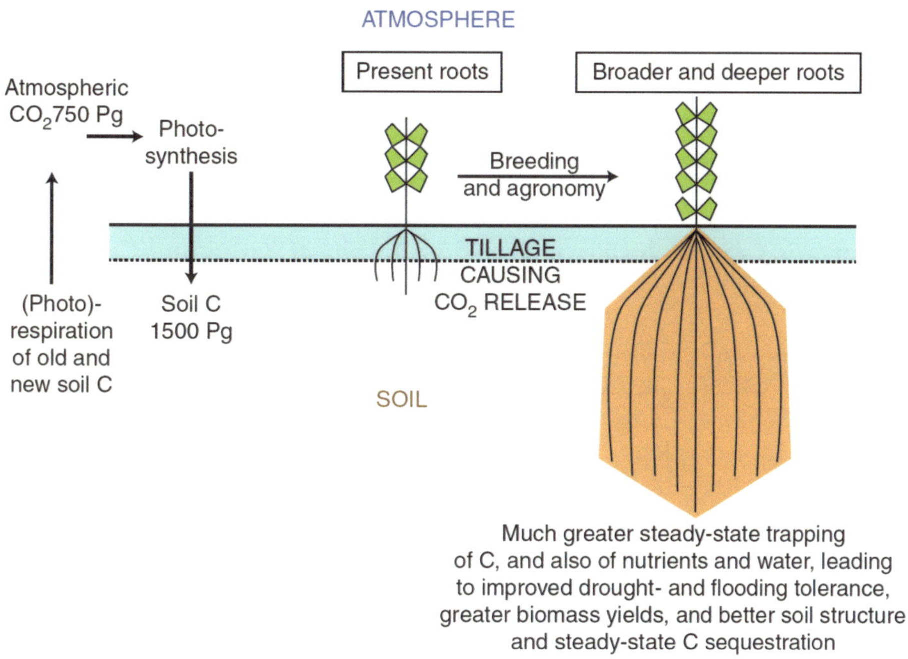

Figure 4. Borrowed from Kell DB, Annals of Botany, pp 1-12.[23]

This calls for ushering a blue revolution [2, 23], the water equivalent of green revolution, where it is envisaged that the water productivity in agriculture is addressed along with equity of water distribution between urban aspirations and rural needs. Finally [24] proposes that roots do much more than supply water to plants, they capture carbon and a well-endowed root system is not only important to the plant but also as a means to mitigate climate change, by trapping carbon in the form of increased microbial activity and dry matter accumulations. Thus, roots not only provide anchor, water, nutrients but also contribute to carbon sequestration and one of the means to mitigate global warming.

Finally, using all shoot and root characters of the plant, be it morphological, physiological, biochemical, phenological, anatomical or responses to environment would provide more opportunities for enhancing drought resistance of the crop. The characters of the plant have to be matched with the appropriate agronomic practices to maximize the expression of the traits. This is a holistic approach to plant breeding for drought resistance and also referred to as 'whole-plant breeding'.

Author details

H.E. Shashidhar[1*], Adnan Kanbar[2], Mahmoud Toorchi[3], G.M. Raveendra[4], Pavan Kundur[4], H.S. Vimarsha[4], Rakhi Soman[4], Naveen G. Kumar[4], Berhanu Dagnaw Bekele[1] and P. Bhavani[4]

*Address all correspondence to: heshashidhar@gmail.com

1 (Genetics and Plant Breeding), Department of Biotechnology, College of Agriculture, UAS, GKVK, Bangalore, India

2 Department of Field Crops, Faculty of Agriculture, University of Damascus, Damascus, Syria

3 Department of Crop Production and Breeding, Faculty of Agriculture, University of Tabriz, Tabriz, Iran

4 Senior Research Fellow, Department of Biotechnology, College of Agriculture, University of Agricultural Sciences, GKVK, Bangalore, India

Department of Biotechnology, University of Gondar, Gondar, Ethiopia

References

[1] Vörösmarty C. J. P, Green J. Salisbury and Lammers. R. B. 2000 Global water resources: Vulnerability from climate change and population growth. Science (289); 284-288.

[2] Blue revolution initiative Strategic framework for Asia and the Near East, Bureau for Asia and the Near East, USAID, May 2006. P 37.

[3] Report of the Fact finding team on Vidharbha, Regional disparities and rural distress in Maharastra with particular reference to Vidharbha, Government of India, Planning Commission. 1 – 244.

[4] Every thirty minutes Farmer suicides, human rights, and the agrarian crisis in India, Center for Human Rights and Global Justice, New York University School of Law1-53,

[5] Suicides and drought in New South Wales in Australia 1970 - 2007, Hanigan IC, Butler CD, Kokic P N, Hutchinson M F, PNAS, August 13, 2012

[6] John C.O'Toole Rice and Water: The final frontier. Paper presented on the occasion of H R H Princess Maha Chakra Sirindhorn's Presentation of the Golden Sickle Award

to Dr. John C. O'Toole for his contribution to the advancement of rice research over the past 30 years. September 1, 2004. Bangkok.

[7] George A, Principles of genetics and plant breeding, Breeding for physiological and morphological traits Chapter 19, 352 -366.

[8] Levitte J, 1972, Response of plants to environmental stresses. Academic press, New York.697 p.

[9] May L. H and Milthrope F. L, 1962, Drought resistance in crop plants Field Crops Abstr. 15: 171-179.

[10] Vavilov, N. The origin, variation immunity and breeding of cultivated plants 1951.ChronicaBotanica 13: 1-366.

[11] ChadraBabu R, Shashidhar H. E, Lilley J. M, Thanh, N. D, Ray J. D, Sadasivam S, Sarkarung, S, Toole J. C, Nguyen H. T. Variation in root penetration ability, osmotic adjustment and dehydration tolerance among accessions of rice adapted to rainfed lowland and upland ecosystems. Plant breeding 120, 233-238.

[12] Shashidhar HE 1990. Studies on drought tolerance in rice. Ph.D Thesis University of Agricultural Sciences, Bangalore

[13] Venuprasad *R*, Shashidhar HE, Hittalmani S, Hemamalini G. S. 2002. Tagging quantitative trait loci associated with *grain yield and root* morphological traits in rice (*Oryza sativa* L.) under contrasting moisture regimes. *Euphytica* 128:293-300

[14] Ceccarelli, S Grando S, Baum M. 2007. Participatory plant breeding in water-limited environments.Expl.Agric 43, 411-435.

[15] Blum, A. 1993. Selection for sustained production in water-deficit environments.*Internat. CropSci.* I. Madison, Wisconsin: Crop Sci. Soc.Am. Pp.343–347.

[16] BidingerF. R., Seeraj, R, Rizvi, S. M. H., Howarth, C, Yadav R. S., Hach C T. 2005 Fiend evaluation ofdrought tolerance QTL effects on phenotype and adaptation in pearl millet (L) R. Br. Top cross hybrids 94 14-32.

[17] Verulkar,. P. Mandal, J. L. Dwivedi, B. N. Singh, P.K. Sinha, R. N. Mahato, P. Dongre, P. N. Singh, L. K. Bose, P. Swain, S. Robin, S. Robin, R. Chandrababu, S. Senthil, A. Jain, H E Shashidhar, S, Hittalmani, C. Vera, Cruz, T. Paris, A, Raman , S. Haefele. R. Serraj, G.Atlin, A, Kumar, 2010 Breeding resilient and productive genotypes adapted to drought prone rainfed ecosystem of India. *Field Crops Research (missing volume and page numbers)*

[18] Champoux M, Wang G, Sarkarung S, Mackill DJ, Toole JC, Huang N, McCouch S, 1996 Locating genes associated with root morphology and drought avoidance in rice via linkage to molecular markers TheorAppl Genet 90: 969-981.

[19] Hemamalini G. S, Shashidar H. E, Hittalmani S. 2000. Molecular marker assisted tagging of morphological and physiological traits under two contrasting moisture regimes at peak vegetative stage in rice (*Oryza sativa* L.) Euphytica (112); 69–78

[20] Steele K. A, A H Price, Shashidhar H. E, Witcombe, J. R. 2006 Marker-assisted selection to introgress QTLs controlling root traits into an Indian upland rice variety, Theor Appl. Genet (2006) 112: 208-221

[21] Gowda V. R, Henry A, Vadez V, Shashidhar H. E and Seeraj R 2012, Water uptake dynamics under progressive drought stress in diverse accession of the OryzaSNP panel of rice (*Oryza sativa* L.) Functional Plant Biology, (PAGE NUMBER)(Missing volume and page numbers)

[22] Banziger M Setimal P. S, Hodson D, Vivek B, Breeding for improved drought tolerance in maize adapted to southern Africa, "New Dimensions for a diverse planet" Proceedings of the International Crop Science Congress. 26th Sept to 1st October 2004.

[23] Kell D. B, Breeding crop plants with deep roots: their role in sustained carbon, nutrient and water sequestration, Annals of Botany 1 – 12, 2011.

[24] Elzabeth P, Plant Genetics; The Blue revolution, drop by drop, gene by gene. News Focus Science 230, 171-173.

Chapter 7

Breeding to Improve Symbiotic Effectiveness of Legumes

Vladimir A. Zhukov, Oksana Y. Shtark,
Alexey Y. Borisov and Igor A. Tikhonovich

Additional information is available at the end of the chapter

http://dx.doi.org/10.5772/53003

1. Introduction

Symbioses with beneficial microorganisms constitute the universal and ecologically highly effective strategy of adaptation of plants towards nearly all types of environmental challenges. Representatives of many groups of fungi and bacteria participate in plant-microbial symbioses (PMS) wherein they can colonize the plant surfaces, tissues or intra-cellular compartments using two basic adaptive strategies: nutritional and defensive. Construction of niches for hosting the symbiotic microbes involves the complicated developmental programs implemented under the joint control by plant and microbial partners and based on the cross-regulation of their genes.

Legume plants (family Fabaceae) are known to form symbioses with extremely broad range of beneficial soil microorganisms (BSM), representing examples of almost all plant-microbe mutualistic systems. Different groups of beneficial microbes improve host mineral nutrition, acquisition of water, promote the plant development and offer protection from pathogens and pests. For ecology and agriculture, the most important beneficial legume symbioses are arbuscular mycorrhiza (AM) and root nodule (RN) symbiosis. These symbioses demonstrate high level of genetic and metabolic integrity, compared with other interactions of legumes with plant growth-promoting rhizosphere bacteria (PGPR) and/or beneficial endophytic bacteria.

High integrity of AM and RN symbioses implies highly specific mutual recognition of partners, formation of special complex symbiotic compartments and integration of partners' metabolic pathways. In the symbioses, legume plant plays a role of the organizing center of the system as it performs functions of coordination and regulation of all developmental processes. During last decade, a significant progress has been achieved in revealing the genetic bases of symbioses formation and functioning, so the knowledge of the plant genetic control over symbioses can effectively facilitate breeding new varieties of legumes that are needed for modern sustainable agriculture. In this chapter, we describe the present state of the developmental genetics of legume symbioses and depict the potential to organize the multi-component symbioses to be used for optimizing the broad spectrum of plant adaptive functions and to improve the sustainability of legume crop production.

2. Mechanisms of positive effect of BSM on the environment and health and yield of the legume plant

2.1. Legume-rhizobia Root-Nodule (RN) symbiosis

Leguminous plants are able to grow in the soil/substrate without any combined nitrogen due to the fixation of atmospheric nitrogen by symbiotic nodule bacteria (collectively called rhizobia). In collaboration with rhizobia, legumes make a large contribution to the global nitrogen balance in natural and agricultural ecosystems [1]. Nitrogen fixation occurs within special plant organs, root nodules (in some associations stem nodules are also formed). Development of these organs represents a well-organized process based on the tightly coordinated expression of specialized symbiotic plant and bacterial genes. The legume nodules provide an ecological niche for bacteria, as well as structure for metabolic/signal exchange between the partners and for the control of symbionts by the hosts [2].

Family Fabaceae contains 17000-19000 species divided between three sub-families (Caesalpinioideae, Mimosoideae and Papilionoideae) and more than 700 genera of world-wide distribution [3]. With a single exception (*Parasponia*: Ulmaceae), the ability for symbioses with rhizobia is restricted to Fabaceae, although in eight related dicotyledonous families (Rosid I clade) an ability to form nodules with the nitrogen-fixing actinomycete *Frankia* is known [4].

By contrast to legumes, their nitrogen-fixing microsymbionts do not constitute a taxonomically coherent group of organisms. The majority of rhizobia belong to the α-proteobacteria assigned into the Rhizobiaceae family solely on the basis of their ability to nodulate the legumes (e.g. *Azorhizobium, Bradyrhizobium, Mesorhizobium, Rhizobium, Sinorhizobium*). Recently some β-proteobacteria (close to *Burkholderia, Cupriavidus, Pseudomonas* and *Ralstonia*) and even some γ-proteobacteria have been discovered that can form nitrogen-fixing nodules with the legumes [5]. All these bacteria vary enormously in their overall genome organization, location of "symbiotic" (*sym*) genes and their molecular organization and regulation [6, 7].

Root-nodule symbiosis is well known as highly specific plant-microbe interaction. According to the early surveys of symbiotic specificity [8], legumes were suggested to comprise a range of taxonomically restricted cross-inoculation groups within which the free cross inoculation occurs, while the species from different groups do not cross-inoculate. The best studied examples of this classification are represented by four cross-inoculation groups: "*Trifolium – Rhizobium leguminosarum* bv. *trifolii*", "*Pisum, Vicia, Lathyrus, Lens –*

R. leguminosarum bv. *viciae*", "*Galega – R. galegae*", "*Medicago, Melilotus, Trigonella – Sinorhizobium meliloti, S. medicae*". However, it was demonstrated later [9, 10] that such strictly defined specificity is limited to the herbage papilionoid legumes growing in temperate zones and representing the "Galegoid complex".

The specificity of legume-rhizobia interactions is expressed just during the pre-infection stage when rhizobia recognize the roots of appropriate host plants and colonize their surfaces. The interaction starts when the root-excreted signals, in particular, flavonoids, activate the rhizobial nodulation genes (*nod/nol/noe*) [11]. These genes control the synthesis of lipochitooligosaccharidic (LCO) nodulation factors (Nod factors, NFs) which induce the early stages of RN symbiosis development [12-14]. NFs represent the unique group of bacterial signal molecules not known outside legume-rhizobia symbiosis. They are among the most potent developmental regulators: their effect is expressed at concentrations of $10^{-8} – 10^{-12}$ M only. The core structure of these molecules, common for all rhizobia species, consists of 3-6 residues of N-acetylglucosamine and of a fatty acid (acyl) chain. The type of symbiotic specificity is dependent mainly on the chemical modifications in NF structures [11]. However, a sufficient role in the host specificity of RN symbiosis may also be implemented by the interactions between bacterial surface molecules (some polysaccharides and proteins) [15, 16] and the lectins located on the root hair surfaces [17].

The main enzyme of nitrogen fixation in nodules is a nitrogenase that has a complex structure [18, 19]. Synthesis of nitrogenase (the enzyme catalysing reduction of N_2 into NH_4^+) and other proteins involved in nitrogen fixation is induced in bacterial cells after they differentiate into a specific form called bacteroids. Bacteroids are embedded into a membrane structure named symbiosome, which formation as well as bacteroid differentiation is induced by plant [20]. These symbiosomes are organelle-like units of plant cell responsible for nitrogen fixation [21, 22]. Peri-bacteroid membrane (PBM) that surrounds bacteroids is an active interface of RN symbiosis where exchange of metabolites between symbionts occurs [23].

A pronounced differentiation is typical for rhizobia-infected plant cells, such as an increase in internal membrane structures participating in the PBM formation and biosynthetic processes. Polyploidization and chromatin decondensation are typical for these cells correlating with an elevated transcription activity [24]. Biochemically plant cell differentiation is expressed as a *de novo* synthesis of many proteins including leghaemoglobin and nodule-specific isozymes of carbon and nitrogen metabolism [25]. Leghaemoglobin binds oxygen actively ensuring its transport towards symbiosomes (which are characterised by the intensive respiration necessary to support energy consuming nitrogen fixation) and microaerobic conditions inside the nodules (required for the nitrogenase activity). The carbon and nitrogen metabolic enzymes responsible for the energy supply to nitrogenase and for the assimilation of fixed nitrogen are nodule specific [26]. Organic nitrogenous compounds formed from N_2 fixation are transported to the upper parts of the plant either as amides (mainly asparagine (Asn), but also glutamine (Gln)) or as ureides (allantoin and allantoate), so that legumes can be classified as amide or ureide exporters according to the compounds they use for the mobilization of fixed nitrogen [27].

Rhizobial cells also undergo differentiation, but its level varies in different legume species. The terminal bacteroid differentiation (when bacteroids increase their size and DNA content and lack the capacity to divide) is specific for legumes belonging to the inverted repeat–lacking clade (IRLC) such as *Medicago, Pisum,* or *Trifolium,* whereas bacteroids in the non-IRLC legumes, such as *Lotus,* show no sign of terminal differentiation as they maintain their normal bacterial size, genome content, and reproductive capacity [28]. The same rhizobia strains that form symbiosis with both IRLC and non-IRLC legumes have different bacteroid differentiation fates in the two legume types. It was demonstrated that in *Medicago* and probably in other IRLC legumes, the nodule-specific NCR peptides act as symbiotic plant effectors to direct the bacteroids into a terminally differentiated state [29]. Possibly, IRLC legumes use nodule-specific NCR peptides to dominate the endosymbionts: NCR peptides interfere with many aspects of the bacteroid metabolism to allow the efficiency of the nitrogen fixation process to be optimized, for example, by stimulation enlargement and polyploidization of bacteroids [30]. Also, the peptides could be part of a mechanism to avoid the "cheating" of rhizobia that could use host resources to accumulate carbon storage compounds instead of fixing nitrogen [29], which is often observed in the non-IRLC legumes but not in the IRLC [30].

It was also found that nodules where terminal bacteroid differentiation takes place are more efficient in terms of energy use. Oono and Denison [31] reported that legume species with terminal bacteroid differentiation (such as peas (*Pisum sativum* L.) and peanuts (*Arachis hypogaea* L.) invest less in nodule construction but have greater fixation efficiency when compared to species with reversible bacteroid differentiation (such as beans (*Phaseolus vulgaris* L.) and cow peas (*Vigna unguiculata* (L.) Walp.). This effect is probably due to genomic endoreduplication of the bacteroids and full contact of single undivided bacteroid with peribacteroid membrane (some reproductive bacteroids can lose contact with PBM after they divide). Still, this is not known if these useful features of terminal bacteroids differentiation in some legumes could be transferred into other legume species. In work of van de Velde et al. [29], expression of NCR genes in nodules of *Lotus japonicus* (Regel.) K. Larsen (with normally reversible bacteroid differentiation) was sufficient to induce bacteroid morphologies reminiscent of terminally differentiated bacteroids of *Medicago truncatula* Gaertn. But, no positive effect on nitrogen fixation efficiency was reported, probably because there are much more regulatory genes needed to make bacteroids work propertly in such a heterologous system.

2.2. Arbuscular Mycorrhiza (AM)

Arbuscular mycorrhiza (AM) is formed by at least 80% of contemporary terrestrial plants with fungi of phylum Glomeromycota. The Glomeromycota are unique as the only monophyletic mycorrhizal fungus lineage that has co-evolved with land plants throughout their history. They are obligate biotrophs that colonize plant roots obtaining photosynthates, such as carbohydrates (hexoses), and niches for both their growth and reproduction. The AM is evolved more than 400 million years ago and was considered to play a decisive role in plants achieving a terrestrial existence [32-34]. The AM is supposed to be "the mother of plant root endosymbioses" [35]. Since legumes originated long after AM, about 60 million years ago [36], it may be assumed that all of them have the potential to produce this type of symbioses. *Lupinus* is the only known genus where this ability had apparently been lost [37-39].

Specificity of AM symbiosis is relatively low [34]. Symbiosis establishment starts with molecular dialogue between the partners. Plant roots release sesquiterpenes (also known as inducers of parasitic plant seed germination) as well as different phenolic compounds, including flavonoids, which induce fungal hypha growth and branching [40, 41]. Similar to rhizobia, AM-fungi produce signal molecules termed Myc factors (mycorrhization factors) [42], which can be recognized by the plant. They are a mixture of several lipochitooligosaccarides, the structure of which is close to that of rhizobial Nod factors, but is presumably more universal for different plant-fungus combinations [43]. Both sesquiterpenes and Myc factors are released constitutively and in the absence of physical contact with symbiotic partner [44].

The AM-fungi penetrate the root to colonize inner cortical cells. Plant plays an active role in fungus hosting inside the root tissues using cellular mechanisms similar to those used during rhizobial invasion, such as nucleus reposition, cytoplasm aggregation, special cytoskeletal tunnel assembly and symbiotic membrane formation (reviewed in: [45]). A special intracellular compartment of AM providing tight metabolic exchange between the partners is arbuscule, which is highly branched fungal hypha surrounded by membrane of plant origin [34] similar to symbiosome of RN symbiosis [35, 46].

Inner-root and outer parts of mycelium remain bound with arbuscules and are a single continuum *via* which the fungus is able to translocate mineral nutrient and water from the soil into the root system [47]. Thus, well developed AM-symbiosis allows plant growing well in nutrient-poor and drought-affected soils, increases its resistance against pathogens and pests and heavy metals, and improves soil structure (see below).

Phosphorous (P) is one of the mineral nutrients essential for the plant growth (constituting up to 0.2% of the dry weight of the plant cell) and development. It plays the diverse regulatory, structural, and energy transfer roles and consequently is required in significant amounts [48, 49]. The plants can acquire soluble forms of phosphorous directly from soil through the plant specific phosphate transporters (PTs). The dominant available forms in soil (orthophosphate ions, P_i) are very poorly mobile because of the abundance of cations such as Ca^{2+}, Fe^{3+} and Al^{3+} [50]. In such environments where inorganic phosphorous is the predominant form in soil, a range of root adaptations, most of them primarily involved in mobilization and assimilation of phosphorous, are described including plant dependence on arbuscular mycorrhizas (see for review: [34, 51]). In most cases there is a preferential uptake *via* fungal hyphae (the mycorrhizal uptake pathway) [52]. Studies employing radioactive tracers to track hyphal P_i uptake from soil have shown considerable AM contributions to phosphorous uptake [53-55]. The process involves several fungal transport systems some of which have an extremely high affinity for P_i [56].

After transporting into hyphae, the major part of P_i is polymerized by polyphosphate kinase into polyphosphates (poly-P), the linear chains of P_i. The granules rich in poly-P together with phosphorous-containing esters are packed into the cylindrical vacuoles which are transported along the hyphae by tubulin fibrils. After reaching the arbuscules, phosphorous compounds are destroyed by phosphatases and the released P_i cross the partners' interface [56-58]. The arbuscule is the site of phosphate transfer from fungus to plant. It is well documented that plants possess many classes of phosphate transport proteins, including those which are expressed only in AM symbiosis [59-61]. It was discovered that five plant and one fungal PT genes are consistently expressed inside the arbusculated cells [60]. A plant phosphate transporter MtPt4 was shown to be expressed specifically on the peri-arbuscular membrane in *Medicago truncatula* [62].

The mycorrhizal P_i uptake pathway is controlled by the plant host. Many results suggest that the plant phosphorous status is a major regulator controlling induction/repression of plant PT genes at both the soil-root interface and the inner-root symbiotic interface [63-65]. It was shown that high phosphorous concentrations counteract the induction of the mycorrhizal P_i transporter genes by phospholipid extracts from mycorrhizal roots containing the mycorrhiza signal lysophosphatidylcholine [65]. The efflux of P_i probably occurs in coordination with its uptake and the fungus, on its side, might exert the control over the amount of P_i delivered to the plant [66].

Although P_i acquisition receives more attention, the important advances in investigations on nitrogen uptake by AM-fungi have been made in recent years. AM-fungi directly uptake ammonium (NH_4^+), nitrate and amino acids [67] with preference to NH_4^+ [68]. The first step in the nitrogen uptake requires the activity of specific transporters located at the interface between the soil and extraradical mycelium. A fungal transporter gene (*GintAMT1*) involved in the process and having high affinity with NH_4^+ was characterized [68].

Inorganic nitrogen that was taken up by the extraradical mycelium should then be incorporated into the amino acids and translocated to the intraradical mycelium, mainly as arginine (Arg) since this is the predominant free amino acid in the external hyphae [69]. The glutamine synthetase/glutamate synthase (GS/GOGAT) cycle is possibly responsible for a subsequent NH_4^+ assimilation in AM extraradical hyphae [70, 71], although the involvement of glutamate dehydrogenase has not been experimentally excluded. Arg similar to Poly-P is stored and is translocated along hyphae in vacuoles and is later released to the plant apoplast [66].

A mycorrhizal-specific NH_4^+ transporter *LjAMT2;2* has been revealed recently in transcriptomic analysis of *Lotus japonicus* roots upon colonization with *Gigaspora margarita*. The gene has been characterized as a high-affinity AMT belonging to the AMT2 subfamily. It is strongly up-regulated and exclusively expressed in the mycorrhizal roots, but not in the nodules, and transcripts have preferentially been located in the arbusculated cells [72].

The plants colonized by AM-fungi have been demonstrated to manifest an increased resistance to attack of some pathogenic microorganisms, such as fungi, nematodes, bacteria, phytoplasma, and plant viruses (reviewed in: [73]) as well as to plant feeding insects [74, 75]. However, it is still unknown whether such increased resistance to pathogens is a consequence of improved plant overall fitness or it is due to the specific defense responses induced by AM-fungi.

Actually, a range of processes occurring as a result of pathogen invasion (plant defense responses) also takes place in mycorrhized root tissues. They include the signal perception, signal transduction and defense-related gene activation [76-80]. The elements of hypersensitive responses have been observed to take place at both compatible and non-compatible combinations of plants with AM-fungi; reactions similar to the "oxidative burst" are typical for AM during fungus penetration into the epidermal cell [81]. In AM, as in other compatible biotrophic interactions, the defense-like response appears to be weak and occurs transitorily during the early phases of colonization, suggesting that the suppression of plant defense responses by the fungal signals may contribute to successful, compatible AM fungal colonization [76, 82]. AM-fungi are known to alter both constitutive and induced defenses in foliar tissues [83-85].

Drought stress is a major agricultural constraint in the semi-arid tropics. In most cases symbiosis with AM-fungi has been shown to increase host plant growth rates during drought stress and plant resistance to drought. Several mechanisms explaining this phenomenon have been proposed: an influence of AM on plant hormone profiles, increasing intensity of gaseous exchange and photosynthesis in leaves, direct water transport via fungal hyphae from soil into the host plant, enhanced water uptake through improved hydraulic conductivity and increasing leaf conductance and photosynthetic activity, nitrate assimilation by fungal hyphae, enhanced activity of plant enzymes involved in defence against oxidative stress, plant osmosis regulation, and changes in cell-wall elasticity (reviewed in: [86-89]).

The AM fungal hyphae grow into the soil matrix and create conditions conducive to the formation of microaggregates and then their packing into macroaggregates due to production copious amounts of the glycoprotein glomalin [90, 91]. Through AM-fungi-mediated effects on soil structure, it seems logical to suggest that AM colonization of a soil might affect its moisture retention properties and, in turn, the behaviour of plants growing in the soil, particularly when it is relatively dry [88].

AM-fungi were found to play an important role in heavy metal detoxification and the establishment of vegetation in strongly polluted areas (see for review: [92]). Fungal strains isolated from old zinc wastes also decrease heavy metal uptake by plants growing on metal rich substrates, limiting the risk of increasing the levels of these elements in the food chain [93]. Phytoremediation of metal contaminated areas attracts the increasing interest as a cheaper alternative to chemical methods, more friendly for environment and nondestructive to soil biota. The effectiveness of the bioremediation techniques depends on the appropriate selection of both the plant and the fungal partners. Plants conventionally introduced in contaminated areas disappear relatively soon, while those appearing during natural succession are better adapted to harsh conditions. Much more stable are plants that appear on the wastes spontaneously, but, it takes a long time till they establish and form stable communities. Symbiotic partners selected on the basis of such research are often the best choice for future phytoremediation technologies [93-96]. Introduction of plants from xerothermic grasslands into the soils contaminated with industrial metal rich wastes is supposed to be a new solution for waste revegetation [97]. Further improvements can be obtained by optimization of diverse microbiota including various groups of rhizospheric bacteria and shoot endophytes [92].

2.3. Associations of roots with Plant Growth-Promoting Rhizobacteria (PGPR)

Plant Growth Promoting Rhizobacteria (PGPR) are the taxonomically diverse group including different bacteria (*Arthrobacter, Azospirillum, Bacillus, Enterobacter, Pseudomonas, Paenibacillus,*

Streptomyces) and even some archaea [98]. The PGPR are inhabitants of soil in the vicinity of plant roots and are dependent on consuming root exudates. Many PGPR are able to attach to root surfaces and to AM and other fungal hyphae. The PGPR provide several benefits affecting the host plant either directly (due to mineral nutrient improvement and stimulation of root development) or indirectly (due to defence of plants from soil-borne pathogens and improving host tolerance to abiotic stresses).

Similar to rhizobia, *Azospirillum* possess nitrogenase and therefore is able to fix atmospheric nitrogen. In the early papers, plant growth promoting activity was attributed mainly to associative nitrogen fixation. A broad distribution of cereal-*Azospirillum* associations was identified (reviewed in: [99]). It was demonstrated later, however, that a partial role in these plant–PGPR associations was due to phytohormone auxin (indole-3-acetic acid, IAA) synthesis [100] which improves the root growth and assimilatory capabilities and hence aids nitrogen uptake by plants. In spite of absence of the visible anatomic differentiation in root-*Azospirillum* associations, its development involves a range of molecular interactions some of which may be common to endosymbiotic associations with rhizobia. Moreover, there is a visible taxonomic relatedness between *Azospirillum* and *Bradyrhizobium* genera. Thus, azospirilla and those slow-growing rhizobia might originate from a common *Azospirillum*-like ancestor (see for review: [101, 102]).

Many PGPR are able to solubilize sparingly soluble phosphates, usually by releasing chelating organic acids. Phosphate solubilizing bacteria (PSB) have been identified, but their effectiveness in the soil-plant system is unclear. The ability of an inoculated PSB to supply phosphopous to plant may be limited, either because the compounds released by PSB to solubilize phosphate are rapidly degraded or because the solubilized phosphate is re-fixed before it reaches the root surface [103].

The best studied examples of bacteria providing efficient defense from phytopathogens are: *Pseudomonas* (*P. fluorescens, P. chlororaphis, P. putida*), *Bacillus* (*B. cereus, B. subtilis*) and some *Serratia* (e.g., *S. marcescens*) species. Many of these bacteria are capable of preventing attacks by pathogenic fungi, nematodes and bacteria [98, 104, 105]. Diverse mechanisms may be involved in host protection offered by PGPR.

The best studied mechanism is the competitive exclusion of pathogens often related to their direct suppression by the bacterial antibiotic substances: phenazine-1-carboxamide, 2,4-diacetylphloroglucinol, kanosamine, oligomycin A, oomycin A, pyoluterin, pyrrolnitrin, xanthobaccin, zwittermycin A, volatile dyes (HCN) and cyclic lipopeptides [98, 104, 105].

An important mechanism for the suppression of pathogens by biocontrol microbes may result from competition for iron or other metals, that involves bacterial siderophores which may possess much greater affinities for ferric ions than those for fungal siderophores [104, 105]. The value of siderophores in biocontrol effects under natural conditions is predominantly associated with their ability to induce forms of systemic resistance in plant [98, 106].

Competitive exclusion of pathogens by PGPR is best achieved when the bacteria exhibit high root-colonizing activity. Application of the technique of genetic labeling with Green Fluorescent Protein (GFP) suggested that these bacteria do not regularly colonize the root interiors, and only rarely they can be observed inside the outer root tissues [98]. Most PGPR cells are concentrated on the root surface where the micro-colonies [98, 104] or bio-films are formed [107]. Since the interactions of plants with root-associated bacteria are not specific, the bacteria will colonize the roots of a broad spectrum of hosts. Specificity of the defensive association may be expressed however, at the point when antimicrobial compounds are being synthesized and this does not always correlate with bacteria taxonomy; many strains of *Bacillus* and *Pseudomonas* which possess plant-protective properties have close relatives amongst phyto-pathogenic types [106, 108, 109].

Microscopic observations demonstrated that suppression of fungi may be correlated with bacterial attachment to pathogen hyphae. As a result of this attachment, some PGPR strains commence their biocontrol functions by behaving as hyper-parasites of pathogenic fungi. This suppression may be related to the production of bacterial enzymes which destroy the pathogen cell walls [104, 105, 110, 111].

Sometimes the biocontrol activities of PGPR do not correlate with intensive colonization of host roots and plant protection results from only a small number of bacteria cells. This occurs when PGPR inoculation induces the systemic resistance mechanisms that make the root non-accessible by pathogens. Initially this effect of PGPR was called ISR (Induced Systemic Resistance) and was attributed exclusively to nonpathogenic systems [112]; SAR (Systemic Acquired Resistance) reactions, by contrast, were considered to be typical for the interactions with plant pathogens. Nevertheless, it was later found that the reactions of both types occur in either pathogen or nonpathogen systems and are distinguished by the nature of their endogenous elicitors (reviewed in: [106, 113]). The conventional SAR reaction is characterized by an accumulation of salicylic acid as signal molecules and pathogenesis-related proteins (PR-proteins), whereas ISR reaction is based on signal transduction pathways regulated by jasmonates and ethylene. The systemic defence responses of both types may be elicited exogenously by PGPR cells attached to the roots or penetrating their outer tissues. Some molecules produced by PGPR (cell wall and cyclic lipopolysaccharides, flagella components, exoenzymes, phytohormones, type III secretion system (TTSS) effectors, siderophores, salicylic acid, and toxins) may be perceived by the plant and elicit a defensive response [106].

It has been reported that PGPR which produce an enzyme which is involved in the catabolism of 1-aminocyclopropane-1-carboxylate (ACC) – the ACC deaminase, can lower ethylene concentration in a developing or stressed plant, protecting it against the deleterious effects of ethylene induced stress and facilitating the formation of longer roots [114, 115]. This demonstrates that ethylene is negative regulator of plant interaction with PGPR.

Despite relatively low specificity of plant associations with PGPR, plant genotype has been shown to influence their effectiveness (i.e. genetic integration exists between the partners), and a series of genome loci (QTL) was identified controlling its quantitative variation [106, 116, 117]. The most pronounced plant species-specificity has been observed in the manifestation of ISR reactions caused by PGPR [118, 119].

Both highly effective direct promotion of plant growth and biocontrol may be due to an ability of the host to regulate PGPR functions by modulating the composition of root exudates. Root-excreted organic acids, but not sugars, are optimal for support of different types of PGPR [120-122]. Additionally, some plants (including the legumes, pea and alfalfa) regulate their PGPR functions by exudating specialised signals from the roots which mimic the bacterial "quorum sensing" regulators required for root colonization and antifungal activities [123]. These observations suggest that improvement of biocontrol functions in root-PGPR associations may be achieved *via* manipulations with the bacterial and plant host genotypes.

2.4. Mutually beneficial associations of plants with endophytic bacteria

Healthy naturally propagated plants grown in the field or in pot cultures are colonized by populations of endophytic bacteria. The spectrum of endophytic bacteria isolated from the roots of various plants covers a wide range of species; representatives of the genera *Pseudomonas, Bacillus* or *Streptomyces* are most frequently encountered as endophytes (reviewed in: [124]). Newly developed molecular methods enable complete analyses of the diversity of culturable and non-culturable bacteria [125]. Most of the known genera include some phytopathogenic endophytes. Endophytes and pathogens both possess many similar virulence factors (reviewed in: [124]).

Some endophytes are seed-borne, but others have mechanisms for colonizing plants that have yet to be elucidated [126]. Although there are occasional poorly substantiated reports of intracellular colonization of bacteria providing a consistent and effective increase in the productivity of crops, it is still considered that the intercellular apoplastic space is the most suitable niche for endophytes [127]. It is suggested that many bacterial 'endophytes' may not colonize the living tissues, but occupy protective niches in dead surface tissues or closely adhering soil of rhizosheaths. Consistent entry of endophytes into living root tissues in the field is supposed to require a bacterial capability to hydrolyse the hydrophobic incrustations of the walls of epidermal, hypodermal, endodermal, and other cortical cells [128].

Plant associations with endophytic bacteria can increase plant growth and promote general development or improve plant resistance to pathogens and other environmental stresses enhancing the host's ability to acquire nutrients, or by production of plant growth-regulating, allelopathic or antibiotic compounds [127, 129]. Sometimes improved plant resistance can be linked to induced systemic resistance caused by bacterial elicitors coming from the endophyte [130].

It is necessary to study the natural associations between bacterial endophytes and their hosts for the purposes of employing such systems most productively in sustainable agriculture [127]. Delivery of endophytes to the environment or agricultural fields should be carefully evaluated to avoid introducing plant, animal and human pathogens [131].

2.5. Synergistic effect of microbes in rhizosphere

Microorganisms in the rhizosphere are under the influence of root exudates and plant as a whole as well as of interspecies interactions with each other. Many fungi including AM-fungi can interact with different bacterial species which frequently attach to fungal mycelium (reviewed in: [103, 132, 133]). For those bacteria known to stimulate mycelial growth of mycorrhizal fungi and/or enhance root mycorrhization the term 'mycorrhiza-helper-bacteria' has been proposed [133, 134]. Particularly, the bacteria may encourage growth of AM-fungi at the perisymbiotic stage of development, which precedes the establishment of a direct contact of the microsymbiont with the plant root [103, 135]. On the other hand, AM-fungi directly modify the environment due to mycelial exudation [136], forming the so-called 'mycorrhizo-sphere' [137]. In addition, the stimulation of root exudation as a result of interactions with AM-fungi leads to qualitative and quantitative changes of the bacterial community in the rhizosphere (reviewed in: [103, 132]).

Synergistic effect between RN and AM symbioses of legumes was described by many authors [95, 138-142]. AM formation is known to promote nodule development and nitrogen fixation by rhizobia, in particular, by means of improvement of mineral (predominantly phosphorous) host plant nutrition (see for review: [103]). AM-fungi also manifest synergism during interactions with PGPR (both indigenous and introduced), which perform biocontrol, nitrogen fixation, and phosphate mobilization during double and complex inoculation [103, 132]. The synergetic effect of plant inoculation by rhizobia and PGPR (*Azospirillum*, *Bacillus*, and *Pseudomonas*) is well known. In particular, it is associated with PGPR production of indole-3-acetic acid, which encourages nodule formation [103, 143]. Triple inoculation of a model legume *Anthyllis cytisoides* with PGPR, AM-fungi and rhizobia was shown to be the most effective approach for revegetation in mediterranean semi-arid ecosystems [94].

Thus, the potential of microbial synergism allows us to speak about high prospects of biotechnologies focused on creation multicomponent symbioses (MCS) that increase the fertility and quality of agricultural legume and nonlegume crops. At the same time, the results of experiments with plant symbioses with AM-fungi, rhizobia and PGPR, including multimicrobial systems, show the important role of physiological and genetic adaptation of microorganisms to local environmental conditions [92, 94, 95, 144]. Hence, during the development of such biotechnologies, it is recommended to use a complex of local microbial isolates adapted to particular environmental conditions.

3. Plant genetic control over development and functioning of mutualistic symbioses of legumes

3.1. Legume genes involved in development of RN and AM symbioses

The complex developmental processes which lead to the formation of intercellular and sub-cellular symbiotic compartments in RN and AM symbioses are controlled by both macro- and microsymbiont. Genetic systems of the symbionts are highly integrated, because some genes and gene products of one partner can switch certain genetic programs in another partner, still the development and function of the symbioses is reliant to the greatest extent on the plant. Developmental genetics of RNS is now well described because both plants and nodule bacteria can be subjected to genetic analysis during nitrogen-fixing nodule formation and functioning. There has been less investigation of AM systems. Mainly this is due to the difficulties encountered in culturing AM-fungi, caused by their obligate symbiotic lifestyle and impossibility of using selective media. Additionally, genetic analysis of AM fungi is more complex because of their heterokaryotic nature and lack of sexual process [34, 145].

The plant genes involved in development of RN and AM symbioses may be divided into two groups, according to approach which was used for the gene identification. The first group, *Sym* genes [146], had been identified with the use of formal genetic analysis (started from selection of plant mutants defective in nodule development). The other group of genes comprises nodulins (from *nodule*) [147], mycorrhizins (from *mycorrhiza*) [148, 149], and symbiosins (from *symbiosis*) [149, 150]. These genes were identified by molecular genetic methods, through identification of proteins and/or RNAs synthesized *de novo* in root nodules (nodulins) or roots colonized by AM fungi (mycorrhizins). The genes whose expression is induced during the development of both endosymbioses, RNS and AM are called symbiosins [150].

Genes of these groups are suspected to play different roles in the processes which may be referred collectively as "management of microsymbionts" inside plant roots. Specifically, the products of some nodulin genes represent the structural elements of newly constructed temporary compartments developed during symbiosis [151]. The other nodulin genes may play essential roles in modulating the hormonal status of the developing nodules [152, 153]. Resently, *in silico* and microarray-based transcriptome profiling approaches have allowed identification of nodulins, mycorrhizins and symbiosins, which are being activated in response to an AM fungal signal, or by either rhizobial or AM fungal stimulus, respectively [149]. Several hundred genes were found to be activated at different stages of either symbiosis, with almost 100 genes being co-induced during nodulation and in AM formation. These co-induced genes representing the common evolutionary bases of AM and nodular symbioses can be associated with those cellular functions which are required for symbiotic efficiency, such as the facilitation of nutrient transport across the perisymbiotic membranes that surround the endosymbiotic bacteroids in root nodules and the arbuscules in AM roots [150]. However, it should be remembered that although most of the nodulins/mycorrhizins/symbiosins were already cloned and sequenced, functions for many of them have been identified only preliminary using the sequence data of the encoding genes and location of the gene products in the symbiotic compartments.

Still, most of nodulins, mycorrhizins and symbiosins seem to play a subordinate role in the regulatory scheme of symbiosis, nevertheless being indispensable for its functionality and stability. In turn, the major, regulatory role in realization of symbiotic programmes is to be assigned to *Sym* genes. These genes, in contrast to nodulin genes, are usually not expressed outside symbiotic structures and there are many examples of the high functional and sequence homologies between them in different legumes. First genes of this group had been identified using the spontaneous mutants from natural legume populations [154] and afterwards using the experimentally induced mutants defective in nodulation or nitrogen fixation (Nod^- and Fix^- phenotypes) [155]. Afterwards, it was demonstrated that mutations in some of these genes also affect the ability of plant to form AM [148]. The presence of such common genes necessary for both AM and RN symbioses development suggested that both endosymbioses were more closely related than it was suspected before. The cloning and sequencing of the common symbiotic genes helped to understand that AM and RN symbioses share the overlapping signaling pathways, which probably were established during evolution the AM symbiosis and was recruited afterwards into the RN symbiosis development [35].

The large sizes of genomes of crop legumes (e.g. soybean *Glycine max* (L.) Merr. and pea) in which the formal genetics of symbioses was initially developed, as well as low capability for genetic transformation, complicate greatly the cloning of symbiotic genes, analysis of their primary structures and the gene manipulations. Therefore, in early 1990s the new legume species, *Lotus japonicus* [156] and *Medicago truncatula* [157, 158] have been introduced in studies as model plants. These species are characterized by small genomes (470 – 500 Mb; [159]) and can easily be genetically transformed [158, 160-162]. In addition, the short lifecycle and high seed productivity made them attractive and convenient model objects for studying molecular bases of RN and AM symbioses.

Genetic analysis in model legumes as well as in crop legumes was started with experimental mutagenesis. Large-scale programs of insertion, chemical and X-rays mutagenesis, performed by different research groups, resulted in generation of numerous symbiotic mutants in *L. japonicus* and *M. truncatula* [163, 164] which allowed researchers to identify and characterize a series of *Sym* genes. The genes involved at the initial stages of nitrogen-fixing symbiosis (early *Sym* genes) were of primary interest, allowing dissection of the mechanisms by which the NF signal is perceived and transduced by host plants [165]. It turned to be that after the perception of NF, the nodulation process follows the same signalling pathway as AM does, with slight differences, though.

3.2. Common Symbiosis Pathway (CSP)

The data obtained during the last fifteen years allowed reconstruction the symbiotic signaling pathway which starts in RN and AM symbioses with recognition the Nod and Myc factors, respectively, and goes on as the signal transduction inside the root. In legumes Nod and Myc factors are most likely perceived by specific receptor complexes [35]. The receptor for NF is considered to be a heterodimer composed of at least two LysM containing receptor kinases [166-168]. Alike, receptor for Myc factor (which is not known yet) also supposed to be consisted of similar receptor kinases, or even include one or more kinases participating in Nod factor signaling [169]. The system of receptor kinases perceiving signal molecules of microsymbionts seems to be complicated, with some receptor complexes being necessary not only for starting the interactions, but also on later stages, during penetration bacteria into the root cortex through root hair. Moreover, some receptor kinases could non-specifically bind Nod and Myc factors, which results in intensified growth of lateral roots [43, 169]. Probably, the diversity of receptor kinases should complement the variability of soil microorganisms and increase the specificity of interactions with mutually beneficial ones.

After the first step of reception of Nod or Myc factor, the symbiotic signal is being transmitted to the common pathway, named Common Symbiosis Pathway [170]. The first player in this pathway is LRR-receptor kinase, or SymRK (symbiotic receptor kinase), which is required for both RN and AM symbioses development [171, 172]. The ligand for this receptor kinase is not known yet. Interestingly, the activity of this kinase is also required for proper progression of late symbiotic stages, at least for rhizobial infection [173]. SymRK kinase domain has been shown to interact with 3-hydroxy-3-methylglutaryl CoA reductase 1 (HMGR1) from *M. truncatula* [174], and an ARID-type DNA-binding protein [175]. These results suggest that SymRK may form protein complex with key regulatory proteins of downstream cellular responses. Symbiotic Remorin 1 (SYMREM1) from *M. truncatula* and SymRK-interacting E3 ligase (SIE3) from *L. japonicus* have also been shown to interact with SymRK [176, 177].

The symbiosis receptor kinase SymRK acts upstream of the Nod and Myc factor-induced Ca^{2+} spiking in the perinuclear region of root hairs within a few minutes after NF application [178]. Perinuclear calcium spiking involves the release of calcium from a storage compartment (probably the nuclear envelope) through as-yet-unidentified calcium channels. To date it is known that the potassium-permeable channels might compensate for the resulting charge imbalance and could regulate the calcium channels in plants [179-183]. Also, nucleoporins NUP85 and NUP133 (to date described only in *Lotus*) are required for calcium spiking, although their mode of involvement is currently unknown. Probably, NUP85 and NUP133 might be a part of specific nuclear pore subcomplex that plays a crucial role in the signal process requiring interaction at the cell plasma membrane and at nuclear and plastid organelle-membranes to induce a Ca^{2+} spiking [184, 185]. Recently, the third constituent of a conserved subcomplex of the nuclear pore scaffold, NENA, was identified as indispensable component of AM and RN endosymbiotic development [186].

The calcium spiking is characteristic for both RN and AM symbioses formation [187]. These Ca^{2+} spikes are supposed to activate a calcium- and calmodulin-dependent protein kinase (CCaMK) that is also required for NF signaling and AM development [188]. This kinase contains an autoinhibition domain, removing of which leads to a spontaneous activation of downstream transcription events and induction of nodule formation in the absence of rhizobia [189]. Thus, CCaMK appears to be a general manager for both symbioses activating different cascades of signaling for N_2-fixing symbiosis and AM in response to different Ca^{2+} spiking, because the next steps of nodulation signaling are independent from those of AM: the mutations in downstream *Sym* genes do not change the mycorrhizal phenotype of the legume. Interestingly, mutations in any *Sym* genes do not influence the defense reactions, suggesting that signaling pathways of mutualistic symbioses and pathogenesis are sufficiently different.

The calcium-calmodulin-dependent protein kinase (CCaMK) is supposed to be also involved in legume interactions with PGPR and/or endophytic bacteria as it was shown using inoculation of *M. truncatula* by *P. fluorescens* that *MtDMI3* gene (encoding for CCaMK) regulates intercellular root colonization by bacteria as well as expression of some plant housekeeping genes known earlier as mycorrhizins [190].

The CCaMK is known to form a complex with CYCLOPS, a phosphorylation substrate, within the nucleus [35]. *cyclops* mutants of *Lotus* severely impair the infection process induced by the bacterial or fungal symbionts, and are also defective in arbuscule development [149]. During RNS, *cyclops* mutants exhibit the specific defects in infection-thread initiation, but not in the nodule organogenesis [191], indicating that CYCLOPS acts in an infection-specific branch of the symbiotic signaling network [35]. *Cyclops* encodes a protein with no overall sequence similarity to proteins with known function, but containing a functional nuclear localization signal and a carboxy-terminal coiled-coil domain.

It is supposed that CCaMK with help of CYCLOPS probably phosphorilates the specific transcription factors already present in cell: NSP1 and NSP2, which influence the changes of expression in several genes related to the symbiosis development [192, 193]. The activity of these proteins leads to the transcriptional changes in root tissues, for instance, increasing the level of early nodulins ENOD40, ENOD11, ENOD12, ENOD5, which are known to be the potential regulators of infection thread growth and nodule primordium formation [165, 194, 195). Also, the changes in cytokinin status of plant are detected, followed by up-regulation of genes encoding for RN symbiosis-specific cytokinin receptors [196-198]. Moreover, transcription regulators NIN and ERN are to be induced specifically downstream of the early NF signaling pathway in order to coordinate and regulate the correct temporal and spatial formation of root nodules [199-202].

The presented genes are responsible for the signal cascade which is aimed to induce the nodulin, mycorrhizin and symbiosin genes responsible for building the symbiotic structures and implementing their biochemical functions. It is supposed that the signaling pathway did not appear *de novo* in legumes when they become able to form nodules, but was developed from already existed system of AM formation into which the novel, nodule-specific genes were recruited. Still, new genes had been involved in RN symbiosis development, especially those encoding the receptors recognizing hormones (e.g. cytokinins) and hormone-like molecules (Nod factors).

3.3. Autoregulation of symbioses formation

Autoregulation of symbiosis development is an important process that takes place after successful mutual partners' recognition and signal exchange. For RN symbiosis, it is considered that legume host controls the root nodule numbers by sensing the external and internal cues. A major external cue is the soil nitrate, whereas a feedback regulatory system in which earlier formed nodules suppress further nodulation through shoot-root communication is an important internal cue. The latter is known as the autoregulation of nodulation (AON), and is believed to consist of two long-distance signals: a root-derived signal that is generated in infected roots and transmitted to the shoot; and a shoot-derived signal that inhibits nodulation systemically [203, 204]. Therefore, AON represents a strategy through which the host plant can balance the symbiotrophic N nutrition with the energetically more "cheap" combined N nutrition.

Recent findings on autoregulation of nodulation suggest that the root-derived ascending signals to the shoot are short peptides belonging to the CLE peptide family [205, 206]. The leucine-rich repeat receptor-like kinase HAR1 of *Lotus* and its homologues in *M. truncatula* and *P. sativum* (*SUNN* and *Sym29*, respectively) mediate AON and also the nitrate inhibition of nodulation, presumably by recognizing the root-derived signal [207-210]. Other genes, like *ASTRAY*, *KLAVIER* and *TML* in *Lotus*, and *RDN1* in *M. truncatula*, are also supposed to play a sufficient role in AON [211-214].

Very little is still known about the plant regulation of mycorrhization process. In split-root systems on alfalfa (*Medicago sativa*), inoculation of one half of a split-root system with the fungus *Glomus mosseae* significantly reduced later AM colonization on the other half. A similar suppressive effect on mycorrhization was observed after inoculation with *Sinorhizobium meliloti* [215]. Furthermore, prior addition of purifed rhizobial Nod factors on one half signifcantly reduced mycorrhization on the other half of the split-root system, and reciprocally, prior mycorrhization on one side suppressed nodule formation on the other side of the split-root system. Together these data point to a common autoregulation circuit for both symbioses [210]. It was suggested that Nod factor signaling, as well as mycorrhizal Myc factor signaling, induces expression or post-translation processing of CLE peptides, which likely function as ascending long-distance signals to the shoot [210]. Also, it was demonstrated that mutations in *HAR1* of *Lotus* and corresponding orthologues in other legumes increase both nodulation and mycorrhization suggesting the shared role of these orthologous genes in controlling the rate of root colonization by microsymbionts. Thereby, not only the local signal transduction (CSP) but the systemic autoregulation is common for the RN and AM symbioses.

3.4. Next stage of development the genetics of symbioses

The next-coming step of development the genetics of symbioses is studying gene networks on intergenomic level, i.e. the coordinated expression of plant and microbe genes. For AM, with use of the new molecular approaches, in particular transcriptomics, a series of AM fungal genes has been identified, having altered expression levels during the AM formation [216-219]. Still it is not well studied at which stages of fungal-plant interaction the complementary partners' genes are induced or repressed, and so the use of plant mutants impaired at different steps of AM development might be a challenging approach to reveal the pattern of plant and fungal genetic cooperation [220]. The same research aimed at identification of plant-rhizobial gene interactions with the use of plant and microbe mutants is also in progress.

It has been recently observed that *Medicago truncatula* showed significantly lower efficiency of nitrogen fixation than its close relative *Medicago sativa* L. [221]. The number of nodules formed on the roots of *M. truncatula* was less than that of *M. sativa*, and the nitrogen fixation measured on plants at the beginning of flowering (as well as specific N_2 fixation ($\mu gN\ h^{-1}\ mg\ nodule^{-1}$)) was significantly lower. The reasons for the low efficiency in nitrogen fixation were partially a result of low relative efficiency (electron allocated to N_2 versus H^+), and slow nitrogen export from nodules in *M. truncatula* when compared to *M. sativa*. This might be connected with a low malate concentration in the nodule tissue of *M. truncatula*, and thus insufficient carbon provision for asparagine formation (fixed nitrogen is to be added to malate to form asparagine) [221]. Therefore, Sulieman and Schulze [221] suggest that improvement the malate formation in *M. truncatula* nodules could help improving the effectiveness of nitrogen fixation.

According to these data, genes encoding for enzymes of malate synthesis should be good candidates for markers to be used as selection and breeding aimed at improvement of symbiotic properties in *M. truncatula*. But, in different species potential markers of symbiotic effectiveness could be found among genes of different functional groups. Our original data on sequencing alleles of symbiotic genes in pea (*Pisum sativum*) varieties with different symbiotic

http://dx.doi.org/10.5772/53003

effectiveness suggest that polymorphism of genes belonging to CSP does not correspond to symbiotic properties of pea varieties analysed (Zhukov V.A., unpublished results). Perhaps, good candidates for markers of symbiotic effectiveness could be found during large-scale screening by transcriptome sequencing in different pea genotypes, which is now underway in our laboratory.

4. New approaches of application of mutually beneficial plant-microbe systems in sustainable agriculture

4.1. Development of multicomponent inocula containing BSM

An existence of plant genes [148, 150, 222] and their molecular products [223] common for both AM and RN symbioses led to a conclusion that system of legume symbiotic genes should be considered as a single whole, controlling the development of a tripartite symbiosis (legume plant + AM fungi + rhizobia). This fact along with the demonstration of synergistic activity in beneficial soil microbes (reviewed in: [103]) and a suggestion that plant genetic systems controling the development of RN and, probably, of some other beneficial plant-microbe associations evolved on the basis of that of AM [35] have great importance for the application of tripartite or even multi-partite symbiotic systems in low-input sustainable environmentally-friendly agrotechnologies.

The use in sustainable agriculture of inocula based on beneficial soil microbes as described above allows the improvement crop productivity with decreased doses of mineral fertilizers and pesticides (reviewed in: [224, 225]). These days the majority of commercial inocula contain pure cultures of single microorganisms and only occasionally multiple combinations. There are several objections to the use of mono-inoculation. Firstly, endemic microbial communities are stable and the introduced microbe may be allowed to occupy a very small niche in the whole community or even get lost in a first week after introduction. Secondly, genetic material in microbes is very plastic, and consequently strains introduced into natural ecosystems can rapidly lose their beneficial traits. Thirdly, the existence of microbial cooperation in the rhizosphere [103] as well as in natural synergistic associations of different microbes including those between AM fungi and their endocellular or superficial symbionts [103, 132] question the possibility and expediency of applying mono-inoculants and even use of the term 'mono-inoculation' itself. Finally, plants possess relatively stable genomes and this fact contributes significantly to the effectiveness of symbiosis [226]. Therefore, for industrial plant production in sustainable systems we should use plants having highly effective interactions with all kinds of beneficial soil microbes, which can encourage the development of multiple niches hosting microbes and regulating their activity. For this it is necessary to develop new multi-component microbial inocula which increase the content and biodiversity of beneficial soil microbes in agricultural land.

There is experimental evidence of the effectiveness of simultaneous inoculation of legumes with AM fungi and nodule bacteria leading to increased productivity and quality of the yield, e.g. groundnut [138], pea [139-141, 227], albaida (*Anthyllis cytisoides*) [95], and soybean [142]. The effect achieved equalled or exceeded that achieved with mineral fertilizers [140, 141, 227]. The effect also exceeded that of mono-inoculation with AM fungi or with rhizobia either in model experiments or under field conditions [139, 140, 142]. In long-term experiments in a desertified Mediterranean ecosystem, it was found that simultaneous inoculation with AM fungi and rhizobia enhanced the establishment of key plant species and increased soil fertility and quality; increased soil nitrogen content, organic matter content, and soil aggregate hydrostability and enhanced nitrogen transfer from nitrogen-fixing to non-fixing species associated with the natural succession of the plants [95].

There is an example of application of triple inoculum (AM fungi, rhizobia and PGPR) to the legume *A. cytisoides* which was successful only when the microorganisms used were isolated from local environment [94]. In collaboration with an innovation company "Bisolbi-Inter" (Russian Federation) the All-Russia Research Institute for Agricultural Microbiology (AR-RIAM), Saint-Petersburg, Russian Federation, has developed technology for the production and application of a new multifunctional biopreparation BisolbiMix [228] containing a complex of the most effective isolates of endosymbiotic microbes (AM fungi and rhizobia) and associative bacteria (PGPR) from the collection held at ARRIAM. A non-sterile substrate-carrier which is derived from washing-filtration by-products of a sugar-beet factory contains its own microbial community including all the above groups of beneficial microbes. The preparation can be formulated into a seed dressing (not effective for all the crop plants tested) or granules. The efficacy of BisolbiMix was demonstrated in field trials with legumes, e.g. pea [227] or non-legumes such as wheat, pumpkin and potato (Chebotar V.K. et al., unpublished results). The use of microbial formulations containing rhizobia for non-legumes seems to be sensible because it is known that nodule bacteria which do not form nodules on a non-host legume as well as non-legume roots can operate as PGPR [229, 230]. Thus, the selection of rhizobia with both PGPR activity and efficient symbiotic nitrogen fixation should be advantageous in crop rotations or intercropping systems using legumes and non-legumes.

It is possible, therefore, to develop effective multi-microbial inoculants, but it is necessary to use local communities of beneficial microbes because this exploits the natural biological and genetical adaptations of the partners to their environment [94, 231].

4.2. Breeding for improving legume symbiotic effectiveness

During development of plant-microbe systems for low-input sustainable ecologically friendly plant cultivation it is necessary to be guided by conclusions of EC experts about global productivity of legumes (http://www.grainlegumes.com/aep/; http://ec.europa.eu/research/biosociety/food_quality/projects/002_en.html) for sustainable agriculture. The use of legumes in agriculture is leading to: improved soil fertility and increased diversity of crops and soil microbial communities; reductions in the use of non-renewable natural resources; decreased negative effects from intensive agrotechnologies on the natural environment due to decreased requirement for mineral fertilizers and pesticides and decreased production of animal protein and associated wastes; local production of pollution-free food and forage; and a more stable income for the agricultural producers. This is why it is necessary to breed legumes which have highly effective interactions with beneficial soil microbes.

For more than twenty five years the authors' laboratory has specialized in the genetics of plant-microbe interactions using pea (*P. sativum* L.) as a model plant. Our experience for improving the effectiveness of beneficial plant-microbe systems with pea is consequently given as an example. At the same time, the authors' team knows only single record of other activity of this nature: genetic variability of onion (*Allium* spp.) has been shown with respect to its responsiveness to AM fungi inoculation which indicate that onion breeding for improving efficacy of associations with AM fungi is possible [232]. The necessity for this sort of plant breeding is also considered, mainly with respect to the effectiveness of RN symbiosis [233-236].

4.3. Analysis of genetic variability of pea with respect to its effectiveness of interactions with beneficial soil microbes

A high level of genetic variability was demonstrated in analyses of the symbiotic effectiveness under double inoculation with AM fungi and nodule bacteria of 99 land-races and outclassed heritage cultivars of *P. sativum* from the collection N.I. Vavilov's All-Russia Research Institute of Plant Industry, Saint-Petersburg, Russian Federation, of different geographical origin [139, 141]. In a few genotypes considerable increases in plant dry weight (about 300 %), seed productivity (more than 650%), phosphorus and nitrogen content (more than 900 and more than 300 %, respectively) were observed. The most promising highly symbiotically effective genotypes and those with low symbiotic potential were included in the Pea Genetic Collection (ARRIAM) to be used for experiments studying the functioning of tripartite/multipartite symbiosis. Types identified as highly symbiotically effective genotypes were involved in breeding programmes to create commercial pea cultivars with great potential for interactions with beneficial soil microbes (in collaboration with All-Russia Institute of Leguminous and Groat Crops (ARILGC), Orel, Russian Federation).

The most promising highly symbiotically effective pea genotypes previously selected and different commercial pea cultivars created without consideration of symbiotic effectiveness were involved in three-year field trials (Orel district) [227]. Seed productivity and plant dry weight were chosen as the main criteria for the evaluation of symbiosis effectiveness in legume crops. The double (actually multiple, see above comments on the nature of AM fungi) inoculation was shown to increase seed productivity and plant dry weight in most of the pea genotypes studied and sometimes this could exceed the effect of mineral fertilizers. The effectiveness of legume breeding to improve the symbiotic potential of legume cultivars was proven therefore under field conditions and the genotypes to be used in such breeding programmes were identified. The genotype K-8274 (non-commercial) was selected as a standard of symbiotic effectiveness. Additionally, it was demonstrated that highly effective genotypes can be also found among commercial pea cultivars created without consideration for effectiveness of interactions with beneficial soil microbes. Taking into account that most commercial legume cultivars have accidentally lost their abilities for symbiotrophic nutrition without selective pressure during breeding of intensive crops, the latter constitutes a very important finding for plant breeders and gives them the possibility for concurrent generation of cultivars with required pea plant architecture, other agriculturally important traits and high effectiveness of interactions with all types of beneficial soil microbes in a single breeding programme.

4.4. Breeding to improve pea symbiotic effectiveness

In order to cultivate plants with improved symbiotic potential a special breeding nursery was created in the experimental trials ground of ARILGC on land where for the 5 years before nursery establishment mineral fertilizers had not been applied. To reduce the incidence and severity of root pathogens a 6-field crop rotation was used where cultivation of winter wheat was followed by peas. The multi-component preparation BisolbiMix was used for the inoculation of test plants.

Using the breeding nursery as well as a breeding protocol developed from long-term collaboration of ARRIAM with ARILGC the first (in the whole history of legume breeding) pea cultivar "Triumph" having increased potential of interactions with beneficial soil microbes was intentionally created [237]. It arose as a result of crossing a commercial cultivar 'Classic' (donor of agriculturally important traits) and the genotype K-8274 (donor of symbiotic effectiveness trait) and subsequent individual selection of genotypes with high productivity and capacity for supporting various beneficial microbes.

The cultivar "Triumph" is of middle stem height, semi-leafless and has stable productivity under different climate conditions, it is comparatively resistant to root rots and pests. Its productivity is not lower than those of the productivity standards for Orel district using the conventional production technologies and 10% greater in comparison with the standard cultivars when inoculated with BisolbiMix. As a result of two-year state trials (2007-2008) the productivity of "Triumph" was shown to be comparable with those of standard regional cultivars enabling recommendation for commercial cultivation in the Central region of Russian Federation (unpublished results). Thus, the innovative concept of the authors' research team for plant breeding (applicable not only for legumes, but also for non-legumes) is bearing its first fruits.

5. Conclusions

Intimate associations of beneficial soil microbes with the host plants described above in detail are applicable in sustainable crop production if taken either separately or in combination. Many authors are now recognizing the need for using the multi-microbial plant inoculants and the advantages of using the indigenous plants (or varieties of local breeding) and microbes.

The authors' team proposes its own concept which offers fundamentally new approaches to plant production. Firstly, it is necessary to consider plant genetic systems controlling interactions with different beneficial soil microbes in unison. Secondly, plants used as a component of this complex plant-microbe system controlling its effectiveness should be bred to improve the effectiveness of interactions with all types of beneficial soil microbes. Increases of plant biomass production due to plant-microbe symbiosis should be used as the main parameter for an evaluation of plant effectiveness in interactions with beneficial soil microbes. The plant production should be done with inoculation composed of multi-component microbial inocula consisting of AM fungi, rhizobia, PGPR and/or beneficial endophytic bacteria. Finally, taking into consideration the importance of legumes for global agriculture, greater emphasis should be placed on plant-microbial systems in the development of low-input agro-biotechnologies enabling wider cultivation of leguminous crops.

Molecular markers are considered to be a convenient tool to facilitate breeding via MAS (marker-assisted selection) approach. But, search for suitable markers that are associated with symbiotic effectiveness trait is rather complicated problem. To our knowledge, there was no direct link between sequences of symbiotic genes and symbiotic effectiveness, and there are only a few examples of successful use of QTL analysis in legumes to trace loci associated with some symbiotic traits in pea [238] and *Lotus* [239]. So there's a gap between molecular genetic bases of symbioses development, from one side, and effective functioning the symbiotic systems in field conditions, from the other side. In our opinion, substantial improvement of methods of molecular genetics and bioinformatics, such as next-generation sequencing and proteome analysis, could help to build a bridge between fundamental and applied science in this area, and to improve the sustainability of the legume crop production.

Key words and abbreviations

arbuscular mycorrhiza (AM),

beneficial soil microorganisms (BSM),

defense of plants from pathogens,

developmental genetics,

endophytic bacteria,

evolution of symbiosis,

Glomeromycota,

leguminous plants,

Lotus japonicus,

Medicago truncatula,

molecular genetics,

mutational analysis,

Nod factor (NF),

phosphate transporter (PT),

Pisum sativum,

plant growth promoting rhizobacteria (PGPR),

plant-microbe symbioses (PMS),

root nodule (RN)

root nodule symbiosis (RNS),

root nodule bacteria (rhizobia),

signal interactions,

symbiosomes,

symbiotrophic plant nutrition,

sustainable agriculture,

systemic regulation

Acknowledgements

We thank Dr. Margarita A. Vishnyakova (N.I. Vavilov All-Russia Research Institute of Plant Industry, St-Petersburg, Russian Federation), Dr. Tatiana S. Naumkina (All-Russia Institute of Legumes and Groat Crops, Orel, Russian Federation) and Dr. Vladimir K. Chebotar ("Bisolbi-Inter" Ltd., St-Petersburg, Russian Federation) for the long-term collaboration in the fields of legume breeding and microbial inocula development. We are also grateful to Victoria Semenova (Komarov Botanical Institute, St-Petersburg, Russian Federation) for critical reading the manuscript. This work was supported by the grants of RFBR (10-04-00961, 10-04-01146, 12-04-01867), Grant to support leading Russian science school (HIII–337.2012.4) and Governmental contracts for research with Ministry of Science and Education of Russian Federation (II1304, 16.512.11.2155, #8109).

Author details

Vladimir A. Zhukov, Oksana Y. Shtark, Alexey Y. Borisov and Igor A. Tikhonovich

*Address all correspondence to: zhukoff01@yahoo.com

All-Russia Research Institute for Agricultural Microbiology, St.-Petersburg, Russia

References

[1] Vance CP. Symbiotic Nitrogen Fixation and Phosphorus Acquisition. Plant Nutrition in the World of Declining Renewable Resources. Plant Physiol 2001;127(2): 390-397.

[2] Brewin NJ. Plant Cell Wall Remodeling in the Rhizobium-Legume Symbiosis. Crit Rev Plant Sci 2004;23: 1-24.

[3] Allen ON, Allen EK. The Leguminosae. A Source Book of Characteristics, Uses and Nodulation. Madison: The University of Wisconsin Press; 1981.

[4] Wall LG. The Actinorhizal Symbiosis. J Plant Growth Regul 2000;19(2): 167-182.

[5] Balachandar D, Raja P, Kumar K, Sundaram SP. Non-Rhizobial Nodulation in Legumes. Biotechnol Molec Biol Rev 2007;2(2): 49-57.

[6] Spaink HP, Kondorosi A, Hooykaas PJJ., editors. The Rhizobiaceae. Molecular Biology of Model Plant-Associated Bacteria. Dordrecht/Boston/London: Kluwer; 1998.

[7] MacLean AM, Finan T, Sadowsky MJ. Genomes of the Symbiotic Nitrogen-Fixing Bacteria of Legumes. Plant Physiol 2007;144(2): 615-622.

[8] Fred EB, Baldwin IL, McCoy E. Root Nodule Bacteria and Leguminous Plants. Madison: Univ Wisconsin Stud Sci; 1932.

[9] Provorov NA. The Interdependence between Taxonomy of Legumes and Specificity of Their Interaction with Rhizobia in Relation to Evolution of the Symbiosis. Symbiosis 1994;17: 183-200.

[10] Broughton WJ, Perret X. Genealogy of Legume-Rhizobium Symbiosis. Curr Opin Plant Biol 1999;2(4): 305-311.

[11] Ovtsyna AO, Staehelin C. Bacterial signals required for the Rhizobium-legume symbiosis. In: Pandalai SG. (ed) Recent Research Developments in Microbiology, Vol 7 (Part II). Trivandrum, India: Research Signpost; 2003. p631-648.

[12] Spaink HP. The Molecular Basis of Infection and Nodulation by Rhizobia: the Ins and Outs of Sympathogenesis. Ann Rev Phytopathol 1995;33: 345-368.

[13] Schultze M, Kondorosi A. Regulation of Symbiotic Root Nodule Development. Annu Rev Genet 1998;32: 33-57.

[14] D'Haeze W, Holsters M. Nod Factor Structures, Responses, and Perception During Initiation of Nodule Development. Glycobiology 2002;12(6): 79-105.

[15] Becker A, Pühler A. Production of Exopolysaccharides. In: Spaink HP, Kondorosi A, Hooykaas PJJ. (eds) The Rhizobiaceae. Molecular Biology of Model Plant-Associated Bacteria. Dordrecht/Boston/London: Kluwer; 1998. p87-118.

[16] Lugtenberg BJJ. Outer Membrane Proteins. In: Spaink HP, Kondorosi A, Hooykaas PJJ. (eds) The Rhizobiaceae. Molecular Biology of Model Plant-Associated Bacteria. Dordrecht/Boston/London: Kluwer; 1998. p45-53.

[17] Jones KM, Sharopova N, Lohar DP, Zhang JQ, VandenBosch KA, Walker GC. Differential Response of the Plant *Medicago truncatula* to its Symbiont *Sinorhizobium meliloti* or an Exopolysaccharide-Deficient Mutant. Proc Natl Acad Sci USA 2008;105(2): 704-709.

[18] Hirsch AM. Developmental Biology of Legume Nodulation. New Phytol 1992;122: 211-237.

[19] Sprent JI. Nodulation in Legumes. Royal Botanical Gardens, Kew: Cromwell Press Ltd; 2001.

[20] Oke V, Long SR. Bacteroid Formation in the Rhizobium-Legume Symbiosis. Curr Opin Microbiol 1999;2(6): 641-646.

[21] Brewin NJ (1998) Tissue and Cell Invasion by Rhizobium: the Structure and Development of Infection Threads and Symbiosomes. In: Spaink HP, Kondorosi A, Hooykaas PJJ. (eds) The Rhizobiaceae. Molecular Biology of Model Plant-Associated Bacteria. Dordrecht/Boston/London: Kluwer; 1998. p417-429.

[22] Tsyganov VE, Voroshilova VA, Herrera-Cervera JA, Sanjuan-Pinilla JM, Borisov AY, Tikhonovich IA, Priefer UB, Olivares J, Sanjuan J. Developmental Down-Regulation of Rhizobial Genes as a Function of Symbiosome Differentiation in Symbiotic Root Nodules of *Pisum sativum* L. New Phytol 2003;159(2): 521-530.

[23] Mylona P, Pawlowski K, Bisseling T. Symbiotic Nitrogen Fixation. Plant Cell 1995;7(7): 869-885.

[24] Pawlowski K, Bisseling T. Rhizobial and Actinorhizal Symbioses: What Are the Shared Features? Plant Cell 1996;8(10): 1899-1913.

[25] Vance CP, Heichel GH. Carbon in N_2 Fixation: Limitation or Exquisite Adaptation? Annu Rev Plant Physiol 1991;42: 373-392.

[26] Fedorova M, Tikhonovich IA, Vance CP. Expression of C-assimilating Enzymes in Pea (*Pisum sativum* L.) Root Nodules. In situ Localization in Effective Nodules. Plant Cell Environ 1999;22(10): 1249-1262.

[27] Schubert KR. Products of Biological Nitrogen Fixation in Higher Plants: Synthesis, Transport, and Metabolism. Annu Rev Plant Physiol 1986;37: 539-574.

[28] Mergaert P, Uchiumi T, Alunni B, Evanno G, Cheron A, Catrice O, Mausset AE, Barloy-Hubler F, Galibert F, Kondorosi A, Kondorosi E. Eukaryotic Control on Bacterial Cell Cycle and Differentiation in the Rhizobium-Legume Symbiosis. Proc Natl Acad Sci USA 2006;103(13): 5230-5235.

[29] Van de Velde W, Zehirov G, Szatmari A, Debreczeny M, Ishihara H, Kevei Z, Farkas A, Mikulass K, Nagy A, Tiricz H, Satiat-Jeunemaître B, Alunni B, Bourge M, Kucho K, Abe M, Kereszt A, Maroti G, Uchiumi T, Kondorosi E, Mergaert P. Plant Peptides Govern Terminal Differentiation of Bacteria in Symbiosis. Science 2010;327(5969): 1122-1126.

[30] Oono R, Denison RF, Kiers ET. Controlling the Reproductive Fate of Rhizobia: How Universal Are Legume Sanctions? New Phytol 2009;183(4): 967-979.

[31] Oono R, Denison RF. Comparing symbiotic Efficiency Between Swollen Versus Nonswollen Rhizobial Bacteroids. Plant Physiol 2010;154(3): 1541-1548.

[32] Schüßler A, Schwarzott D, Walker C. A New Fungal Phylum, the Glomeromycota: Phylogeny and Evolution. Mycol Res 2001;105: 1413-1297.

[33] Brundrett MC Coevolution of Roots and Mycorrhizas of Land Plants. New Phytol 2002;154: 275-304.

[34] Smith SE, Read DJ. Mycorrhizal Symbiosis (3rd ed.). London: Academic Press; 2008.

[35] Parniske M. Arbuscular Mycorrhiza: the Mother of Plant Root Endosymbioses. Nat Rev Microbiol 2008;6(10): 763-775.

[36] Lavin M, Herendeen PS, Wojciechowski MF Evolutionary Rates Analysis of Leguminosae Implicates a Rapid Diversification of Lineages during the Tertiary. Syst Biol 2005;54: 574-594.

[37] Sprent JI. Evolving Ideas of Legume Evolution and Diversity: A Taxonomic Perspective on the Ocurrence of Nodulation. New Phytologist 2007;174: 11-25.

[38] Sprent J. Evolution and Diversity of Legume Symbiosis. In: Dilworth MJ, James EK, Sprent JI, Newton WE (eds) Nitrogen-Fixing Leguminous Symbioses. Dordrecht: Springer; 2008. P 363-394.

[39] Sprent JI, James EK. Legume Evolution: Where Do Nodules and Mycorrhizas Fit in? Plant Physiol 2007;144: 575-581.

[40] Akiyama K, Matsuzaki K, Hayashi H. Plant Sesquiterpenes Induce Hyphal Branching in Arbuscular Mycorrhizal Fungi. Nature 2005;435: 824-827.

[41] Nagahashi G, Douds DD, Ferhatoglu Y. Functional Categories of Root Exudate Compounds and their Relevance to AM Fungal Growth. In: Koltai H, Kapulnik Y (eds) Arbuscular Mycorrhizas: Physiology and Function. Dordrecht: Springer; 2010. P 33-56.

[42] Kosuta S, Chabaud M, Lougnon G, Gough C, Denarie J, Barker DG, Becard G. A Diffusible Factor From Arbuscular Mycorrhizal Fungi Induces Symbiosis-Specific *Mtenod11* Expression in Roots of *Medicago truncatula.* Plant Physiol 2003;131: 952-962.

[43] Maillet F, Poinsot V, André O, Puech-Pagès V, Haouy A, Gueunier M, Cromer L, Giraudet D, Formey D, Niebel A, Martinez EA, Driguez H, Bécard G, Dénarié J. Fungal Lipochitooligosaccharide Symbiotic Signals in Arbuscular Mycorrhiza. Nature 2011;469(7328): 58-63.

[44] Navazio L, Moscatiello R, Genre A, Novero M, Baldan B, Bonfante P, Mariani P. A Diffusible Signal From Arbuscular Mycorrhizal Fungi Elicits a Transient Cytosolic Calcium Elevation in Host Plant Cells. Plant Physiol 2007;144: 673-681.

[45] Genre A, Bonfante P. The Making of Symbiotic Cells in Arbuscular Mycorrhizal Roots. In: Koltai H, Kapulnik Y (eds) Arbuscular Mycorrhizas: Physiology and Function. Dordrecht: Springer; 2010. P 57-81.

[46] Parniske M. The *Lotus japonicus* LjSym4 Gene is Required for the Successful Symbiotic Infection of Root Epidermal Cells. Molec Plant-Microbe Iinteract 2000;13: 1109-1120.

[47] Genre A, Bonfante P. Building a Mycorrhiza Cell: How to Reach Compatibility Between Plants and Arbuscular Mycorrhizal Fungi. J Plant Interact 2005;1: 3-13

[48] Bieleski RL Phosphate Pools, Phosphate Transport and Phosphate Availability. Annu Rev Plant Physiol 1973;24: 225-252.

[49] Schachtman DP, Reid RJ, Ayling SM. Phosphorus Uptake by Plants: From Soil to Cell. Plant Physiol 1998;116: 447-453.

[50] Tinker PB, Nye PH. Solute Movement in the Rhizosphere. Oxford, UK: Oxford University Press; 2000.

[51] Neumann E, George E. Nutrient Uptake: The Arbuscular Mycorrhiza Fungal Symbiosis as a Plant Nutrient Acquisition Strategy In: Koltai H, Kapulnik Y (eds) Arbuscular Mycorrhizas: Physiology and Function. Dordrecht: Springer; 2010. P 137-167.

[52] Smith SE, Smith FA, Jakobsen I. Mycorrhizal Fungi Can Dominate Phosphate Supply to Plants Irrespective of Growth Responses. Plant Physiol 2003;133: 16–20

[53] Schweiger P, Jakobsen I. Laboratory and Field Methods for Measurement Of Hyphal Uptake of Nutrients in Soil. Plant Soil 2000;226: 237–244.

[54] Nielsen JS, Joner EJ, Declerck S, Olsson S, Jakobsen I. Phospho-Imaging as a Tool for Visualization and Noninvasive Measurement of P Transport Dynamics in Arbuscular Mycorrhizas. New Phytol 2002;154: 809–820.

[55] Rufyikiri G, Declerck S, Thiry Y. Comparison of 233U and 33P Uptake and Translocation by the Arbuscular Mycorrhizal Fungus *Glomus intraradices* in Root Organ Culture Conditions. Mycorrhiza 2004;14: 203–207.

[56] Ezawa T, Smith SE, Smith FA. P Metabolism and Transport in AM Fungi. Plant Soil 2002;244: 221–230.

[57] Ashford A. Tubular Vacuoles in Arbuscular Mycorrhizas. New Phytol 2002;54: 545–547.

[58] Ezawa T, Cavagnaro TR, Smith SE, Smith FA, Ohtomo R. Rapid Accumulation of Polyphosphate in Extraradical Hyphae of an Arbuscular Mycorrhizal Fungus as Revealed by Histochemistry and a Polyphosphate Kinase/Luciferase System. New Phytol 2003;161: 387–392.

[59] Karandashov V, Bucher M. Symbiotic Phosphate Transport in Arbuscular Mycorrhizas. Trends Plant Sci 2005;10: 22-29.

[60] Balestrini R, Gomez-Ariza J, Lanfranco L, Bonfante P. Laser Microdissection Reveals that Transcripts for Five Plant and One Fungal Phosphate Transporter Genes are Contemporaneously Present in Arbusculated Cells. Molec Plant-Microbe Interact 2007;20: 1055-1062.

[61] Javot H, Pumplin N, Harrison MJ. Phosphate in the Arbuscular Mycorrhizal Symbiosis: Transport Properties and Regulatory Roles. Plant Cell Environ 2007;30: 310-322

[62] Harrison MJ, Dewbre GR, Liu J. A Phosphate Transporter from *Medicago truncatula* Involved in the Acquisition of Phosphate Released by Arbuscular Mycorrhizal Fungi. Plant Cell 2002;14: 2413–2429.

[63] Maeda D, Ashida K, Iguchi K, Chechetka SA, Hijikata A, Okusako Y, Deguchi Y, Izui K, Hata S. Knockdown of an Arbuscular Mycorrhiza-Inducible Phosphate Transporter Gene of *Lotus japonicus* Suppresses Mutualistic Symbiosis. Plant Cell Physiol 2006;47: 807-817.

[64] Javot H, Penmetsa RV, Terzaghi N, Cook DR, Harrison MJ. A *Medicago truncatula* Phosphate Transporter Indispensable For The Arbuscular Mycorrhizal Symbiosis. Proc. Natl. Acad. Sci. USA 2007;104: 1720-1725.

[65] Nagy R, Drissner D, Amrhein N, Jakobsen I, Bucher M. Mycorrhizal Phosphate Uptake Pathway in Tomato Iis Phosphorusrepressible and Transcriptionally Regulated. New Phytol 2009;181: 950–959.

[66] Bonfante P, Balestrini R, Genre A, Lanfranco L. Establishment and Functioning Of Arbuscular Mycorrhizas. In: Deising H (ed) The Mycota V. Plant Relationship (2nd ed.). Berlin, Heidelberg: Springer-Verlag; 2009. P 259-274.

[67] Hawkins HJ, Johansen A, George E. Uptake and Transport of Organic and Inorganic Nitrogen by Arbuscular Mycorrhizal Fungi. Plant Soil 2000;226: 275-285.

[68] Lopez-Pedrosa A, Gonzalez-Guerrero M, Valderas A, Azcon-Aguilar C, Ferrol N. *GintAMTi* Encodes a Functional High-Affinity Ammonium Transporter that is Expressed in the Extraradical Mycelium of *Glomus intraradices*. Fungal Genet Biol 2006;43: 102-110.

[69] Jin H, Pfeffer PE, Douds DD, Piotrowski E, Lammers PJ, Shachar-Hill Y. The Uptake, Metabolism, Transport and Transfer of Nitrogen in an Arbuscular Mycorrhizal Symbiosis. New Phytol 2005;168: 687-696.

[70] Johansen A, Finlay RD, Olsson PA. Nitrogen Metabolism of External Hyphae of the Arbuscular Mycorrhizal Fungus *Glomus intraradices*. New Phytol 1996;133: 705-712.

[71] Breuninger M, Trujillo CG, Serrano E, Fischer R, Requena N. Different Nitrogen Sources Modulate Activity but not Expression of Glutamine Synthetase in Arbuscular Mycorrhizal Fungi. Fungal Genet Biol 2004;41: 542–552.

[72] Guether M, Neuhauser B, Balestrini R, Dynowski M, Ludewig U, Bonfante P. A Mycorrhizal-Specific Ammonium Transporter from Lotus japonicus Acquires Nitrogen Released by Arbuscular Mycorrhizal Fungi. Plant Physiol 2009;150: 73–83.

[73] Akhtar MS, Siddiqui ZA. Arbuscular Mycorrhizal Fungi as Potential Bioprotectants Against Plant Pathogens. In: Siddiqu ZA et al (eds) Mycorrhizae: Sustainable Agriculture and Forestry. Dordrecht: Springer; 2008. P 61–97.

[74] Koricheva J, Gange AC, Jones T. Effects of Mycorrhizal Fungi on Insect Herbivores: a Metaanalysis. Ecology 2009;90: 2088–2097.

[75] Currie AF, Murray PJ, Gange AC. Is a Specialist Root-Feeding Insect Affected by Arbuscular Mycorrhizal Fungi? Appl Soil Ecol 2011;47: 77–83.

[76] Harrison MJ. Molecular and Cellular Aspects of the Arbuscular Mycorrhizal Symbiosis. Ann Rev Plant Physiol Plant Mol Biol 1999;50: 361-389.

[77] Blilou I, Bueno P, Ocampo JA, Garcia-Garrido JM. Induction of Catalase And Ascorbate Peroxidase Activities in Tobacco Roots Inoculated with the Arbuscular Mycorrhizal Fungus *Glomus mossea*. Mycol Res 2000;104: 722-725.

[78] Blilou I, Ocampo JA, Garcia-Garrido JM. Resistance of Pea Roots to Endomycorrhizal Fungus or *Rhizobium* Correlates with Enhanced Levels of Endogenous Salicylic Acid. J Exp Bot 1999;50: 1663-1668.

[79] Lambais MR. Regulation of Plant Defence-Related Genes in Arbuscular Mycorrhizae. In: Podila GK, Douds DD (eds) Current Advances in Mycorrhizae research The American Phytopathological Society, Minnesota; 2000. P 45-59.

[80] Bonanomi A, Wiemken A, Boller T, Salzer P. Local Induction of a Mycorrhiza-Specific Class III Chitinase Gene in Cortical Root Cells of *Medicago truncatula* Containing Developing or Mature Arbuscules. Plant Biol 2001;3: 94-199.

[81] Salzer P, Corbiere H, Boller T. Hydrogen Peroxide Accumulation in *Medicago Truncatula* Roots Colonized by the Arbuscular Mycorrhiza-Forming Fungus *Glomus mosseae*. Planta 1999;208: 319-325.

[82] Garcia-Garrido JM, Ocampo JA. Regulation of the Plant Defence Response in Arbuscular Mycorrhizal Symbiosis. J Exp Bot 2002;53: 377-1386

[83] Liu J, Maldonado-Mendoza I, Lopez-Meyer M, Cheung F, Town CD, Harrison MJ. Arbuscular Mycorrhizal Symbiosis is Accompanied by Local and Systemic Alterations in Gene Expression and an Increase in Disease Resistance in the Shoots. Plant J 2007;50: 529-544.

[84] Bennett AE, Bever JD, Bowers MD. Arbuscular Mycorrhizal Fungal Species Suppress Inducible Plant Responses and Alter Defensive Strategies Following Herbivory. Oecologia 2009;160: 711–719.

[85] Kempel A, Schmidt AK, Brandl R, Schadler M. Support from the Underground: Induced Plant Resistance Depends on Arbuscular Mycorrhizal Fungi. Funct Ecol 2010;24: 293–300.

[86] Quilambo OA. The Vesicular-Arbuscular Mycorrhizal Symbiosis. African J Biotechnol 2003;2: 539-546.

[87] Augé RM. Water Relations, Drought and Vesicular-Arbuscular Mycorrhizal Symbiosis Mycorrhiza 2001;11: 3-42.

[88] Augé RM, Moore JL, Sylvia DM, Cho K. Mycorrhizal Promotion of Host Stomatal Conductance in Relation to Irradiance and Temperature. Mycorrhiza 2004;14: 85-92.

[89] Ruiz-Lozano JM, Aroca R. Host Response to Osmotic Stresses: Stomatal Behaviour and Water Use Efficiency of Arbuscular Mycorrhizal Plants. In: Koltai H, Kapulnik Y (eds) Arbuscular Mycorrhizas: Physiology and Function. Dordrecht: Springer; 2010. P 239-256.

[90] Celik I, Ortas I, Kilic S. Effects of Compost, Mycorrhiza, Manure and Fertilizer on Some Physical Properties of a Chromoxerert Soil. Soil and Tillage Res 2004;78: 59-67.

[91] Rillig MC. Arbuscular Mycorrhizae, Glomalin and Soil Aggregation. Can J Soil Sci 2004;84: 355-363.

[92] Turnau K, Ryszka P, Wojtczak G. Metal Tolerant Mycorrhizal Plants: A Review from the Perspective on Industrial Waste in Temperate Region In: Koltai H, Kapulnik Y (eds) Arbuscular Mycorrhizas: Physiology and Function. Dordrecht: Springer; 2010. P 257-279.

[93] Ryszka P, Turnau K. Arbuscular Mycorrhiza of Introduced and Native Grasses Colonizing Zinc Wastes: Implications for Restoration Practices. Plant Soil 2007;298: 219–229.

[94] Requena N, Jimenez J, Toro M, Barea JM. Interactions Between Plant-Growth-Promoting Rhizobacteria (PGPR), Arbuscular Mycorrhizal Fungi and *Rhizobium* spp. in the Rhizosphere of *Anthyllis cytisoides*, a Model Legume for Revegetation in Mediterranean Semi-Arid Ecosystems. New Phytologist 1997;136(4): 667-677.

[95] Requena N, Perez-Solis E, Azcón-Aguilar C, Jeffries P, Barea JM. Management of Indigenous Plant-Microbe Symbioses Aids Restoration of Desertified Ecosystems. Appl Environ Microbiol 2001;67(2): 495-498.

[96] Turnau K, Orlowska E, Ryszka P, Zubek S, Anielska T, Gawronski S, Jurkiewicz A. Role of Mycorrhizal Fungi In Phytoremediation and Toxity Monitoring of Heavy Metal Rhich Industrial Wastes in Southern Poland. In: Twardowska I, Allen HE, Häggblom MM, Stefaniak S (eds) NATO Science Series. Soil and Water Pollution Monitoring, Protection and Remediation. Dordrecht: Springer; 2007;69: 533-551.

[97] Turnau K, Anielska T, Ryszka P, Gawroński S, Ostachowicz B, Jurkiewicz A. Establishment of Arbuscular Mycorrhizal Plants Originating from Xerothermic Grasslands on Heavy Metal Rich Industrial Wastes – New Solution for Waste Revegetation. Plant Soil 2008;305: 267–280.

[98] Bloemberg G, Lugtenberg BJJ. Molecular Basis of Plant Growth Promotion and Biocontrol by Rhizobacteria. Curr Opin Plant Biol 2001; 4: 343–350

[99] Dobereiner J Isolation and Identification of Root Associated Diazotrophs. Plant Soil 1988;110: 207-212.

[100] Costacurta A, Vanderleyden J. Synthesis of Phytohormones by Plant-Associated Bacteria. Crit Rev Microbiol 1995;21: 1-18.

[101] Provorov NA, Vorobyov NI. Evolutionary Genetics of Plant-Microbe Symbioses. New York: NOVA Science Publishers; 2010.

[102] Shtark O., Provorov N., Mikić A., Borisov A., Ćupina B., Tikhonovich I. Legume Root Symbioses: Natural History and Prospects For Improvement. Ratarstvo i povrtarstvo (Field and Vegetable Crops Research) 2011;48: 291-304.

[103] Barea JM, Pozo MJ, Azcon R, Azcon-Aguilar C. Microbial Cooperation in the Rhizosphere. J Exp Botany 2005;56(417): 1761-1778.

[104] Haas D, Defago G. Biological Control of Soil-Borne Pathogens by Fluorescent Pseudomonads. Nature Rev Microbiol. AOP, doi:10.1038/nrmicro1129 (accessed 10 March 2005).

[105] Siddiqui ZA. PGPR: Prospective Biocontrol Agents of Plant Pathogens. In: Siddiqui ZA (ed) PGPR: Biocontrol and Biofertilization. Dordrecht: Springer; 2005. P 111–142.

[106] Preston GM Plant Perceptions of Plant Growth-Promoting Pseudomonas. Phil Trans R Soc Lond B 2004;359: 907-918.

[107] O'Toole GA, Kolter R. Initiation of Biofilm Formation in *Pseudomonas fluorescens* WCS365 Proceeds via Multiple, Convergent Signalling Pathways: a Genetic Analysis. Mol Microbiol 1998;28(3): 449-61.

[108] Stephens C, Murray W. Pathogen Evolution: How Good Bacteria go Bad. Curr Biol 2001;11: 53-56.

[109] Catara V. *Pseudomonas corrugata*: Plant Pathogen and/or Biological Resource? Mol Plant Pathol 2007;8: 233-244.

[110] Bolwerk A, Lagopodi AL, Wijfjes AHM, Lamers GEM, Lugtenberg BJJ, Bloemberg GV. Interactions between *Pseudomonas* Biocontrol Strains and *Fusarium oxysporum* f.sp. *radicis-lycopersici* in the Tomato Rhizosphere. In: Tikhonovich IA, Lugtenberg BJJ Provorov NA (eds) Biology of Plant-Microbe Interactions. IS-MPMI, St.-Petersburg 2004;4: 323-326.

[111] Popova EV, Khatskevich LK. In: Tikhonovich IA, Lugtenberg BJJ Provorov NA (eds) Biology of Plant-Microbe Interactions. IS-MPMI, St.-Petersburg 2004;4: 315-318.

[112] Van Loon LC, Bakker PA, Pieterse CMJ. Systemic Resistance Induced by Rhizosphere Bacteria. Annu Rev Phytopathol 1998;36: 453-483.

[113] Vallad E, Goodman RM. Systemic Acquired Resistance and Induced Systemic Resistance in Conventional Agriculture. Crop Sci 2004;44: 1920-1934.

[114] Penrose DM, Glick BR. Methods for Isolating and Characterizing ACC Deaminase-Containing Plant Growth-Promoting Rhizobacteria. Physiol Plantarum 2003;118: 10-15.

[115] Glick BR. The Role of Bacterial ACC Deaminase in Promoting the Plant Growth. In: Tikhonovich IA, Lugtenberg BJJ Provorov NA (eds) Biology of Plant-Microbe Interactions. IS-MPMI, St.-Petersburg 2004;4: 557-560.

[116] Wu P, Zang G, Ladha JK, McCouch SR, Huang N. Molecular-Marker-Facilitated Investigation on the Ability to Stimulate N_2 Fixation in the Rhizosphere by the Irrigated Rice Plants. Theor Appl Genet 1995;91: 1177-1183.

[117] Smith KP, Goodman RM. Host Variation for Interactions with Beneficial Plant-Associated Microbes. Annu Rev Phytopathol 1999;37: 473-491.

[118] Liu L, Kloepper JW, Tuzun S. Induction of Systemic Resistance in Cucumber by Plant Growth-Promoting Rhizobacteria: Duration of Protection and Root Colonization. Phytopathol 1995;85: 1064-1068.

[119] Van Wees SCM, Pieterse CMJ, Trijssenaar A, van Westende TAM, Hartog F, van Loon LC. Differential Induction of Systemic Resistance in *Arabidopsis* by Biocontrol Bacteria. Mol Plant-Microbe Interact 1997;10: 716-724.

[120] Kravchenko LV, Leonova EI. Use of Tryptophane from Root Exometabolites for Biosynthesis of Indolil-3-Acetic Acid by the Root-Associated Bacteria. Russian J Microbiol 1993;62: 453–459.

[121] Shtark OY, Shaposhnikov AI, Kravchenko LV. The Production of Antifungal Metabolites by *Pseudomonas chlororaphis* Grown on Different Nutrient Sources. Russian J Microbiol 2003;72(5): 574–578.

[122] Kamilova F, Kravchenko LV, Shaposhnikov AI, Makarova N, Lugtenberg B. Effect of Tomato Pathogen *Fusarium oxysporum* f. sp. *radicis-lycopersici* and Biocontrol Bacterium *Pseudomonas fluorescens* WCS635 on the Composition of Organic Acids and Sugars in Tomato Root Exudates. Mol. Plant-Microbe Interact 2006;19: 1121-1126.

[123] Teplitski M, Robinson JB, Bauer WD. Plants Secrete Substances that mimic Bacterial N-Acyl Homoserine Lactone Signal Activities and Affect Population Density-Dependent Behaviors in Associated Bacteria. Mol Plant-Microbe Interact 2000;13: 637-648.

[124] Hallmann J, Berg G. Spectrum and Population Dynamics of Bacterial Root Endophytes. In: Schulz B, Boyle S, Sieber T (eds) Microbial Root Endophytes. Dordrecht: Springer; 2006. P 15-32.

[125] Van Overbeek LS, van Vuurde J, van Elsas JD. Application of Molecular Fingerprinting Techniques to Explore the Diversity of Bacterial Endophytic Communities. In: Schulz B, Boyle S, Sieber T (eds) Microbial Root Endophytes. Dordrecht: Springer; 2006. P 337-354.

[126] Schulz B, Boyle S, Sieber T. What are Endophytes? In: Schulz B, Boyle S, Sieber T (eds) Microbial Root Endophytes. Dordrecht: Springer; 2006. P 1-14.

[127] Sturz AV, Christie BR, Nowak J. Bacterial Endophytes: Potential Role in Developing Sustainable Systems of Crop Production. Cr Rev Plant Sci 2000;19(1): 1-30.

[128] McCully ME Niches for Bacterial Endophytes in Crop Plants: a Plant Biologists's View. Aust J Plant Physiol 2001;28: 983-990.

[129] Berg G, Hallmann J. Control of Plant Pathogenic Fungi with Bacterial Endophytes. In: Schulz B, Boyle S, Sieber T (eds) Microbial Root Endophytes. Dordrecht: Springer; 2006. P 53–70.

[130] Kloepper JW, Ryu CM. Bacterial Endophytes as Elicitors of Induced Systemic Resistance. In: Schulz B, Boyle S, Sieber T (eds) Microbial Root Endophytes. Dordrecht: Springer; 2006. P 33-52.

[131] Rosenblueth M, Martinez-Romero E. Bacterial Endophytes and their Interactions with Hosts. Mol Plant-Microbe Interact 2006;19: 827-837.

[132] Artursson V, Finlay RD, Jansson JK. Interactions between Arbuscular Mycorrhizal Fungi and Bacteria and Their Potential for Stimulating Plant Growth. Environ Microbiol 2006;8(1): 1-10.

[133] Frey-Klett P, Garbaye J, Tarkka M. The Mycorrhiza Helper Bacteria Revisited. New Phytol 2007;176: 22–36.

[134] Garbaye J. Helper Bacteria: a New Dimension to the Mycorrhizal Symbiosis. New Phytol 1994;128: 197-210.

[135] Hildebrandt U, Ouziad F, Marner FJ, Bothe H. The Bacterium *Paenibacillus validus* Stimulates Growth of the Arbuscular Mycorrhizal fungus *Glomus intraradices* up to the formation of Fertile Spores. FEMS Microbiol Lett 2006;254: 258-267.

[136] Toljander JF, Lindahl BD, Paul LR, Elfstrand M, Finlay RD. Influence of Arbuscular Mycorrhizal Mycelial Exudates on soil Bacterial Growth and Community Structure. FEMS Microbiol Ecol 2007;61: 295–304.

[137] Rambelli A. The Rhizosphere of Mycorrhizae. In: Marks, G.L., and Koslowski, T.T. (eds) Ectomycorrhizae. New York, USA: Academic Press; 1973. P 299–343.

[138] Ibrahim KK, Arunachalam V, Rao PSK, Tilak KVBR. Seasonal Response of Groundnut Genotypes to Arbuscular Mycorrhiza – *Bradyrhizobium* Inoculation. Microbiol Res 1995;150: 218-224.

[139] Jacobi LM, Kukalev AS, Ushakov KV, Tsyganov VE, Provorov NA, Borisov AY, Tikhonovich IA. Genetic Variability of Garden Pea (*Pisum sativum* L.) for Symbiotic Capacities. Pisum Genetics 1999;31: 44-45.

[140] Borisov AY, Tsyganov VE, Shtark OY, Jacobi LM, Naumkina TS, Serdyuk VP, Vishnyakova MA. Pea (Symbiotic effectiveness). In: Tikhonovich IA, Vishnyakova MA. (eds) The Catalogue of World-Wide Collection. Issue 728. Saint Petersburg: VIR; 2002.

[141] Borisov AY, Shtark OY, Danilova TN, Tsyganov VE, Naumkina TS. Effectiviness of Combined Inoculation of Field Peas with Arbuscular Mycorrhizal Fungi and Nodule Bacteria. Russian Agricultural Sciences (Doklady Rossiiskoi Akademii Sel'skohozyaistvennykh Nauk) 2004;4: 5-7.

[142] Labutova NM, Polyakov AI, Lyakh VA, Gordon VL. Influence of Inoculation with Nodule Bacteria and Endomycorrhizal Fungus *Glomus intraradices* on Yield and Seed

Protein and Oil Content of Different Soybean Cultivars. Russian Agricultural Sciences (Doklady Rossiiskoi Akademii Sel'skohozyaistvennykh Nauk) 2004;4(2): 2-4.

[143] Bakker PAHM, Raaijmakers JM, Bloemberg G et al (eds). New Perspectives and Approaches in Plant Growth-Promoting Rhizobacteria Research (Reprinted from Eur J Plant Pathol 2007;119(2)). Dordrecht: Springer; 2007.

[144] Andronov EE, Petrova SN, Chizhevskaya EP, Korostik EV, Akhtemova GA, Pinaev AG. Influence of Introducing the Genetically Modified Strain *Sinorhizobium meliloti* ACH-5 on the Structure of the Soil Microbial Community. Russian J Microbiol 2009;78(4): 474–482.

[145] Pawlowska TE, Taylor JW. Organization of Genetic Variation in Individuals of Arbuscular Mycorrhizal Fungi. Nature 2004;427(6976): 733-737.

[146] Lie TA. Temperature-Dependent Root-Nodule Formation in Pea cv. Iran. Plant Soil 1971;34(3): 751-752.

[147] van Kammen A. Suggested Nomenclature for Plant Genes Involved in Nodulation and Symbiosis. Plant Mol Biol Rep 1984;2: 43-45.

[148] Gianinazzi-Pearson V. Plant Cell Responses to Arbuscular Mycorrhizal Fungi: Getting to the Roots of the Symbiosis. Plant Cell 1996;8(10): 1871-1883.

[149] Kistner C, Winzer T, Pitzschke A, Mulder L, Sato S, Kaneko T, Tabata S, Sandal N, Stougaard J, Webb KJ, Szczyglowski K, Parniske M. Seven *Lotus japonicus* Genes Required for Transcriptional Reprogramming of the Root During Fungal and Bacterial Symbiosis. Plant Cell 2005;17(8): 2217-2229.

[150] Küster H, Vieweg MF, Manthey K, Baier MC, Hohnjec N, Perlick AM. Identification and Expression Regulation of Symbiotically Activated Legume Genes. Phytochemistry 2007;68(1): 8-18.

[151] Albrecht C, Geurts R, Lapeyrie F, Bisseling T. Endomycorrhizae and Rhizobial Nod Factors Both Require SYM8 to Induce the Expression of the Early Nodulin Genes PsENOD5 and PsENOD12A. Plant J 1998;15(5): 605-614.

[152] Kumagai H, Kinoshita E, Ridge RW, Kouchi H. RNAi Knock-Down of ENOD40s Leads to Significant Suppression of Nodule Formation in *Lotus japonicus*. Plant Cell Physiol 2006;47(8): 1102-1111.

[153] Wan X, Hontelez J, Lillo A, Guarnerio C, van de Peut D, Fedorova E, Bisseling T, Franssen H. *Medicago truncatula* ENOD40-1 and ENOD40-2 Are Both Involved in Nodule Initiation and Bacteroid Development. J Exp Bot 2007;58(8): 2033-2041.

[154] Nutman PS. Genetical Factors Concerned in the Symbiosis of Clover and Nodule Bacteria. Nature 1946;157: 463-465.

[155] Jacobsen E. Modification of Symbiotic Interaction of Pea (*Pisum sativum* L.) and *Rhizobium leguminosarum* by Induced Mutations. Plant Soil 1984;82(3): 427-438.

[156] Handberg K, Stougaard J. *Lotus japonicus*, an Autogamous, Diploid Legume Species for Classical and Molecular Genetics. Plant J 1992;2: 487-496.

[157] Barker D, Bianchi S, Blondon F, Dattee Y, Duc G, Essad S, Flament P, Gallusci P, Genier G, Guy P, Muel X, Tourneur J, Denarie J, Huguet T. *Medicago truncatula*, a Model Plant for Studying the Molecular Genetics of the Rhizobium-Legume Symbiosis. Plant Mol Biol Rep 1990;8: 40-49.

[158] Cook DR. *Medicago truncatula* – a Model in the Making. Curr Opin Plant Biol 1999;2(4): 301-304.

[159] Young ND, Mudge J, Ellis THN. Legume Genomes: More Than Peas in a Pod. Curr Opin Plant Biol 2003;6(2): 199-204.

[160] Cook DR, Vandenbosch K, de Brujin FJ, Huguet T. Model Legumes Get the Nod. Plant Cell 1997;9: 275-281.

[161] Udvardi MK. Legume Models Strut Their Stuff. Mol Plant Microbe Interact 2001;14(1): 6-9.

[162] Stougaard J. Genetics and Genomics of Root Symbiosis. Curr Opin Plant Biol 2001;4(4): 328-335.

[163] Penmetsa RV, Cook DR. A Legume Ethylene-Insensitive Mutant Hyperinfected By Its Rhizobial Symbiont. Science 1997;275(5299): 527-530.

[164] Schauser L, Handberg K, Sandal N, Stiller J, Thykjaer T, Pajuelo E, Nielsen A, Stougaard J. Symbiotic Mutants Deficient in Nodule Establishment Identified After T-DNA Transformation of *Lotus japonicus*. Mol Gen Genet 1998;259(4): 414-423.

[165] Albrecht C, Geurts R, Bisseling T. Legume Nodulation and Mycorrhizae Formation; Two Extremes in Host Specificity Meet. EMBO J 1999;18(2): 281-288.

[166] Radutoiu S, Madsen LH, Madsen EB, Felle HH, Umehara Y, Gronlund M, Sato S, Nakamura Y, Tabata S, Sandal N, Stougaard J. Plant Recognition of Symbiotic Bacteria Requires Two LysM Receptor-Like Kinases. Nature 2003;425(6958): 585-592.

[167] Madsen EB, Madsen LH, Radutoiu S, Olbryt M, Rakwalska M, Szczyglowski K, Sato S, Kaneko T, Tabata S, Sandal N, Stougaard J. A Receptor Kinase Gene of the LysM Type Is Involved in Legume Perception of Rhizobial Signals. Nature 2003;425(6958): 637-640.

[168] Limpens E, Franken C, Smit P, Willemse J, Bisseling T, Geurts R. LysM-domain Receptor Kinases Regulating Rhizobial Nod Factor-Induced Infection. Science 2003;302(5645):630-633.

[169] Op den Camp R, Streng A, De Mita S, Cao Q, Polone E, Liu W, Ammiraju JS, Kudrna D, Wing R, Untergasser A, Bisseling T, Geurts R. LysM-type Mycorrhizal Receptor Recruited for Rhizobium Symbiosis in Nonlegume Parasponia. Science 2011;331(6019): 909-912.

[170] Banba M, Gutjahr C, Miyao A, Hirochika H, Paszkowski U, Kouchi H, Imaizumi-Anraku H. Divergence of Evolutionary Ways Among Common Sym Genes: CASTOR

and CCaMK Show Functional Conservation Between Two Symbiosis Systems and Constitute the Root of a Common Signaling Pathway. Plant Cell Physiol 2008;49(11): 1659-1671.

[171] Endre G, Kereszt A, Kevei Z, Mihacea S, Kalo P, Kiss GB. A Receptor Kinase Gene Regulating Symbiotic Nodule Development. Nature 2002;417(6892): 962-966.

[172] Stracke S, Kistner C, Yoshida S, Mulder L, Sato S, Kaneko T, Tabata S, Sandal N, Stougaard J, Szczyglowski K, Parniske M. A Plant Receptor-Like Kinase Required for Both Bacterial and Fungal Symbiosis. Nature 2002;417(6892): 959-962.

[173] Limpens E, Mirabella R, Fedorova E, Franken C, Franssen H, Bisseling T, Geurts R. Formation of Organelle-Like N_2-fixing Symbiosomes in Legume Root Nodules Is Controlled by DMI2. Proc Natl Acad Sci USA 2005; 102(29): 10375-10380.

[174] Kevei Z, Lougnon G, Mergaert P, Horvath GV, Kereszt A, Jayaraman D, Zaman N, Marcel F, Regulski K, Kiss GB, Kondorosi A, Endre G, Kondorosi, E-Ané JM. 3-Hydroxy-3-methylglutaryl Coenzyme A Reductase 1 Interacts with NORK and Is Crucial for Nodulation in *Medicago truncatula*. Plant Cell 2007;19(12): 3974-3989.

[175] Zhu H, Chen T, Zhu M, Fang Q, Kang H, Hong Z, Zhang Z. A Novel ARID DNA-binding Protein Interacts with SymRK and Is Expressed During Early Nodule Development in *Lotus japonicus*. Plant Physiol 2008;148(1): 337-347.

[176] Lefebvre B, Timmers T, Mbengue M, Moreau S, Herve C, Tóth K, Bittencourt-Silvestre J, Klaus D, Deslandes L, Godiard L, Murray JD, Udvardi MK, Raffaele S, Mongrand S, Cullimore J, Gamas P, Niebel A, Ott T. A Remorin Protein Interacts with Symbiotic Receptors and Regulates Bacterial Infection. Proc Natl Acad Sci USA 2010;107(5): 2343-2348.

[177] Yuan S, Zhu H, Gou H, Fu W, Liu L, Chen T, Ke D, Kang H, Xie Q, Hong Z, Zhang Z. A Ubiquitin Ligase of Symbiosis Receptor Kinase Involved in Nodule Organogenesis. Plant Physiol 2012; DOI:10.1104/pp.112.199000.

[178] Wais RJ, Galera C, Oldroyd G, Catoira R, Penmetsa RV, Cook D, Gough C, Dénarié J, Long SR. Genetic Analysis of Calcium Spiking Responses in Nodulation Mutants of *Medicago truncatula*. Proc Natl Acad Sci USA 2000;97(24): 13407-13412.

[179] Ané JM, Kiss GB, Riely BK, Penmetsa RV, Oldroyd GE, Ayax C, Lévy J, Debellé F, Baek JM, Kalo P, Rosenberg C, Roe BA, Long SR, Dénarié J, Cook DR. *Medicago truncatula* DMI1 Required for Bacterial and Fungal Symbioses in Legumes. Science 2004;303(5662): 1364-1367.

[180] Imaizumi-Anraku H, Takeda N, Charpentier M, Perry J, Miwa H, Umehara Y, Kouchi H, Murakami Y, Mulder L, Vickers K, Pike J, Downie JA, Wang T, Sato S, Asamizu E, Tabata S, Yoshikawa M, Murooka Y, Wu GJ, Kawaguchi M, Kawasaki S, Parniske M, Hayashi M. Plastid Proteins Crucial for Symbiotic Fungal and Bacterial Entry into Plant Roots. Nature 2005;433(7025):527-531.

[181] Edwards A, Heckmann AB, Yousafzai F, Duc G, Downie JA. Structural Implications of Mutations in the Pea SYM8 Symbiosis Gene, the DMI1 Ortholog, Encoding a Predicted Ion Channel. Mol Plant Microbe Interact 2007;20(10): 1183-1191.

[182] Riely BK, Lougnon G, Ané JM, Cook DR. The Symbiotic Ion Channel Homolog DMI1 Is Localized in the Nuclear Membrane of *Medicago truncatula* Roots. Plant J 2007;49(2): 208-216.

[183] Peiter E, Sun J, Heckmann AB, Venkateshwaran M, Riely BK, Otegui MS, Edwards A, Freshour G, Hahn MG, Cook DR, Sanders D, Oldroyd GE, Downie JA, Ané JM. The *Medicago truncatula* DMI1 Protein Modulates Cytosolic Calcium Signaling. Plant Physiol 2007;145(1): 192-203.

[184] Kanamori N, Madsen LH, Radutoiu S, Frantescu M, Quistgaard EMH, Miwa H, Downie JA, James EK, Felle HH, Haaning LL, Jensen TH, Sato S, Nakamura Y, Tabata S, Sandal N, Stougaard J. A Nucleoporin Is Required for Induction of Ca^{2+} Spiking in Legume Nodule Development and Essential for Rhizobial and Fungal Symbiosis. Proc Natl Acad Sci USA 2006;103(2): 359-364.

[185] Saito K, Yoshikawa M, Yano K, Miwa H, Uchida H, Asamizu E, Sato S, Tabata S, Imaizumi-Anraku H, Umehara Y, Kouchi H, Murooka Y, Szczyglowski K, Downie JA, Parniske M, Hayashi M, Kawaguchi M. NUCLEOPORIN85 Is Required for Calcium Spiking, Fungal and Bacterial Symbioses, and Seed Production in *Lotus japonicus*. Plant Cell 2007;19(2): 610-624.

[186] Groth M, Takeda N, Perry J, Uchida H, Draxl S, Brachmann A, Sato S, Tabata S, Kawaguchi M, Wang TL, Parniske M. NENA, a *Lotus japonicus* Homolog of Sec13, is Required for Rhizodermal Infection by Arbuscular Mycorrhiza Fungi and Rhizobia But Dispensable for Cortical Endosymbiotic Development. Plant Cell 2010;22(7): 2509-2526.

[187] Oldroyd GE, Downie JA. Calcium, Kinases and Nodulation Signalling in Legumes. Nat Rev Mol Cell Biol 2004;5(7): 566-576.

[188] Catoira R, Galera C, de Billy F, Penmetsa RV, Journet EP, Maillet F, Rosenberg C, Cook D, Gough C, Denarie J. Four Genes of *Medicago truncatula* Controlling Components of a Nod Factor Transduction Pathway. Plant Cell 2000;12(9): 1647-1665.

[189] Gleason C, Chaudhuri S, Yang T, Munoz A, Poovaiah BW, Oldroyd GE. Nodulation Independent of Rhizobia Induced by a Calcium-Activated Kinase Lacking Autoinhibition. Nature 2006;441(7097): 1149-1152.

[190] Sanchez L, Weidmann S, Arnould C, Bernard AR, Gianinazzi S, Gianinazzi-Pearson V. *Pseudomonas fluorescens* and *Glomus mosseae* Trigger *DMI3*-Dependent Activation of Genes Related to a Signal Transduction Pathway in Roots of *Medicago truncatula.* Plant Physiol 2005;139(2): 1065-1077.

[191] Yano K, Yoshida S, Muller J, Singh S, Banba M, Vicker K. CYCLOPS, a Mediator of Symbiotic Intracellular Accommodation. Proc Natl Acad Sci USA 2008;105(51): 20540-20545.

[192] Kaló P, Gleason C, Edwards A, Marsh J, Mitra RM, Hirsch S, Jakab J, Sims S, Long SR, Rogers J, Kiss GB, Downie JA, Oldroyd GE. Nodulation Signaling in Legumes Requires NSP2, a Member of the GRAS Family of Transcriptional Regulators. Science 2005;308(5729): 1786-1789.

[193] Smit P, Raedts J, Portyanko V, Debellé F, Gough C, Bisseling T, Geurts R. NSP1 of the GRAS Protein Family Is Essential for Rhizobial Nod Factor-Induced Transcription. Science 2005;308(5729): 1789-1791.

[194] Heckmann AB, Lombardo F, Miwa H, Perry JA, Bunnewell S, Parniske M, Wang TL, Downie JA. *Lotus japonicus* Nodulation Requires Two GRAS Domain Regulators, One of Which Is Functionally Conserved in a Non-Legume. Plant Physiol 2006;142(4): 1739-1750.

[195] Murakami Y, Miwa H, Imaizumi-Anraku H, Kouchi H, Downie JA, Kawasaki KMS. Positional cloning identifies *Lotus japonicus* NSP2, a Putative Transcription Factor of the GRAS Family, Required for NIN and ENOD40 Gene Expression in Nodule Initiation. DNA Res 2006;13: 255-265.

[196] Gonzalez-Rizzo S, Crespi M, Frugier F. The *Medicago truncatula* CRE1 Cytokinin Receptor Regulates Lateral Root Development and Early Symbiotic Interaction with *Sinorhizobium meliloti*. Plant Cell 2006;18(10): 2680-2693.

[197] Murray JD, Karas BJ, Sato S, Tabata S, Amyot L, Szczyglowski K. A Cytokinin Perception Mutant Colonized by *Rhizobium* in the Absence of Nodule Organogenesis. Science 2007;315(5808): 101-104.

[198] Tirichine L, Sandal N, Madsen LH, Radutoiu S, Albrektsen AS, Sato S, Asamizu E, Tabata S, Stougaard J. A Gain-of-Function Mutation in a Cytokinin Receptor Triggers Spontaneous Root Nodule Organogenesis. Science 2007;315(5808): 104-107.

[199] Schauser L, Roussis A, Stiller J, Stougaard J. A Plant Regulator Controlling Development of Symbiotic Root Nodules. Nature 1999;402(6758): 191-195.

[200] Borisov AY, Madsen LH, Tsyganov VE, Umehara Y, Voroshilova VA, Batagov AO, Sandal N, Mortensen A, Schauser L, Ellis N, Tikhonovich IA, Stougaard J. The *Sym35* Gene Required for Root Nodule Development in Pea Is an Ortholog of *Nin* from *Lotus japonicus*. Plant Physiol 2003;131(3): 1009-1017.

[201] Marsh JF, Rakocevic A, Mitra RM, Brocard L, Sun J, Eschstruth A, Long SR, Schultze M, Ratet P, Oldroyd GE. *Medicago truncatula* NIN Is Essential for Rhizobial-Independent Nodule Organogenesis Induced by Autoactive Calcium/Calmodulin-Dependent Protein Kinase. Plant Physiol 2007;144(1): 324-335.

[202] Middleton PH, Jakab J, Penmetsa RV, Starker CG, Doll J, Kalo P, Prabhu R, Marsh JF, Mitra RM, Kereszt A, Dudas B, VandenBosch K, Long SR, Cook DR, Kiss GB, Oldroyd GE. An ERF Transcription Factor in *Medicago truncatula* That Is Essential for Nod Factor Signal Transduction. Plant Cell 2007;19(4): 1221-1234.

[203] Caetano-Anolles G, Gresshoff PM. Plant Genetic Control of Nodulation. Annu Rev Microbiol 1991;45: 345-382.

[204] Ferguson BJ, Indrasumunar A, Hayashi S, Lin MH, Lin YH, Reid DE, Gresshoff PM. Molecular Analysis of Legume Nodule Development and Autoregulation. J Integr Plant Biol 2010;52(1): 61-76.

[205] Okamoto S, Ohnishi E, Sato S, Takahashi H, Nakazono M, Tabata S, Kawaguchi M. Nod Factor/Nitrate-Induced CLE Genes That Drive HAR1-Mediated Systemic Regulation of Nodulation. Plant Cell Physiol 2009;50(1): 67-77.

[206] Mortier V, Den Herder G, Whitford R, Van de Velde W, Rombauts S, D'Haeseleer K, Holsters M, Goormachtig S. CLE Peptides Control *Medicago truncatula* Nodulation Locally and Systemically. Plant Physiol 2010;153(1): 222-237.

[207] Krusell L, Madsen LH, Sato S, Aubert G, Genua A, Szczyglowski K, Duc G, Kaneko T, Tabata S,de Bruijn F, Pajuelo E, Sandal N, Stougaard J. Shoot Control of Root Development and Nodulation Is Mediated by a Receptor-Like Kinase. Nature 2002;420(6914): 422-426.

[208] Nishimura R, Hayashi M, Wu GJ, Kouchi H, Imaizumi-Anraku H, Murakami Y, Kawasaki S, Akao S, Ohmori M, Nagasawa M, Harada K, Kawaguchi M. HAR1 Mediates Systemic Regulation of Symbiotic Organ Development. Nature 2002;420(6914): 426-429.

[209] Schnabel E, Journet EP, de Carvalho-Niebel F, Duc G, Frugoli J. The *Medicago truncatula* SUNN Gene Encodes a CLV1-like leucine-Rich Repeat Receptor Kinase That Regulates Nodule Number and Root Length. Plant Mol Biol 2005;58(6):809-822.

[210] Staehelin C, Xie ZP, Illana A, Vierheilig H. Long-Distance Transport of Signals During Symbiosis: Are Nodule Formation and Mycorrhization Autoregulated in a Similar Way? Plant Signal Behav 2011;6(3): 372-377.

[211] Nishimura R, Ohmori M, Fujita H, Kawaguchi M. A *Lotus* Basic Leucine Zipper Protein with a RING-Finger Motif Negatively Regulates the Developmental Program of Nodulation. Proc Natl Acad Sci USA 2002;99(23): 15206-15210.

[212] Oka-Kira E, Tateno K, Miura K, Haga T, Hayashi M, Harada K, Sato S, Tabata S, Shikazono N, Tanaka A, Watanabe Y, Fukuhara I, Nagata T, Kawaguchi M. klavier (klv), a Novel Hypernodulation Mutant of *Lotus japonicus* Affected in Vascular Tissue Organization and Floral Induction. Plant J 2005;44(3): 505-515.

[213] Magori S, Oka-Kira E, Shibata S, Umehara Y, Kouchi H, Hase Y, Tanaka A, Sato S, Tabata S, Kawaguchi M. Too Much Love, a Root Regulator Associated with the Long-Distance Control of Nodulation in *Lotus japonicus*. Mol Plant Microbe Interact 2009;22(3): 259-268.

[214] Schnabel EL, Kassaw TK, Smith LS, Marsh JF, Oldroyd GE, Long SR, Frugoli JA. The ROOT DETERMINED NODULATION1 Gene Regulates Nodule Number in Roots of

Medicago truncatula and Defines a Highly Conserved, Uncharacterized Plant Gene Family. Plant Physiol 2011;157(1): 328-340.

[215] Catford JG, Staehelin C, Lerat S, Piché Y, Vierheilig H. Suppression of Arbuscular Mycorrhizal Colonization and Nodulation in Split-Root Systems of Alfalfa after Pre-Inoculation and Treatment with Nod Factors. J Exp Bot 2003;54(386): 1481-1487.

[216] Grunwald U, Nyamsuren O, Tarnasloukht M, Lapopin L, Becker A, Mann P, Gianinazzi-Pearson V, Krajinski F, Franken P. Identification of Mycorrhiza-Regulated Genes with Arbuscule Development-Related Expression Profile. Plant Mol Biol 2004;55(4): 553-566.

[217] Gianinazzi-Pearson V, Brechenmacher L. Functional Genomics of Arbuscular Mycorrhiza: Decoding the Symbiotic Cell Programme. Canad J Bot 2004;82(8): 1228-1234.

[218] Seddas PMA, Arnould C, Tollot M, Arias CM, Gianinazzi-Pearson V. Spatial Monitoring of Gene Activity in Extraradical and Intraradical Developmental Stages of Arbuscular Mycorrhizal Fungi by Direct Fluorescent in situ RT-PCR. Fungal Gen Biol 2008;45(8): 1155-1165.

[219] Seddas PM, Arias CM, Arnould C, van Tuinen D, Godfroy O, Benhassou HA, Gouzy J, Morandi D, Dessaint F, Gianinazzi-Pearson V. Symbiosis-Related Plant Genes Modulate Molecular Responses in an Arbuscular Mycorrhizal Fungus During Early Root Interactions. Mol Plant Microbe Interact 2009;22(3): 341-351.

[220] Kuznetsova E, Seddas-Dozolme PM, Arnould C, Tollot M, van Tuinen D, Borisov A, Gianinazzi S, Gianinazzi-Pearson V. Symbiosis-Related Pea Genes Modulate Fungal and Plant Gene Expression During the Arbuscule Stage of Mycorrhiza with *Glomus intraradices*. Mycorrhiza 2010;20(6): 427-443.

[221] Sulieman S, Schulze J. The Efficiency of Nitrogen Fixation of the Model Legume *Medicago truncatula* (Jemalong A17) Is Low Compared to *Medicago sativa*. J Plant Physiol 2010;167(9): 683-692.

[222] Duc G, Trouvelot A, Gianinazzi-Pearson V, Gianinazzi S. First Report of Non-Mycorrhizal Plant Mutants (Myc$^-$) Obtained in Pea (*Pisum sativum* L.) and Faba Bean (*Vicia faba* L.). Plant Sci 1989;60(2): 215-222.

[223] Frühling M, Roussel H, Gianinazzi-Pearson V, Pühler A, Perlick AM. The *Vicia faba* Leghemoglobin Gene VfLb29 Is Induced in Root Nodules and in Roots Colonized by the Arbuscular Mycorrhizal Fungus *Glomus fasciculatum*. Mol Plant Microbe Interact 1997;10(1): 124-131.

[224] Xavier IJ, Holloway G, Leggett M Development of Rhizobial Inoculant Formulations. Crop Management (Online) 2004; doi:10.1094/CM-2004-0301-06-RV.

[225] Rai MK., editor. Handbook of microbial biofertilizers. New York: Haworth Press, Technology & Engineering; 2006.

[226] Tikhonovich IA, Provorov NA. Cooperation of Plants and Microorganisms: Getting Closer to the Genetic Construction of Sustainable Agro-Systems. Biotechnol J 2007;2(7): 833-848.

[227] Shtark OY, Danilova TN, Naumkina TS, Vasilchikov AG, Chebotar VK, Kazakov AE, Zhernakov AI, Nemankin TA, Prilepskaya NA, Borisov AY, Tikhonovich IA. Analysis of Pea (*Pisum sativum* L.) Source Material for Breeding of Cultivars with High Symbiotic Potential and Choice of Criteria for Its Evaluation. Ecological genetics ("Ekologicheskaja genetika") 2006;4(2): 22-28 (In Russian).

[228] Chebotar VK, Kazakov AE, Erofeev SV, Danilova TN, Naumkina TS, Shtark OY, Tikhonovich IA, Borisov AY. Method of Production of Complex Microbial Fertilizer. Patent No 2318784. 2008.

[229] Prévost D, Antoun H. Potential Use of Rhizobium as PGPR with Non-Legumes: Abstracts from the Inoculant Forum, March 17-18, 2005. Saskatoon, Saskatchewan, Canada.

[230] Hossain MS, Mårtensson A. Potential Use of *Rhizobium* spp. to Improve Fitness of Non-Nitrogen-Fixing Plants. Acta Agriculturae Scandinavica, Section B – Plant Soil Science 2008;58(4): 352-358.

[231] Gentili F, Jumpponen A. Potential and Possible Uses of Bacterial and Fungal Biofertilizers. In: Rai MK. (ed.) Handbook of Microbial Biofertilizers. New York: Haworth Press, Technology & Engineering; 2006. p1-28.

[232] Galvan GA, Burger-Meijer K, Kuiper TW, Kik C, Scholten OE. Breeding for Improved Responsiveness to Arbuscular Mycorrhizal Fungi in Onion. Proceedings of 3rd International Congress of the European Integrated Project Quality Low Input Food (QLIF) Congress, Hohenheim, Germany, March 20–23, 2007. (Online) http://orgprints.org/view/projects/int_conf_qlif2007.html

[233] Herridge D, Rose I. Breeding for Enhanced Nitrogen Fixation in Crop Legumes. Field Crops Res 2000;65: 229-248.

[234] Rengel Z. Breeding for Better Symbiosis. Plant Soil 2002;245(1): 147-162.

[235] Graham PH, Hungria M, Tlusty B. Breeding for Better Nitrogen Fixation in Grain Legumes: Where Do the Rhizobia Fit In? Crop Management 2004; doi:10.1094/CM-2004-0301-02-RV.

[236] Howieson JG, Yates RJ, Foster KJ, Real D, Besier RB. Prospects for the Future Uses of Legumes. In: Dilworth MJ, James EK, Sprent JI, Newton WE. (eds) Nitrogen Fixing Leguminous Symbioses. Berlin/Heidelberg: Springer Science+Business Media BV; 2008. p363-394.

[237] Borisov AY, Danilova TN, Shtark OY, Solovov II, Kazakov AE, Naumkina TS, Vasilchikov AG, Chebotar VK, Tikhonovich IA. Tripartite Symbiotic System of Pea (*Pisum sativum* L.): Applications in Sustainable Agriculture. In: FD Dakora, BM Chimphango,

AJ Valentine, C Elmerich, WE Newton (eds) Biological Nitrogen Fixation: Towards Poverty Alleviation Through Sustainable Agriculture. Proceedings of 15th International Congress on Nitrogen Fixation & 12th International Conference of the African Association for Biological Nitrogen Fixation. Berlin/Heidelberg: Springer Science and Business Media BV; 2008. p15-17.

[238] Bourion V, Rizvi SM, Fournier S, de Larambergue H, Galmiche F, Marget P, Duc G, Burstin J. Genetic Dissection of Nitrogen Nutrition in Pea Through a QTL Approach of Root, Nodule, and Shoot Variability. Theor Appl Genet 2010;121(1): 71-86.

[239] Tominaga A, Gondo T, Akashi R, Zheng SH, Arima S, Suzuki A. Quantitative Trait Locus Analysis of Symbiotic Nitrogen Fixation Activity in the Model Legume *Lotus japonicus*. J Plant Res 2012;125(3): 395-406.

Chapter 8

Opium Poppy: Genetic Upgradation Through Intervention of Plant Breeding Techniques

Brij Kishore Mishra, Anu Rastogi, Ameena Siddiqui, Mrinalini Srivastava, Nidhi Verma, Rawli Pandey, Naresh Chandra Sharma and Sudhir Shukla

Additional information is available at the end of the chapter

http://dx.doi.org/10.5772/53132

1. Introduction

Opium poppy (*Papaver somniferum* L.) has its importance as a plant based natural pain reliever from the time dating back to early civilization till today. Its pain relieving properties had been described in various books of unani, allopathy and ayurvedic medication system. Today our pharmaceutical industries solely depend on opium poppy for their crude resources for manufacturing of pain killing drugs. The medical practitioners around the world routinely prescribe important life saving drugs, are the secondary metabolites produced as a result of complex plant metabolism. The important life saving drugs are mostly derived from five major alkaloids viz., morphine, codeine, thebaine, noscapine and papaverine which are present in opium latex in ample amount [1]. According to a report from an international organization i.e. WHO (World Health Organization), about 85% of the population in developing countries depend on herbal plants for curatives, medicinal and other medico related applications. India being one of the twelve mega biodiversity centers of the world is fully fledged with diverse array of herbal and medicinal plants which makes it "Botanical Garden of World". About 10,000 different medicinal plant species are found in India among which opium poppy occupies the highest place in terms of food (seeds) and pharmaceuticals (alkaloids). These valuable alkaloids are mainly extracted in India from green unripe capsules by making incision upto 1-2 mm in the epidermal wall of the capsule (Figure 1), but globally it is extracted from the dried capsule which is called CPS (Concentrated poppy straw) system. In CPS system, the dried capsules along with eight inches of peduncle are harvested and seeds are threshed. The remaining husk is used to extract various alkaloids. The whole plant parts of opium poppy are valuable in terms of food, medicine, vegetable and as brewages. The seeds of opium poppy are highly nutritious as it contains protein upto 24% and other vital nutrients beneficial for human health. The leaves of the plant are used as vegetable in some places in the world. The seed oil of poppy is also important for health point of view due to having high percentage of linoleic acid (68%) which helps in lowering blood cholesterol level in human body and is also used in the treatment of cardiovascular diseases in human system [2,3].

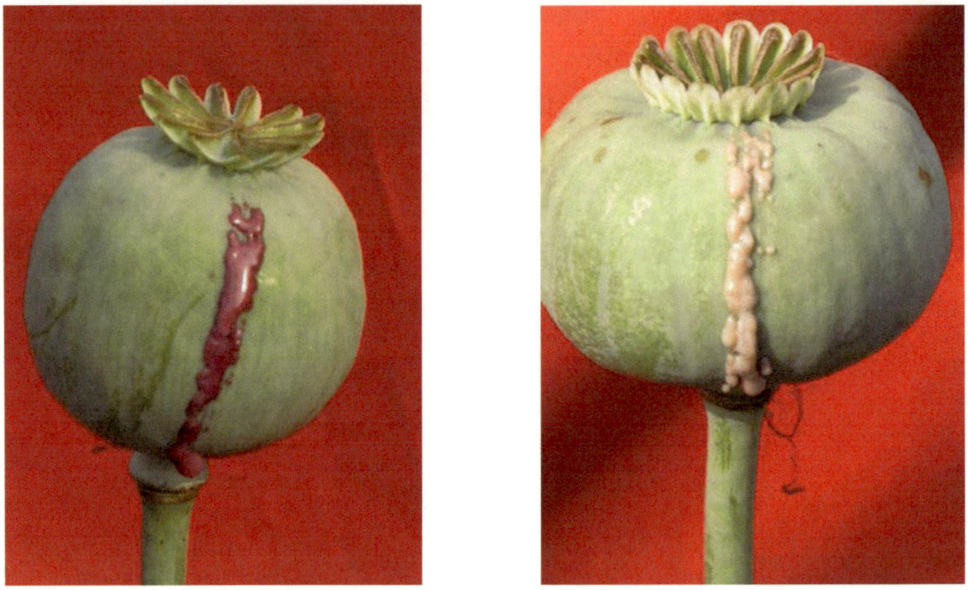

Red Latex Pink Latex

Figure 1. Capsule having brown and pink latex in opium poppy.

2. Geographical distribution

In India, the main opium cultivating areas are divided into 12 divisions including Madhya Pradesh, Uttar Pradesh and Rajasthan while in other parts minor cultivation is also practiced (Figure 2). In Uttar Pradesh, the opium cultivation belt is around Barabanki, Shahjahanpur, Faizabad and Bareilly while Ratlam, Mandsaur and Neemuch in Madhya Pradesh are major opium producing areas. Kota, Chittorgarh and Jhalawar in Rajasthan are the areas producing opium. The opium poppy is distributed in the temperate and subtropical regions of the old world extending from 60° North West Soviet Union whereas the southern limit reach almost the tropics. Legally it is cultivated in India, China, USSR, Egypt, Yugoslavia, Czechoslovakia, Poland, Germany, Netherland, Japan, Argentina, Spain, Bulgaria, Hungary and Poland [4, 5]. India is the largest opium producing and exporting country in the world. Globally the licit opium poppy cultivation is under the strict control of Central Bureau of

Narcotics with its headquarter at Vienna, Austria. But at some places illegal cultivation is also being practiced which include Golden Crescent (Iran, Afghanistan and Pakistan) and Golden Triangle (Thailand, Burma, Myanmar). In Afghanistan, illegal cultivation of opium poppy to a large extent is the reason for very high drug trafficking compared with other illegal cultivating areas. Eleven other countries i.e. Australia, Austria, France, China, Hungary, the Netherlands, Poland, Slovenia, Spain, Turkey and Czech Republic also cultivate opium poppy, but they do not extract gum. They cut the bulb with 8" of the stalk (CPS system) for processing to extract alkaloids (Described earlier).

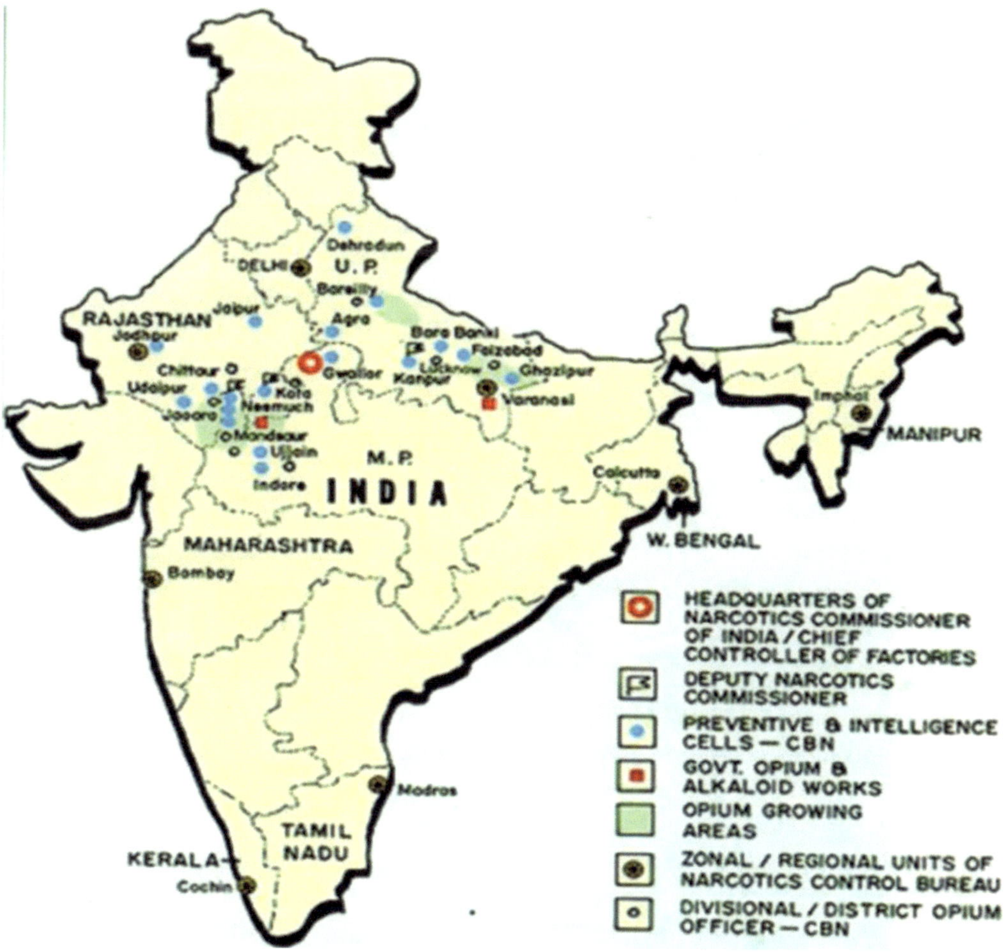

Figure 2. Opium cultivating areas in India and different offices of Narcotics Deptt. Cited from: http://www.uwmc.uwc.edu/academics/departments/political_science/opiumprod.html#map

3. Economic importance of opium poppy and its derivatives

Opium poppy belongs to the family Papaveracae and has been attracting the interest of researchers because of its pharmaceutical, decorative and alimentary attributes. Scientists have been able to identify 2500 different compounds in opium poppy belonging to different biochemical groups used in pharmaceutical industries. Among the various drugs of medicinal importance, opioids are an important class of compounds produced by opium poppy which are used in medicine as a pain reliever. These opioids interact with the opioid receptor present in the central nervous system and gastro-intestinal tract [6]. However, several of these medicinal compounds can be made synthetically but alkaloids belonging to various groups viz., Phenanthredene (Morphine, Codeine, Thebaine), the true Benzylisoquinilone (Papaverine) and Phthalideisoquinilone (Narcotine) are only obtained from opium which place opium poppy at the highest place among the diverse array of medicinal plants [7]. The most important and potent alkaloid is morphine which can be used for both short term as well as long term pain control, is widely used in many prescriptions of pain medications. The drug occurs as a white crystalline powder or colorless crystals and is available for legal medical use. Recently, scientists at the University of Pennsylvania have noticed complication in patient with hepatitis C disease due to withdrawal of morphine as it suppresses IFN-alpha-mediated immunity and enhances virus replication. This disease is common among intravenous drug users. Due to the interactive role of morphine with hepatitis C disease, interest has been developed in determining the effect of drug abuse, especially morphine and heroin on progression of the disease. The discovery of the association between two would certainly help in the treatment of both HCV infection and drug abuse [8]. Morphine is also beneficial for immediate relief in reducing the symptoms of shortness of breath caused due to cancer and non-cancerous incident [9, 10]. Morphine is widely available in market as tablets, modified release-tablets, capsules, oral liquid and sachets of modified-release oral liquid, injections and suppository [11]. There are however, many serious side effects of morphine which includes shallow breathing, slow heartbeat, stiff muscles, seizure (convulsions), unusual thoughts or behavior, severe weakness, constipation etc.

Another important alkaloid is codeine which is considered as a prodrug because it is converted into morphine and codeine-6-glucuronide (C6G) in *in vivo* [12, 13]. Codeine is a natural isomer of morphine and is formulated as 3-methyl morphine. In *in vivo* system, 5-10% of codeine is metabolized into morphine, while remaining is left free or in conjugated system as codeine-6-glucuronide (~70%), or it is converted into norcodeine (~10%) and hydromorphone (~1%). Codeine is less effective and has lower dependence-liability than morphine [13]. Similar to all other opioids, continuous use of codeine induces physical dependence and it can be psychologically addictive. However, mild effects are caused due to its withdrawal, so is less addictive than other opiates. Codeine is also used as antitussive drug against coughing and widely used in the treatment of severe diarrhea and diarrhea predominant bowel syndrome. The most frequently used drug forms are "loperamide, diphenoxylate, paregoric and laudanum [14, 15]. In addition to analgesic and antitussive effect there are some side effects of codeine which includes euphoria, itching, drowsiness, vomiting, orthostatic hypotension, urinary retention, depression and constipation [16]. One of the most serious adverse effects includes respiratory depression [17]. Another alkaloid thebaine is also produced which is non-narcotic in nature can also be used as an analgesic. It is used for the production of oxycodone and other semi-synthetic analgesic opiates [18, 19]. Higher doses of thebaine cause convulsions similar to that of strychnine poisoning [20]. Another important constituent in opium latex is noscapine which is used in relieving cough and headache. Researchers are continuously investigating of its use in treatment of several cancers and hypoxic ischemia in stroke patients. In the treatment of cancers, noscapine appears to interfere with the functioning of microtubule and thus in division of cancer cells while in treatment of stroke patients, noscapine seems to block the bradykinine β-2 receptors which help in recovery from the disease. Early studies in the treatment of prostate cancer are very promising [21]. Scientists have found a noticeable decrease in mortality in patients treated with noscapine [22]. Noscapine is non-addictive, widely available, has low incidence of side effect and can be easily administered orally, prompting a huge potential for its use in developing countries. An important member of Benzylisoquinilone group 'Papaverine' is also an important alkaloid produced by opium poppy. Papaverine is used in the treatment of spasms of the gastrointestinal tract, bile ducts and ureter. It is also used as a cerebral and coronary vasodilator in subarachnoid hemorrhage (combined with balloon angioplasty) and coronary artery bypass surgery [21, 23-25]. Papaverine is also used as an erectile dysfunction drug alone or sometimes in combination with phentolamine [26, 27]. During microsurgery, papaverine is used as a smooth muscle relaxant and is directly applied to blood vessels [28, 29]. It is also applied in cryopreservation of blood vessels along with other glycosaminoglycans and protein suspensions [21, 30]. Papaverine also functions as a vasodilator during cryopreservation when used in conjunction with verapamil, phentolamine, nifedipine, tolazoline or nitroprusside [22, 31]. Scientists are continuously investigating for its use as a topical growth factor in tissue expansion with some success [23]. All these effects of papaverine are attributed to its inhibitory effect on phosphodiesterases [32]. Though papaverine has such extra ordinary attributes but has some common side effects which include polymorphic ventricular tachycardia, constipation, increased transaminase levels, increased alkaline phosphatase levels, somnolence and vertigo. The area under poppy cultivation varied according to the total demand of opium put through the United Nation. India is one of the largest producer and exporter of licit opium and produces about half the opium utilized by the world's pharmaceutical industries.

Keeping in mind, the enormous importance of opium poppy among the diverse array of medicinal plants, researchers were encouraged to work for its genetical improvement. Researchers engaged in opium poppy researches are continuously working to develop designer plants having all specific alkaloids in latex in large quantities. Previously, both conventional and molecular approaches have been applied to develop varieties rich in specific alkaloids. This chapter deals a detailed account (in different subheadings) of the conventional breeding techniques applied to upgrade the latex and alkaloid status along with its nutritional content in opium poppy.

4. Breeding objectives

Since, opium poppy is widely and commonly used for dual purpose i.e. food (seed) and pharmaceuticals (alkaloids) so the major emphasis has been given for its genetical upgradation on both these aspects. The different breeding objectives are depicted in following subheadings.

4.1. Breeding for modified opium yield, seed yield and specific alkaloid variety

Due to ever increasing global demand of opium latex raised by the pharmaceutical industries for manufacturing of life saving drugs, scientists/plant breeders took the challenge of developing high opium yielding varieties. However, they have been able to develop several high opium yielding varieties, but yet it is not able to fulfill the pressure created due to enhance global demand raised as a consequence of population growth. At present our scientists have been able to discover more than 80 alkaloids of immense medicinal importance. Despite of their best possible efforts to identify more and more alkaloids, the demand for five major alkaloids i.e. morphine, codeine, thebaine, narcotine and papaverine have elevated due to major application in medical field. The importance of these five major alkaloids has been discussed earlier. Previously, morphine being the main pain killer was in high demand, for which our scientist made great success in development of high morphine containing varieties. But now a days, the demand for specific alkaloids i.e. thebaine, codeine, narcotine and papaverine have arisen due to their specific use in different medical treatments. The scientists are now trying to develop varieties with specific alkaloid in opium latex through conventional and molecular techniques. Opium poppy is a narcotic crop, due to the presence of morphine (narcotic constituent) in major proportion of opium latex. In recent days, scientists are working to develop low morphine or morphine less varieties to check its illegal cultivation. The development of low morphine or morphine less varieties can also help Narcotics Department, as it will not require issuing license for growing opium poppy to the cultivators. Globally, different group of researchers are engaged in this direction using both conventional and molecular approaches.

Poppy seeds having high nutritive values are also in high demand and major emphasis has been given for the development of food grade poppy which can only be possible, if opiumless poppy varieties can be developed. Both conventional and molecular approaches are being applied aiming at this target, fortunately a variety "Sujata" has been developed by Central Institute of Medicinal and Aromatic Plants, Lucknow [33]. The development of such varieties can assist opium cultivators to grow food grade poppy without any restriction or permission in form of license. Seeds of opium poppy have high value in global market which puts a great pressure on plant breeders to develop high seed yielding varieties that can substantiate the ever increasing global demands. The importance of poppy seeds has been described earlier in details. However, many high seed yielding varieties have been developed but since global population is increasing at an enormous rate, plant breeders are continuously putting their best possible efforts to capture this ever increasing demand.

4.2. Breeding for disease resistant variety, causal organism and their management

Diseases are major problem in cultivation of any crop. The development of multiple disease resistant varieties is in need from very long time in opium poppy. A number of diseases occur which ruins the entire crop and ultimately the opium products. Several researchers especially plant breeders have faced many challenges during specific breeding objectives due to severe disease in opium poppy. Our scientists have put their best possible efforts and continuously trying to develop such varieties resistant to major diseases through molecular and conventional tools. One of the major hindrances in any successful breeding program is the prevalence of certain fungal, bacterial, insect borne diseases etc., which cause an unexpected loss in terms of productivity. Opium poppy crop is highly susceptible to certain diseases but the most contagious diseases are caused by fungus results high losses in yield.

Some commonly found fungal, bacterial, viral and pest related diseases in opium poppy are summarized below:-

Downy Mildew: The causal agent for this most serious and widely spread disease of opium poppy is *Peronospora arborescens*. The symptoms include hypertrophy and curvature of the stem and flower stalks. The infection starts spreading upwards from the lower leaves and the entire leaf surface gets covered by brown powder. The plants dies prematurely as the stem, branches and even capsules are also attacked by this causal organism. In India, the disease appears annually on the crop from seedling to maturity stage mainly in the areas of Madhya Pradesh, Uttar Pradesh and Rajasthan. Capsule formation is also adversely affected due to infection causing significant reduction in opium yield. The primary inoculum of the pathogen is oospore which is present in infested soil and leaf debris introgresses through underground plant parts and infects the plant giving rise to stunting and chlorotic syndrome etc in the fields of opium poppy [34]. The major control measures of the disease include disinfection and spraying of the seed beds with 0.5% Bordeaux mixture and different copper containing fungicides. Some other control measures include use of Bisdithane (0.15%) followed by Benlate (0.05%), Gramisan, dusting with Thiram. **Powdery Mildew:** This disease is caused by *Erysiphae polygoni* and causes severe losses in opium production. It caused severe damage to poppy in Rajasthan in 1972. The symptoms appear in late stages of plant growth with white powder on the surface of leaves and capsules. The control measures include field sanitation along with spray of Spersul (0.5%) and seed disinfection. **Collar Rot disease:** This is one of the most severe fungal diseases of opium poppy caused by *Rhizoctonia solani* Kühn. Decline in seed yield, premature death of infected plant appears with the progress of disease in plants [35].

Seed borne diseases: Seed borne diseases are also a curse to opium poppy crop both in terms of production and yield. The major effect of seed borne disease is on capsules and seeds only, which results reduction in germination percentage and seedling delays. Some commonly spreading seed borne diseases have been discussed. **Leaf Blight** (causal agent - *Pleospora calvescens*): Symptoms include defused yellow spots followed by premature drying of infected leaves. During the course of pathogenesis, toxins are released by the parasites enabling it to assimilate the requisite nutrient. High temperature and heavy rainfall favors the disease. **Seedling Blight** (causal agents - *Phytium ultimum* and *Phytium mamimmatum*): Few studies undertaken on characterization of the disease revealed that the disease affects physiological process in poppy. However, no control measures could be found with total control effects. **Leaf Spots** (causal agent - *Helminthosporium sps.*): The main symptoms include dechlorosis of the leaves accompanied by curling. The disease is not of much importance, but due to correlation between opium alkaloids and leaf spot, it may be considered harmful. Several control measures to control the disease include seed disinfection or spraying of seed beds with 0.5% Bordeaux or any other copper fungicides, incorporation of lime as $CaCO_3$ at 285 kg/ha, Systox, Ogranol, borate and manganese superphosphate, germisan, Gramisan and spray of Bavistin. **Wilt & Root Rot** (causal agent - *Fusarium semitectum*): This is another major problem in poppy cultivation where plants in advance stage rapidly wilt due to desiccation. The infection appears at the stem base followed by damping of roots. The disease causes reduction in opium yield and can be controlled only by the removal of infected plants.

Diseases caused by bacteria: It would be worthwhile if there is a lack of description of bacterial disease in opium poppy. Since the bacteria are ubiquitous in nature, opium poppy is also not left by bacterial infection where heavy losses occur. Systemic infection prevails with the entry of bacterium through stomata and aquapores in later stage of growth. Multiplication of the bacterium starts in vascular system. Seeds are malformed and discolored as a result of infection. Plant parts are also damaged due to bacterial infection.

Diseases caused by viruses: There are certain viral diseases in opium poppy which are caused by Cabbage ring spot virus, beat yellow virus etc., which are transmitted through beans, sap, aphids etc. The symptoms include yellowing of plants, elongation of stem, irregular chlorotic bands along the veins, stunting etc. These viral disease cause heavy losses to poppy crop in terms of seed and opium yield and sometimes the whole plant dies results total loss of crop.

Diseases caused by insect and pests: Apart from different diseases caused by fungus, bacteria, viruses etc., some insects are also known to damage poppy crop. The most common among them are those damaging roots i.e. Root Weevil, damaging leaf and stem i.e. Aphids, floral damage i.e. thrips and sawfly, capsule damage by head gall fly, capsule weevil, capsule borer etc. A brief description of these are summarized here. **Root weevil** (causal agent - *Sternocarus fuliginosus*): This pest is known for maximum damage to poppy crop by boring into upper parts of the roots which ultimately turns blackish and leaves wither due to chlorosis while the larva mines the leaf lamina. The control measures include dusting of BHC (12%) along with superphosphate. However, the application of lindane 1.3D @10kg/acre in soil before sowing is beneficial. **Cutworm** (causal agent - *Agrotis spp.*): The larva of this pest is dark brown with red colour head, active at night and remains hidden in cracks in the ground. It mostly targets young plants destroying basal part of the stem while the adult, brown in color and dark color spots on wings also destroys the crop severely. The control measures include hand picking of the caterpillars and spraying of NSKE 5%. Additionally, poison bait with rice bran, jiggery and carbonyl can also be used as preventive measures. **Aphid** (causal agent - *Myzus persicae)*: This is also another major pest of opium poppy crop. The nymphs and adults suck the leaf sap results damage of leaf and consequently whole plant. The adults are yellowish green rarely reddish. The control measures include spray of neem oil 0.5% or NSKE 5%. However, natural enemies like coccinellid beetle can also be encouraged. **Capsule borer** (causal agent - *Helicoverpa armigera)*: The capsule borer is also a serious pest in opium poppy which harms capsule to a maximum extent. It destroys whole capsule eating up the floral head and seeds. The larva is greenish with dark grey lines along the sides of the body. The control measures include hand picking of the larvae along with pheromone traps is recommended while spray of NPV 250 lit/ha is also beneficial. The use of Bt spray formulation @ 2g/2ml per litre of water and use of egg parasitoids *Trichogramma chilonis* @ 5cc/ha is also found effective.

4.3. Breeding for growing conditions:

The opium poppy is an environmental sensitive crop. The temperature, photoperiod, rain, wind etc., majorly affects on its proper growth and ultimately yield. The poppy crop requires a maximum temperature upto 20°C at the time of germination while dry weather at the maturity. The humidity in the air is the major problem which posses maximum damage to crop by insect pests. Most of the fungal diseases also prevail in damp climatic conditions. The rains are also a big problem to poppy as heavy rains enhance the growth of plants and at the time capsules are ready to lance, the crops lay down resulting in heavy opium losses. Rains at the time of lancing also damages the yield as the latex is washed away by the rain water. Mist and frost increases the amount of latex and ease in collection. Since the poppy cultivation requires enormous irrigation, wet soil during the time of sowing can result in low germination percentage. The most preferred soil type for poppy is medium loamy textured sandy loam to loam with good aeration, soil conductivity, well drained and properly ploughed and pulverized. The best time for sowing is the first fortnight of November with temperature ranging from 20 to 25°C. However, the delay in sowing can cause poor germination and growth and hence poor yield. The quantity of seeds required for sowing depends on the mode of sowing with 6-7 kg/ha required for broadcasting and 5-6 kg/ha for row sowing with spacing 25-30cm apart. The plant density of 3.30 lakh plants/ha should be maintained. Recommended cultural practices should be followed for a good stand which include pre sowing addition of farmyard manure @ 10 t/ha, 5-6 t/ha neem cake and 30, 50, 40 kg /ha N, P, and K respectively as basal dressing. The recommended application of 60 kg/ha N in two split after 30 and 60 days after sowing as top dressing and spray of the fungicide diethelene biscarbamate (dithane M-45 0.2%) at 45 and 60 days after sowing [36] should be followed for obtaining maximum returns.

Germination in opium poppy requires optimal soil moisture which ensures good germination percentage. The first irrigation in given 20-25 days after sowing followed by frequent light irrigation at an interval of 15-20 days as the weather conditions prevail. A total of 6-8 irrigation is required for a good stand which includes last irrigation before the start of lancing. Weeding and hoeing are also necessary for providing poppy seedling a better chance to grow. The first weeding is done 20-25 days after sowing followed by 15-20 days interval. The optimum spacing between the plants should be maintained at a distance of 10cm apart. In India, lancing is done by cutting of the superficial layer of the capsule wall from which the latex oozes out. The mature green capsule is lanced with an instrument called "Nastar" having 3-4 small blades designed to ensure uniformity in depth of incisions. Generally 3-4 lancing is done in each capsule with parallel longitudinal cuts which is performed after mid day and allow the latex to remain overnight on the capsules for coagulation. In the following morning the latex is collected from the capsule walls with blunt edge of small iron scoop. The opium is kept in small plastic box or earthen pot or copper bowls. The latex colour varies from dark to light brown to pink based on the variety. The depth of incision should not be more than 1.2 mm. After collection of opium, lanced capsules are left to dry over plants for next 15-20 days for harvesting of seeds.

5. Conventional breeding strategies applied for genetic upgradation of opium poppy

The conventional breeding approaches are a step by step procedure to develop desired plant type. The important steps involved in opium poppy breeding program are described in following subheadings:-

5.1. Plant Introduction

Conventional plant breeding programs require distinct plant genotypes with specific characteristics to initiate any hybridization technique. The distinctness in the base material ensures higher percentage of success through breeding programme. The collection of diverse germplasm from different geographical regions can be the best approach for initiation of any breeding programme with specific objectives. The foremost step to initiate any crop breeding program is plant introduction. The procedure of growing a variety or a species into an area where it has not been grown earlier is termed as Plant Introduction. However, bringing plant material from one environmental condition to another within a country or continents is also called as plant introduction. Plant introduction and germplasm collection thus becomes one of the richest sources of creation of variability [37, 38].

In India, researches on opium poppy are confined at some agricultural and scientific institutes viz., Central Institute of Medicinal and Aromatic Plants, Lucknow, National Botanical Research Institute, Lucknow, Jahawarlal Nehru Krishi Vishwavidalaya-College of Agriculture, Jabalpur, Narendra Dev University of Agriculture and Technology, Faizabad, National Bureau for Plant Genetic Resources, New Delhi, Rajasthan Agricultural University, Udaipur. These centers have been working on genetic upgradation of opium poppy for the last four to five decades. Khanna and Singh [39] bought 190 strains from Russia, Hungary, Poland, U.K. and other temperate countries and evaluated these strains at NBRI, Lucknow. They noticed that most of the cultivars belonging to European countries require long photoperiod, hence were unsuitable in Indian climatic conditions. However, the cultivars of Iran were only possible to cultivate in India by introduction. Similarly, Prajapati et al. [40] screened capsule husk of a set of 115 Indian land races of opium poppy (*Papaver somniferum* L.) for papaverine, reticuline, narcotine, thebaine, codeinone, codeine, morphine and oripavine at CIMAP,

Lucknow. These germplasms were grouped into four clusters on the basis of alkaloid profile. Based on the study of alkaloid profiles of these germplasm and correlations between alkaloids in all the four groups of accessions, they concluded that in Indian genetic resources of *P. somniferum* (a) morphine is synthesized from codeine rather than oripavine, (b) net alkaloid content was low under narcotine deficiency, and (c) accumulation of morphine and codeine was in limited upstream of codeinone and morphinone. It was also depicted from their study that the accessions identified based on alkaloid profiles, harboring genetic blocks in phenanthrene and benzylisoquinoline biosynthetic pathways can be useful for understanding the genetic control of secondary metabolism in opium poppy.

In continuation of plant introduction, Shukla et al. [41] studied alkaloid spectrum in 1470 individual plants belonging to 98 germplasm which has been collected from different sources and maintained at NBRI, Lucknow for several years. Based on alkaloid profiles, the content of different alkaloids were categorized into class interval exhibiting maximum number of plants and accessions for morphine fall in group of 10–15% followed by 15–20%, for codeine in group of 2–4% followed by 4–6%, for thebaine in 1–2% followed by 2–4%, for narcotine in 5–10% followed by 10–15% and for papaverine content 0–2%, while 24 germplasm lines had morphine content above 16.0%. Based on distinctness in morphological and agronomical characteristics, 1,000 distinct poppy germplasm lines were provided by Agriculture faculty, Ankara University from which 99 poppy lines were evaluated in terms of alkaloid analysis in *in vitro* [42]. They observed the range of different alkaloids in poppy husk (CPS) viz., morphine, thebaine, codeine, papaverine and noscapine from 0.110 to 1.140%, 0.005 to 0.134%, 0.005 to 0.27%, 0.001 to 0.440% and 0.006 to 0.418%, respectively. Dittbrenner et al. [43] evaluated 300 accessions of opium poppy for 35 morphological and agronomic traits collected from all over the world at IPK Gene Bank, Gatersleben, Germany. Based on their study on five major alkaloids taken for two years, they concluded highly significant correlation between total alkaloid content and morphine. However, four other major alkaloids i.e. codeine, thebaine, noscapine and papaverine did not show any correlation between them or with total alkaloid content. Additionally they also noticed that there is no important correlation between morphological traits and alkaloid content. They also determined the chromosome number in each accession and found that the subspecies *setigerum* was natural tetraploid while the rest of the subspecies were diploid. They finally concluded that none of the studied morphological traits could be used for prediction of alkaloid content which may give erroneous information in breeding programmes.

6. Diversity analysis through conventional tools

One of the foremost steps in the genetical improvement of any crop through conventional breeding program is to study the genetic diversity available in the introduced plant/crop material. To conduct any breeding program judiciously, diversity analysis based on morphological and biochemical traits is prerequisite. In opium poppy, several of the exotic collections at different research institutes have been evaluated for genetic diversity. Few studies on genetic diversity undertaken so far in opium poppy are summarized here. Singh et al. [44] studied genetic divergence using 101 germplasm lines of different ecogeographical origin for seed and opium yield per plant and its 8 component traits following multivariate and canonical analysis. They grouped the germplasm into 13 clusters on the basis of multivariate analysis which was also confirmed by canonical analysis. 68% genotypes were found genetically close to each other and grouped in 6 clusters while apparent diversity was noticed for 32 percent of the genotypes who diverged into rest 7 clusters. They concluded that the genotypes in clusters IX, X, XI and XII had greater potential as breeding stock by virtue of high mean values of one or more component characters and high statistical distances among them. Yadav et al. [45] made an effort to study the genetic divergence in a genetically distinct new stock of opium poppy using cluster and principle component analysis. They found that a large amount of variability exists among the accessions and formed 8 clusters from which some accessions were recommended which can be used in hybridization programme to get desirable transgressive segregants. Similarly, Yadav et al. [46] assessed genetic divergence in 110 population (20 parents and 90 F_1 hybrids) using multivariate analysis. All the entries were grouped into 14 clusters which indicated substantial diversity among parental genotypes which had potential to release considerable variation in their crosses. Similarly, Brezinova et al. [47] evaluated 404 genotypes of poppy from world collection to assess genetic diversity over the selected traits based on their morphological characteristic to create a digitalized visual documentation. On the basis of morphometric analysis, the important diversity in observed traits were recognized in agro-climatic conditions of Slovakia, documented by statistical characteristics and by digitalized documentation of accessions. Diversity based on alkaloid spectrum in 122 accessions of indigenous opium poppy was undertaken by Shukla et al. [48]. They obtained 11 clusters based on extent of correlation between five major alkaloids i.e. morphine, codeine, thebaine, narcotine and papaverine. Mostly the clusters comprised of accessions with different possible combinations of alkaloids comprising high in one alkaloid with high or low of another. Generally the percentage of morphine content was higher than the sum of four other alkaloids except in one cluster where narcotine content was slightly higher than morphine. Based on their study they concluded that successful breeding for specific alkaloids or a combination of alkaloids could be achieved by using these accessions in hybridization programme.

7. Creation of variability through hybridization

A breeding programme focused to develop improved varieties requires knowledge about the genetic variability that exists for the concern trait. It is documented that sufficient variation for composition and content of secondary metabolites occurs in a number of medicinal plant. Several studies have been carried out in opium poppy to study the existing variability in different set of materials which showed varying results for composition of secondary metabolites and other chemical compounds along with morphological variations. Singh et al. [49] found that F_8 genotypes obtained through interspecific cross between *Papaver somniferum* and *Papaver setigerum* had higher oil (>40%) and fatty acid concentration than respective parental species. They also obtained varying results for linoleic (68%-74.4%) and oleic acid

(13.6%-20.3%) content in F_8 genotypes. High oleic desaturation ratio and C18 polyunsaturated fatty acid with very low linolenic (18:3) acid (0.37%) indicated the possibility of using poppy oil for edible purposes. However, oleic (18:1) acid was not correlated with other fatty acids, except for significant negative correlation with linoleic (C18:2) acid. Ozturk and Gunlu [50] conducted correlation and path coefficient analysis for qualitative and quantitative traits in four poppy cultivars in Central Anatolia. They found statistically significant differences for all the studied traits among all the four genotypes. Positive and significant correlation of morphine yield with morphine content, seed yield, capsule yield, oil yield; capsule yield with oil yield; seed yield with capsule yield, oil yield were noticed. Through path analysis, it was noticed that morphine content, capsule yield, seed yield and oil yield had positive direct effect on morphine yield. Yadav et al. [51] analyzed F_1 and F_2 generations of a twenty parents fractional diallel cross in opium poppy (*P. somniferum* L.) to estimate the combining ability of the crosses based on ten quantitative and five qualitative (alkaloids) traits. The results indicated that significant differences exists among the parents for all the traits and GCA (General Combining Ability) and SCA (Specific Combining Ability) components of variances were also significant for all the traits. However, SCA component of variance (σ^2s) was predominant which indicated the preponderance of non-additive gene effect for all the traits except for leaves/plant and papaverine in F_1 hybrids. The average degree of dominance (σ ^{2}s/ σ ^{2}g) was more than unity indicated over dominance and also confirmed the non-additive mode of gene action. They suggested that the inclusion of good general combiners in a multiple crossing program or an intermating among the population involving all possible crosses subjected to biparental mating can be expected to offer maximum promise in breeding for higher opium and seed yield and alkaloid content. In an another study, Yadav et al. [52] examined combining ability for yield and its component traits along with morphine content to elucidate the inheritance pattern governing these traits and also to identify potential genotypes which could be further exploited in breeding programmes. They noticed that most of the traits were governed by non-additive gene action while additive gene action was also important for some other traits. They found three best parents viz., BR-232, BR-245 and BR-234 as good general combiners which could be used in hybridization programme aiming at maximum gain. Similarly, Kumar and Patra [53] also studied inheritance pattern for quantitative traits in four single crosses in opium poppy. They found that simple additive, dominance and epistatic genetic components were significant for inheritance of the traits under study. They also noticed differential gene actions with differential magnitude for different traits and concluded that following biparental mating followed by recurrent selection for desired recombinants may be utilized for genetic upgradation of opium poppy crop. Mishra et al. [54] evaluated progenies of randomly selected individuals from 14 promising hybrids over F_2 to F_6 generations for opium and seed yield and their contributing traits for the formulation of effective selection strategy in opium poppy (*P. somniferum* L.). They observed that in general heritability and genetic gain declined from generation to generation. They obtained a cross MOP541 x BR241 which showed similar pattern for genetic gain in all the traits. The values of broad sense heritability decreased from F_2 to F_6 generation for most of the traits. Matyasova et al. [55] evaluated 57 cultivars of opium poppy comparing the groups of values representing the indicators of production-significant morphologic and agricultural traits and morphine content in husk in relation to ideotype, which in these indicators represents 100% of the value. They observed lower values of morphine in husk of white coloured seeds while high morphine in blue to grey seeds. They observed that these cultivars achieved very good values in the morphological indicators and average value in the economic indicators. Based on their results they concluded that these results will be used in selection and classification of suitable genetic resources of poppy as industrial forms. Nemeth-Zambori et al. [56] conducted a hybridization experiment between five parents with different chemotypes namely Minoan, Medea, Korona, Przemko and Kozmosz and studied the alkaloid profile for F_1 to F_3 generations. They observed that in some cross combinations with high alkaloid containing parents, the content of total alkaloid, morphine and thebaine showed significant increase in hybrid generation which persisted upto F_3 generation. However, the concentration of narcotine was lesser than mid parent value and also showed decreasing trend over generations. As a matter of fact, homogenous strains started to accumulate at F_3 generation. In contrast to the high alkaloid parents, the cross combinations with low alkaloid parents exhibited considerable heterosis for total alkaloid content in F_1 while low alkaloid containing recessive individuals segregated in F_2 and stabilized in F_3 generation. They finally concluded that their experiment reflected well with the effects of genetic regulation at three levels of enzymatic processes during the alkaloid biosynthesis. The morphinans and narcotine was controlled by complex polygenic effects so, the selection for fixing of very low content of narcotine may be effective in early F_2 generation as narcotine was found lesser than mid parent value. However, selection for morphinane alkaloids which are in major proportion is not worthy before F_3 generation. Yadav et al. [57] investigated inheritance pattern for different quantitative traits through generation mean analysis using five parameter model on five cross combinations with five generations i.e. parents, F_1s, F_2s, and F_3s selected from an extensive hybridization programme carried out in partial mating design. They found that additive x additive and dominance x dominance was higher in magnitude than combined main effect of additive and dominance effect for all the traits in all five crosses. However, dominance x dominance effect was predominant over additive x additive for all the traits except for few. They also observed substantial amount of realized heterosis, residual heterosis and high broad sense heritability with moderate genetic advance and significant correlation among important traits in positive direction. Based on their study they finally advised selective diallel mating and biparental mating in early generations followed by recurrent selection which can be used for genetic upgradation of opium poppy. Kumar and Patra [58] undertook a study to understand the gene action involved in the inheritance of opium yield and its component traits (plant height, leaves per plant, peduncle length, capsule index, seed and straw yield per plant and morphine content) in two families viz., VG26 x VG20 and SG35II x VE01 of opium poppy. They found significant additive, dominance and epistatic genetic components for the inheritance of different traits and concluded that biparental mating followed by recurrent selection involving desired recombinants may be utilized for genetic upgradation of opium poppy through components traits.

8. Screening and evaluation for oil and fatty acids

One of the important aspects of breeding programmes is selection which is based on several factors and requires experience and command to observe. Selection can be based on maturity period, disease resistance, lodging, withering and yield etc. Investigation about oil yield, fatty acid compositions and total protein content of three varieties of Turkish poppy were done by Azcan et al. [59] who found that solvent extraction of yellow seed gave highest oil yield upto 49.2%, while white seed had 36.8% and blue seed 33.6% which was considerably low. Fatty acid compositions of oils were determined by GC/MS in which major components were of linoleic (56.4–69.2%), oleic (16.1–19.4%), and palmitic (10.6–16.3%) acid depending on the color of the seeds. Similar investigation on volatile compounds of several seed oil samples from *Papaver somniferum* L. using solid phase micro extraction (SPME) with DVB/ Carboxen/PDMS Stable-Flex fiber was done by Krist et al. [60]. They identified 1-Pentanol (3.3-4.9%), 1-hexanal (10.9-30.9%), 1-hexanol (5.3-33.7%), 2-pentylfuran (7.2-10.0%), and caproic acid (2.9-11.5%) as the main volatile compounds in all examined poppy seed oil samples. Furthermore, the TAG (Triglyceride) composition of these oils was analyzed by MALDI-TOF and ESI-IT-MS/MS. The predominant TAG components were found to be composed of linoleic, oleic and palmitic acid, comprising 70% of the oil. Similarly, Ozcan and Atalay [61] investigated physical and chemical properties of seven poppy varieties. Weight of 1000 seeds, moisture, crude protein, crude ash, crude fibre, HCl-insoluble ash, crude energy and crude oil content of all seven varieties of poppy seeds were 0.29-0.429 g, 3.39-4.76 %, 11.94-13.58 %, 4.92-6.25 %, 22.63-30.08 %, 0.72-1.68 %, 6367.0-6740.5 kcal/100g and 32.43-45.52 % respectively. The poppy seed oil contained an appreciable amount of beta-tocopherol (309.5 ppm-567.3 ppm). Poppy seed oil also contained stearic, palmitic, oleic, linoleic and linolenic acid as the main constituent of fatty acids. Linoleic acid was established as the dominant fatty acid in all varieties. Similar investigation were also done by Hakan et al. [62] who investigated fatty acid, tocopherol and sterol content of the oil of several poppy seeds. They found that the main fatty acids in poppy seed oil were linoleic, oleic and palmitic acid while oil contained an appreciable amount of gamma-tocopherol and alpha-tocopherol. The concentrations of total sterol ranged from 1099.84 mg kg^{-1} to 4816.10 mg kg^{-1}. The major sterols were beta-sitosterol ranged from 663.91 to 3244.39 mg kg^{-1}; campesterol ranged from 228.59 to 736.50 mg kg^{-1} and delta (5)-avenasterol ranged from 103.90 to 425.02 mg kg^{-1}.

9. Stability analysis for identification of stable and adaptable varieties

The analysis of genotype x environmental interaction, which indicates the stability of genotypes has always been part of plant breeding programmes before release of any variety for commercial cultivation. To study the GxE interaction, several methods have been proposed to analyze it i.e. univariate methods such as Francis and Kannenberg's coefficient of variability [63], Plaisted and Peterson's mean variance component for pair-wise GE interactions [64], Wricke's ecovalence [65], Shukla's stability variance [66], Finlay and Wilkinson's regression coefficient [67], Perkins and Jinks's regression coefficient [68] and Eberhart and Russell's sum of square deviations from regression [69]. Simultaneously, two other stability models based on graphical representation of the genotypes in different environments are available i.e. Yan's GGE Biplot model and AMMI model. Yadav et al. [70] investigated stability for seed yield, opium yield and morphine content in 11 advanced breeding lines over five years in opium poppy. Combined ANOVA showed that both main effects and interactions were significant, indicating the presence of genotype x environment interactions. Yadav et al. [19, 36] studied phenotypic and genotypic variability, broad sense heritability, genetic advance under selection and interrelationship of traits in 74 and 122 accessions of opium poppy respectively. They found high variations among the accessions along with broad sense heritability and genetic advance. Genetic correlation analysis revealed negative correlation between opium yield and morphine and papaverine content while other alkaloids showed positive correlation. The 11 genotypes of opium poppy were evaluated on the basis of non-parametric model by Yadav et al. [71] for opium yield and morphine content over 5 environments to identify stable and promising genotypes which can sustain adverse environmental conditions. Several of the evaluated genotypes were found to be stable in all the environmental conditions and were stable for both the traits i.e. opium yield and morphine content. Yadav et al. [72] evaluated 22 strains of opium poppy to find out variability and suitable selection indices for opium and seed yield. The discriminant functions based on single character were less efficient while on the basis of combination it was in general more efficient. The comparison of different functions revealed that capsule weight/plant, capsule length, plant height were major yield components and thus practicing selection for attainment of high opium and seed yielding lines, maximum weightage should be given to these characters. The positive association of opium and seed yield suggested that by adopting suitable component breeding and selection, a dual-purpose variety (opium and seed yield) can be developed. Singh et al. [44] investigated the extent of genetic variability, heritability, correlation and path analysis for opium yield, seed yield and eight component traits in a group of 101 germplasm lines of different ecogeographical origins. They noticed high heritability coupled with high genetic advance and coefficient of variability for most of the traits. Path coefficient analysis indicated that capsule per plant had high direct path towards opium yield followed by four other traits.

10. Mutation breeding approaches

Besides, different hybridization programs, mutation breeding program was also flourished and encouraging results were obtained all over the world. An era of mutation breeding came into existence due to significant achievements obtained in many crops of pharmaceutical, industrial and food interest. In opium poppy also scientists obtained fascinating results. A mutation breeding experiment was carried out using physical and chemical mutagens to develop non-narcotic opium poppy from narcotic crop [73]. They isolated two families containing twenty latex less/opium-less and twelve partial latex bearing plants in M_1 generation which gave similar observations in M_2 generations also. The best mutant genotype, LL-34 of family C[1]-Comb-113-2 with 5.66 g seeds/capsule had 52.6% oil was designated as cv. 'Sujata'. This was the world's first opiumless and alkaloid free seed poppy cultivar, offers a cheap and permanent (fundamental) solution to the global problem of opium-linked social abuse. Simultaneously, it serves as a food grade crop with proteinacious seeds along with healthy unsaturated seed oil. Similarly Chatterjee et al. [74] studied induced mutation through gamma rays, EMS and their combined doses in two varieties of opium poppy (NBRI-1 and NBRI-5) to create new genetic variability for isolation of high yielding genotypes along with specific alkaloids. The genetic coefficient of variability (GCV), heritability and genetic advance was noticed higher for opium and seed yield and capsule weight for all the doses in both the varieties with some exception. They finally concluded that the criteria for selection of plants should be based on capsule weight and capsule number which can provide ideal plant type with enhanced yield potential. Chatterjee et al. [75] also found a variant plant of opium poppy (*Papaver somniferum* L.) having high thebaine content. The M_2 seeds of variant plant were subjected to *in vitro* studies to investigate the prospects of thebaine production through tissue culture. Consequently, alkaloid profile of variants showed higher thebaine in stem followed by leaf callus, stem callus and cotyledons. From the same mutation breeding experiment Chatterjee et al. [76] made an effort of identify appropriate dose of the mutagens for the enhancement of specific alkaloid especially thebaine and also studied correlation between cytological aberrations and their effects on alkaloid quantity in two stable high yielding varieties of opium poppy i.e. NBRI-1 and NBRI-5. They found that NBRI-1 was more sensitive than NBRI-5 and that the mutagen EMS was most potent in creating chromosomal abnormalities. They concluded that two doses i.e. kR 10 + 0.2% EMS and 0.2% EMS was most effective for getting fruitful results. The dose kR 10 + 0.2% EMS possessed high chiasms frequency while 0.2% EMS in combinations with all doses of gamma was effective in enhancing the total alkaloid as well as specific alkaloids. In continuation of their study Chatterjee et al. [77] also tried to broaden the genetic variability and to evaluate the advance generations for different agronomic and chemotypic traits in the experimental high yielding varieties i.e. NBRI-1 and NBRI-5 through induced mutations. Here, they noticed that the dose kR30 and kR10 + 0.4% EMS gave highest positive results for genotypic coefficient of variability, heritability and genetic advance (%) for seven traits in NBRI-1 and ten traits in NBRI-5 respectively. They further concluded that their study confirmed that the morphinan and phthalideisoquinilone pathway bifurcated at lower combined doses i.e. kR30 and kR10 + 0.4% EMS which was effective in causing micromutation in morphinan and phthalideisoquinilone pathways respectively.

A mutant variety known as 'TOP 1' ('thebaine oripavine poppy 1') in opium poppy (*Papaver somniferum*) was developed by Tasmania Company. In this mutant the morphinan pathway is blocked at thebaine results in absence of codeine and morphine. The major loss of this blockage is on the end product i.e. morphine which is absent in this mutant [84]. This mutant was developed by a mutagen treatment to seeds of commercial poppy cultivar (*P. somniferum*). Phenotypically the mutation is visible in the form of pigmented latex than normal white. In TOP 1 mutant, one possibility is that the gene responsible for an enzyme 6-O demethylase which act on thebaine and oripavine might be affected at its transcriptional level or modified protein structure. It may be possible that there is an alteration occurs in transport component that blocks the entry of substrates (thebaine and oripavine) of the enzyme to the subcellular compartment for 6-O demethylation. These mutant plants are very important since the production of thebaine is only amenable which can help in checking of drug trafficking. However, identification of the candidate genes which has been blocked can be identified and characterized. The complex mechanism involved in morphinane biosynthesis can also be elucidated. These morphine free plants can be beneficial for the treatment of opioid addiction. But there is a slight risk with this mutant for licit to illicit uses (by conversion of non-narcotic alkaloids to narcotic alkaloids). The Tasmania drug industry has been using TOP 1 mutants since 1998 for production of various analgesic drugs viz. buprenorphine, oxycodone, naloxone and naltrexone.

11. Polyploidy approaches

The event of polyploidization has been observed long back as most of our cultivated and wild species are polyploids as a result of diploidization or cross pollination among various ploidy levels. This has been an important aspect in conventional breeding programs. Basically, polyploidy is of two types i.e. auto- and allo- ploidy, wherein the auto polyploids arises due to duplication in same genomic content in a species whereas in case of allopolyploidy, there is chromosome complementation i.e. two different chromosomal content from different species combine to form allopolyploid. Few studies on polyploidization in opium poppy have been undertaken so far. Polyploids are beneficial in many aspects viz., organism can resort to higher number of genes and higher number of allelic variants which may lead to substantial increase in the ultimate product. One of the recent study was undertaken on ploidy aspect of opium poppy [78]. They aimed to understand the phenotypic, genetic and genomic consequences of induced polyploidy and to enhance total alkaloid content along with specific alkaloid using colchicine. They observed that the induced auto-tetraploidy did not show any significant differences in phenotypic level while stomatal and chromosomal studies confirmed the tetraploidy. They also noticed differential gene expression of the diploids and autotetraploids which led to the elucidation of dosage regulated gene expression leading significant enhancement in morphine content in tetraploid plants. Their study in auto-tetraploids opens avenues towards the development of hexaploids and amphidiploids which can give multifold increase in specific alkaloids. This study also opens a new vista towards understanding of ploidy level changes in term of phenotypic, genetic and genomic and a better understanding of the complex mechanism involved in polyploidization.

12. Other conventional approaches

Apart from different conventional breeding strategies applied for genetic upgradation of opium poppy, several researchers with similar aim carried out several studies in opium poppy. A unique study was carried out on honey bees foraging on plant flowers [79]. They noticed significantly higher foraging response of honeybees (*Apis mellifera*) manifesting honeybee's preference towards specific plant morphotypes in genetically divergent plant of opium poppy (*Papaver somniferum*). Furthermore the genotype specific for foraging response of honeybees could be attributed to physico-chemical properties of opium poppy flowers. This could have implications for the development of opium alkaloid fortified honey for novel pharmaceuticals and isolation of natural spray compounds to attract honeybee pollinators for promoting crossing and sustainable hybridity in crops. Since the seed of opium poppy is widely used as food in almost all parts of the world, several researchers tried different ways to develop plants producing nutritionally rich seeds. Losak and Richter [80] studied the effect of nitrogen supplementation to cultivar 'Opal' of opium poppy plant in a pot experiment. They applied ammonium nitrate in single dose at two stages of plant growth i.e. at the beginning of growing season and at the stage of flowering. They observed that the increasing dose of nitrogen increased number of capsules per plant, morphine content and the capsule volume irregularly. However, an optimum dose of nitrogen i.e. 0.9 g N/pot showed statistically significant positive effect on seed yield. The effect of varying concentration of CO_2 (300, 400, 500, 600 μ mol mol^{-1}) was examined on various morphological traits such as number of capsules, capsule weight and latex-yield in *Papaver setigerum*. A significant positive effect of increasing CO_2 concentration on various morphological traits was noticed with an increase of 3.6, 3.0 and 3.7 times, respectively on per plant basis. Significant and positive response of secondary metabolites especially morphine, codeine, narcotine and papaverine was also noticed to CO_2 enrichment. However, the major alkaloid i.e. morphine was significantly increased by 10.4, 11.7, 12.9 and 12.4%, respectively at each dose (300, 400, 500 and 600 μmol mol^{-1}) of CO_2 [81]. Szabo et al. [82] investigated the effects of water stress on the alkaloid production and content at three different developmental stages i.e. Rosette, Flowering and Lancing in opium poppy. They used four types of water conditions i.e. control, withdrawal, 50% water supply and inundation and found that leaves responded significantly to water stress conditions. They further concluded that constant water supply is beneficial for the accumulation of alkaloids in poppy capsules. In many parts of the world, seeds of opium poppy are widely used as food and efforts are continuously made to develop nutritionally rich poppy seeds. In Central European countries, the content of selenium is very low in poppy seeds. Hence, with the aim of supplementing opium poppy plants with selenium (a trace element), Skarpa and Richter [83] tried to explore the effect of foliar application of this element on seed yield, selenium content in seeds and its uptake by the roots. They applied a single dose of selenium of 300 g/ha at two different stages i.e. during the stage of the end of elongation growth and after the fall of blossoms. They found that seed yield was reduced by 11.5% and 11.8% after both stages of application respectively but the content of selenium increased significantly from 139 μg/kg to 757 μg/kg of seeds. However, the uptake of selenium also increased significantly upto 4.8 times.

Since for the last few decades, scientific researchers have been continuously contributing for the genetic upgradation of opium poppy through various approaches including conventional breeding methodologies, mutation breeding and molecular techniques with breeding and it is a matter of high enthusiasm for the development of varieties, hybrids, synthetics and GMO in opium poppy till date. At present few varieties have been developed through conventional approaches that can be grouped as-

12.1. Varieties developed by National Botanical Research Institute, Lucknow

In due course of time many breeding approaches have been applied in opium poppy for the development of new high yielding and disease resistant varieties. These varieties are now stabilized and suited for different agro-climatic conditions. A brief characteristic description of the varieties are given below -

- **BROP-1**:- In this variety the plants are medium sized having 3-4 capsules/plant and capsules are of three types viz. oily, parrot coloured and black peduncle. Flowers are white. It is a synthetic variety stabilized after hybridization/intermating between three high yielding cultivars viz. kali dandi (black peduncle), suga pankhi (parrot color) and sufaid dandi (white peduncle) followed by selection. The average opium yield, seed yield and morphine content are up to 54kg/ha, 1000-1200kg/ha and 13% respectively. Geographically it can be cultivated mainly in Northern Indian plains.
- **NBRI-1**:- This variety is developed through selection. The plants are medium tall having large fringed leaves and white flowers. The average opium yield, seed yield and morphine content are up to 52kg/ha, 1000kg/ha and 12-13% respectively. Geographically it can be cultivated mainly in Northern Central India.
- **NBRI-2**:- This variety has intermediate tall plants, thick stem, broad leaves, long peduncle with big capsules and flowers are white. This variety is also developed through selection amongst local collection having above characters. Average opium yield, seed yield and morphine content are up to 52 kg/ha, 1200kg/ha and 15%respectively. Northern Central part of India is recommended for its cultivation.
- **NBRI-6**:- In this variety, plants are medium tall with narrow leaves and white flowers. It is developed by hybridization between two germplasm lines BR007 and BR008 (BR007 x BR008) followed by rigorous selection generation after generation up to eight generations. Average opium yield, seed yield and morphine content are up to 55kg/ha, 1200kg/ha and 13-14% respectively. Geographically Northern Indian plains are mainly recommended for its cultivation.
- **NBRI-9**:- In this variety, plants are intermediate sized with white flowers and large capsules. The variety is high yielding (seed yield) and is developed by hybridization between germplasm lines S-10 x S-18 followed by rigorous selection until the variety is stabilized (up to eight generations). It's average opium yield, seed yield and morphine content is upto 52kg/ha, 1400kg/ha and 12% respectively. For the cultivation of the variety, Northern Indian Plains are recommended as most suitable.
- **NBRI-10**:- The plants in this variety are medium tall, having dark green leaves and white flowers. The development of variety was done through hybridization germplasm lines (IC-30 x S-10) followed by rigorous selection up to eight generations. Average opium yield, seed yield and morphine content are up to 50kg/ha, 1200kg/ha and 12% respectively. Geographically Northern Central plains are recommended for its cultivation.

http://dx.doi.org/10.5772/53132

- **Madakini**:- It is a high yielding variety for opium poppy, have multiple disease resistance and is granted US patent no.7,442,854B2 in 2009. The variety is developed by hybridization germplasm lines (BR007 x BR008) followed by rigorous selection. Plants of the variety are vigorous having dark green leaves, white flowers with blackish flowering stalk at the bottom of capsule at maturity. Average opium yield, seed yield and morphine content are up to 64kg/ha, 1200kg/ha and 15% respectively. Northern Central India is recommended for its cultivation (Figure 3).

- **High thebaine lines**:- As we know that thebaine is a non-narcotic alkaloid and can be used in making pain killing drugs. Thus for fulfilling the increasing worldwide demand of thebaine, with the help of interspecific hybridization (*P. somniferum* x *P. setigerum*) and mutation breeding experiments NBRI has succeeded in the development of few stable high thebaine lines. Thebaine content in these lines ranges 8-10% which is much higher than pre-existing varieties and germplasm (Figure 4).

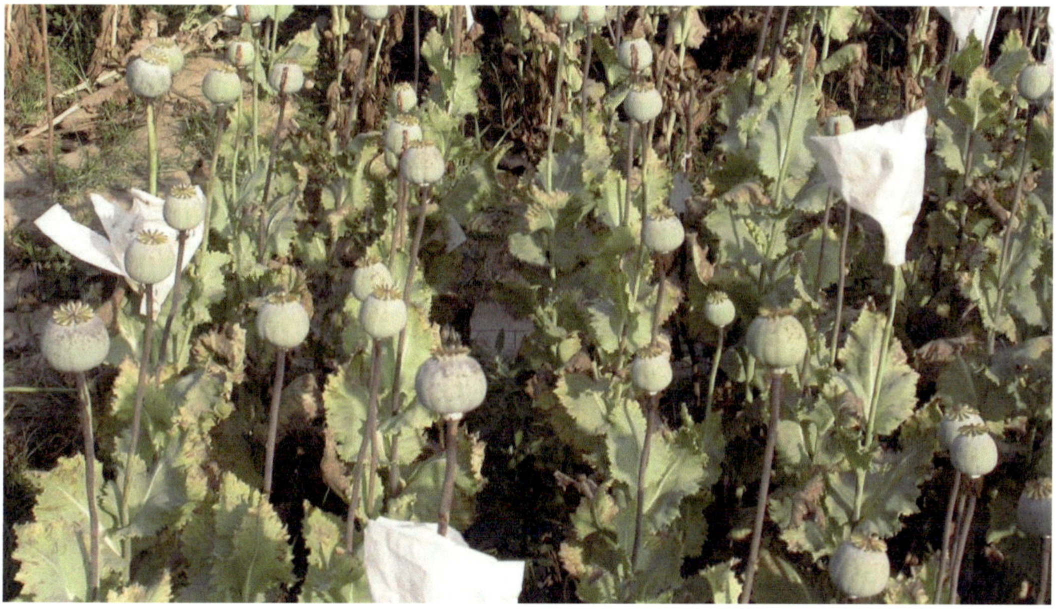

Figure 3. Field view of developed high yielding variety "Madakini".

12.2. Varieties developed by Central Institute of Medicinal and Aromatic Plants, Lucknow

- **Rakshit**:-It is a disease resistant and morphine rich variety in CPS (concentrated poppy straw). The plants are 106-112 cm tall with 20-26 cm long green peduncle and oblong capsules with waxy surface. The variety is developed by hybridization and selection generation after generation up to eight generations. Average seed yield and straw yield of the variety are up to 1200-1400kg/ha and 900-1100kg/ha respectively.

- **Sanchita**:- In this high yielding variety, plants are 107 cm tall and have 2-3 capsules/plant. The average seed yield and straw yield are 840kg/ha and 640kg/ha respectively. Morphine content of this variety is very low in CPS (approx. 0.74%).
- **Vivek**:- The plants of this variety are 112 cm tall with 2-3 capsules/plant. It is also a high yielding variety having seed yield and straw yield up to 840kg/ha and 760kg/ha respectively. Morphine content of this variety is also very low in husk (approx. 0.73%).
- **Sweta**:- It is high yielding variety with 66.5kg/ha opium yield and about 18% morphine content in latex.
- **Subhra**:- In this variety plants are medium sized having 3-4 capsules/plant. The average seed yield and husk yield of the variety are approx. 910kg/ha and 790kg/ha respectively. The morphine percentage in husk is approx. 0.77%.
- **Shyama**:- In this variety plants are 105 cm tall with black peduncle and also has erect incised leaves. It is a high yielding variety having seed yield, husk yield and morphine content up to 720kg/ha, 650kg/ha and 0.75% respectively.
- **Sujata**:- In this variety plants are 80-100 cm tall having 3-4 flat glabrous capsules with 18-20 cm long erratic black peduncle. It is an opium less, alkaloid less and non narcotic variety.

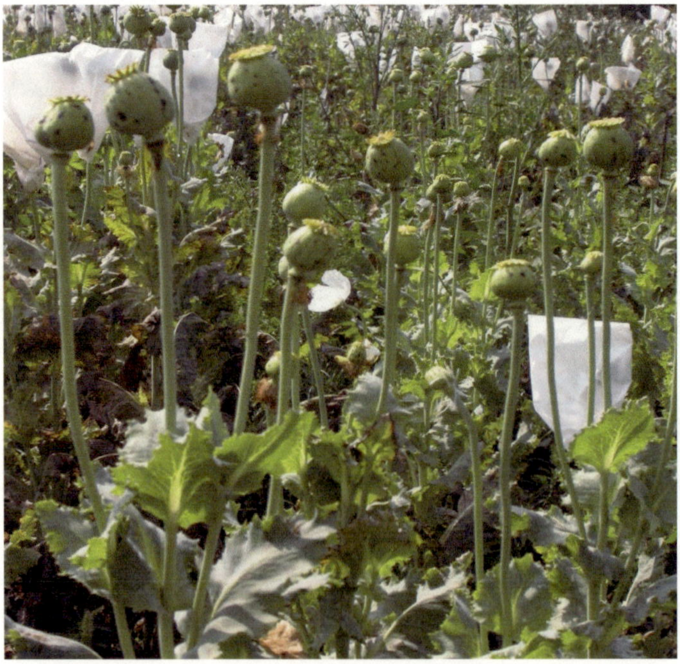

Figure 4. Field view of developed high thebaine lines.

Narendra Dev University of Agriculture and Technology, Faizabad has developed a downy mildew resistant variety by selection and named Kirtiman (NOP-4). The plants of this variety are quite tall having white flowers and 1-2 oval capsules. Opium yield, seed yield and morphine content of the variety ranges 35-46kg/ha, 900-1100kg/ha and up to 12% respectively. Eastern U.P. region is best suited for its cultivation.

National Bureau of Plant Genetic Resources, New Delhi developed a variety Trishna (IC 42) for resistance to frost, root rot and downy mildew through inbreeding and selection. The plants of the variety are tall with 5-7 capsules/plant and pink flowers. Opium yield, seed yield and morphine content ranges up to 49-53kg/ha, 1000kg/ha and 12-14.78% respectively.

Rajasthan Agricultural University, Udaipur has developed a resistant variety to disease and lodging and named it as **Chetak (UO 285)**. The plants of this variety are average tall with big capsules. Flowers are white with smooth petals. Opium yield, seed yield and morphine content ranges up to 54kg/ha, 1000-1200kg/ha and 12% respectively. Geographically Rajasthan is most suitable for its cultivation.

Jawaharlal Nehru Krishi Vishwavidalaya, College of Agriculture, Jabalpur (M.P.) has also succeeded in developing a downy mildew resistant variety by pure line selection and named as Jawahar Aphim 16 (JA-16). Plants of this variety are tall having white flowers and 1-3 big capsules/plant. The variety has opium yield, seed yield and morphine content up to 45-54kg/ha, 900-1000kg/ha and 12% respectively. Madhya Pradesh is geographically recommended for its cultivation.

13. Future prospects

The medicinal uses of opium poppy are innumerable and also its value as food grade crop is significant. The genetic upgradation process in opium poppy cannot be ended until and unless it is able to meet the ever increasing global demand for opium alkaloids and nutritious seeds. The genetic upgradation process needs to be continued for the development of varieties rich in total alkaloid content. The conservation of germplasm and creation of genetic variability through the intervention of conventional, mutational, polyploidy and molecular approaches is essential to carry forward future breeding programmes aiming to develop designer plants in opium poppy. At present the indigenous poppy germplasm has very narrow genetic base, we need to concentrate on broadening of its genetic base through the intervention of above strategies. The prospects of mutation breeding and interspecific hybridization has proved useful in creation of genetic variability and development of varieties rich in specific alkaloid with high yield needs further efforts to enhance the total alkaloid content.

The opium poppy crop is highly sensitive to several diseases caused by biological agents. The development of multiple disease resistant varieties is another major challenge in opium poppy. Very few studies have been done on this aspect, so, further studies are required to develop resistant varieties in poppy against fungus, bacteria, viruses, insects, pests etc, which causes severe damage to the crop. The genes responsible for disease resistant can be identified and characterized through molecular techniques, so, efforts should be made in the direction of developing disease resistant transgenic plants, from which the candidate gene could be transferred through back crossing program into our high yielding varieties.

Another important aspect is that the opium poppy is highly sensitive to varied environmental conditions. Although a number of high yielding varieties have been developed, but the development of photoperiod insensitive, stable and adaptable varieties for different climatic conditions are still required. This can be achieved by transferring the genes of interest from the cultivars of different countries into our indigenous varieties in green houses. However, the development of morphine less or opium less varieties, which can check drug trafficking and allows the farmers to grow poppy without any restriction or necessity of obtaining license, is still a challenging task. Different molecular techniques such as virus induced gene silencing, RNA interference (RNAi) technology etc., can help in the development of opium less and morphine-less varieties. Till to date, 17 genes have been identified and characterized involved in alkaloid biosynthesis, but the genes involved in other benzylisoquinoline and pthalideisoquinoline pathways are still unknown. So, the efforts should be done to explore all the genes involved in alkaloid biosynthesis which may help in development of desired designer plants in opium poppy.

Author details

Brij Kishore Mishra[1], Anu Rastogi[1], Ameena Siddiqui[1], Mrinalini Srivastava[1], Nidhi Verma[1], Rawli Pandey[1], Naresh Chandra Sharma[2] and Sudhir Shukla[1*]

*Address all correspondence to: s_shukla31@rediffmail.com

1 Deptt. of Genetics and Plant Breeding, National Botanical Research Institute, Lucknow, U.P., U.P. India

2 Deptt. of Biochemistry and Genetics, Barkatullah University, Bhopal, M.P., U.P. India

References

[1] Frick Susanne, Kramell R, Schmidt J, Fist AJ and Kutchan TM. Comparative qualitative and quantitative determination of alkaloids in narcotic and condiment *Papaver somniferum* cultivars. Journal of Natural Products 2005; 68 666-673.

[2] Vos E and Cunnne SC. A-Linolenic acid, Linoleic acid, Coronary heart diseases and overall mortality. American Journal of Clinical Nutrition 2003; 72(2) 521-522.

[3] Sacks FM and Campos H. Polysaturated fatty acids, inflammation and cardiovascular diseases: Time to widen our view of the mechanism. Clinical Endocrinology Metabolism 2006; 91(2) 398-400.

[4] Vesselovskaya MA. The poppy, Amerind Publishing Co. Pvt. Ltd. 1976; (Translated from Russian).

[5] Singh SP, Khanna KR, Shukla S, Dixit BS and Banerjee R. Prospects of breeding opium poppies (*P. somniferum* L.) as a high linoleic acid crop. Journal of Plant Breeding 1995; 114 89-91.

[6] Aniszewski T. Alkaloids-secrets of life: Alkaloid chemistry, biological significance, applications and ecological role. Elsevier, Amsterdam 2007.

[7] Pienkny S, Brandt W, Schmidt J, Kramell R and Ziegler J. Functional characterization of a novel benzylisoquinoline O-methyltransferase suggests its involvement in papaverine biosynthesis in opium poppy (*Papaver somniferum* L). The Plant Journal 2009; 60(1) 56-67.

[8] Wang CQ, Li Y and Douglas SD. Morphine withdrawal enhances hepatitis C virus replicon expression. American Journal of Pathology 2005; 167(5) 1333-1340.

[9] Schrijvers D and van Fraeyenhove F. Emergencies in palliative care. Cancer Journal 2010; 16(5) 514-520.

[10] Naqvi F, Cervo F and Fields S. Evidence-based review of interventions to improve palliation of pain, dyspnea, depression. Geriatrics 2009; 64(8) 8–10.

[11] British National Formulary, 60th Edition. British Medical Association and Royal Pharmaceutical Society of Great Britain, London 2010.

[12] Srinivasan V, Wielbo D and Tebbett IR. Analgesic effects of codeine-6-glucuronide after intravenous administration. Europran Journal of Pain 1997; 1(3) 185–90.

[13] Vree TB, Van-Dongen RT and Koopman-Kimenai PM. Codeine analgesia is due to codeine-6-glucuronide, not morphine. International Journal of Clinical Practices 2000; 54(6) 395–398.

[14] Chung KF. Drugs to suppress cough. Expert Opinion on Investigational Drugs 2005; 14 19–27.

[15] Guandalini S and Vaziri H. Diarrhea: Diagnostic and Therapeutic Advances, Humana Press, New York, USA. 2010; pp. 452.

[16] Australian Medicinal Handbook. Rossi S. (Ed.) Adelaide: Australian Medicines Handbook, Australian Medicines Handbook 2004.

[17] Armstrong SC and Cozza KL. Pharmacokinetic drug interactions of morphine, codeine, and their derivatives: theory and clinical reality, Part II. Psychosomatics 2003; 44(6) 515-520.

[18] Shukla S and Singh SP. Exploitation of interspecific crosses and its prospects for developing novel plant type in opium poppy (*P. somniferum* L.). In: Trivedi PC (Ed.) Herbal drugs and biotechnology. Pointer Publishers, Jaipur 2004; 210-239.

[19] Yadav HK, Shukla S and Singh SP. Character association and genetic variability for quantitative and qualitative traits in opium poppy (*Papaver somniferum* L). Journal of Genetics and Breeding 2005; 59 303–312.

[20] Aceto MD, Harris LS, Abood ME and Rice KC. Stereoselective mu- and delta- opioid receptor-related antinociception and binding with (+)-thebaine. European Journal of Pharmacology 1999; 365(2-3) 143-147.

[21] Ebrahini SA, Zareie, Rostami P and Mahmoudian M. Interaction of noscapine with the bradykinin mediation of the cough response. Acta Physiologia Hungarica 2003; 90 147-155.

[22] Mahmoudian M and Rahimi-Moghaddam P. The anti-cancer activity of noscapine: A review. Recent Patents on Anti-Cancer Drug Discovery 2009; 4 92-97.

[23] Tang Y, Luan J and Zhang X. Accelerating tissue expansion by application of topical papaverine cream. Plastic and Reconstructive Surgery 2004; 114(5) 1166–1169.

[24] Siuciak JA, Chapin DS and Harms JF. Inhibition of the striatum-enriched phosphodiesterase PDE10A: a novel approach to the treatment of psychosis. Neuropharma 2006; 51 (2) 386–396.

[25] Brisman JL, Eskridge JM and Newell DW. Neuro interventional treatment of vasospasm. Neurological Research 2006; 28 769-776.

[26] Desvaux P. An overview of the management of erectile disorders. Press Medicals 2005; 34(13 suppl) 5-7.

[27] Bella AJ and Brock GB. Intracavernous pharmacotherapy for erectile dysfunction. Endocrine 2004; 23(2-3) 149-155.

[28] Sato Y, He JX, Nagai H, Tani T and Akao T. Isoliquiritigenin, one of the antispasmodic principles of Glycyrrhiza ularensis roots, acts in the lower part of intestine. Biological and Pharmceutical Bulletin 2007; 30 145-149.

[29] Thomas JA. Pharmacological aspects of erectile dysfunction. The Japanese Journal of Pharmacology 2002; 89 101–112.

[30] Müller-Schweinitzer E and Ellis P (). Sucrose promotes the functional activity of blood vessels after cryopreservation in DMSO-containing fetal calf serum. Naunyn Schmiedeberg's Archives of Pharmacology 1992; 345(5) 594–597.

[31] Giglia JS, Ollerenshaw JD, Dowson PE, Black KS and Abbott WM. Cryopreservation prevents arterial allograft dilation. Annals of Vascular Surgery 2002; 16(6) 762-767.

[32] Boswell-Smith V, Spina D and Page CP. Phosphodiesterase inhibitors. British Journal of Pharmacology 2006; 147(1) S252–S257.

[33] Sharma JR, Lal RK, Gupta AP, Misra HO, Pant V, Chandra R and Rashid Md. Opiumless and alkaloid-free non-narcotic opium poppy (*Papaver somniferum* L.) variety "Sujata". United States Patent No. 6730838B1, 2004.

[34] Borrego MM, Landa BB, Cortes-Navas JA, Ledesma-Munoz FJ, Diaz-Jimenez. Role of oospores as primary inoculum for epidemics of downy mildew caused by Peronospora arborescens in opium poppy crops in Spain. Plant Pathology 2009; 58 1092–1103.

[35] Trivedi M, Tiwari RK, Dhawan OP. Genetic parameters and correlations of collar rot resistance with important biochemical and yield traits in opium poppy (*Papaver somniferum* L.). Journal of Applied Genetics 2006; 47(1) 29–38.

[36] Yadav HK, Shukla S and Singh SP. Genetic variability and interrelationship among opium and its alkaloids in opium poppy (*Papaver somniferum* L.). Euphytica 2006; 150 207–214.

[37] Khanna KR and Gupta RK. An assessment of germplasm and prospects for exploitation of heterosis in opium poppy (*P. somniferum* L.). Contemporary Trends in Plant Sciences; Verma SC (Ed.), Kalyani Publishers, New Delhi 1981; pp. 368-381.

[38] Bhandari MM. Preliminary evaluation of opium poppy (*Papaver somniferum* L.) collections from Kota district. Journal of Current Biology 1989; 6(10) 9-15.

[39] Khanna KR and Singh UP. Genetic effects of irradiation in opium poppy. Proceeding Ist Indian Congress of Cytology and Genetics, Chandigarh 1975; pp, 274.

[40] Prajapati S, Bajpai S, Singh D, Luthra R, Gupta MM and Kumar S. Alkaloid profiles of the Indian land races of the opium poppy (*Papaver somniferum* L.). Genetic Resources and Crop Evolution 2002; 49(2)183-188.

[41] Shukla S, Singh SP, Yadav HK and Chatterjee A. Alkaloid spectrum of different germplasm lines in opium poppy (*Papaver somniferum* L.). Genetic Resources and Crop Evolution 2006; 53 533–540.

[42] Gumuscu A, Arslan N and Saran EO. Evolution of selected poppy (*Papaver somniferum* L.) lines by their morphine and other alkaloid contents. European Food Research and Technology 2008; 226(5) 1213-1220.

[43] Dittbrenner A, Mock HP, Borner A and Lohwasser U. Variability of alkaloid content in *Papaver somniferum* L. Journal of Applied Botany and Food Quality-Angewandte Botanik 2009; 82(2) 103-107.

[44] Singh SP, Shukla S and Yadav HK. Multivariate analysis in relation to breeding system in opium poppy (*Papaver somniferum* L.). Genetika 2004; 36 111-120.

[45] Yadav HK, Shukla S, Rastogi A and Singh SP. Assessment of diversity in new genetic stock of opium poppy (*Papaver somniferum* L.). Indian Journal of Agricultural Sciences 2007; 77(8) 537–539.

[46] Yadav HK, Shukla S and Singh SP. Genetic divergence in parental genotypes and its relation with heterosis, F_1 performance and general combining ability (GCA) in opium poppy (*Papaver somniferum* L.). Euphytica 2007; 157 123–130.

[47] Brezinova B, Macak M and Eftimova J. The morphological diversity of selected traits of world collection of poppy genotypes (Genus *Papaver*). Journal of Central European Agriculture 2009; 10(2) 183–190.

[48] Shukla S, Yadav HK, Rastogi A, Mishra BK and Singh SP. Alkaloid diversity in relation to breeding for specific alkaloids in opium poppy (*Papaver somniferum* L.). Czech Journal of Genetics and Plant Breeding 2010; 46(4) 164-169.

[49] Singh SP, Shukla S, Dixit BS and Banerji R. Variation of major fatty acids in F_8 generation of opium poppy (*Papaver somniferum* L). Journal of the Science of Food and Agriculture 1998; 76 168–172.

[50] Ozturk O and Gunlu H. Determining relationships amongst morphine, capsule and oil yield using path coefficient analysis in poppy (*Papaver somniferum* L.). Asian Journal of Chemistry 2008; 20(4) 2979-2988.

[51] Yadav HK, Maurya KN, Shukla S and Singh SP. Combining ability of opium poppy genotypes over F-1 and F-2 generations of 8x8 diallel cross. Crop Breeding and Applied Biotechnology 2009; 9(4) 353-360.

[52] Yadav HK, Shukla S and Singh SP. Genetic combining ability estimates in the F1 and F2 generations for yield, its component traits and alkaloid content in opium poppy (*Papaver somniferum* L.) Euphytica 2009; 168 23-32.

[53] Kumar B and Patra NK. Genetic analysis of capsule and its associated traits in opium poppy (*Papaver somniferum* L.). Journal of Heredity 2010; 101(5) 657-660.

[54] Mishra BK, Shukla S, Rastogi A and Sharma A. Study of heritability and genetic advance for effective selection in opium poppy (*Papaver somniferum* L.). Indian Journal of Agricultural Science 2010; 80(6) 470–476.

[55] Matyasova E, Novak J, Stranska I, Hejtmankova A, Skalicky M, Hejtmankova K and Hejnak V. Production of morphine and variability of significant characters of *Papaver somniferum* L. Plant Soil and Environment 2011; 57(9) 423-428.

[56] Nemeth-Zambori E, Jaszberenyi C, Rajhart P and Bernath J. Evaluation of alkaloid profiles in hybrid generations of different poppy (*Papaver somniferum* L.) genotypes. Industrial Crops and Products 2011; 33(3) 690-696.

[57] Yadav HK and Singh SP. Inheritance of quantitative traits in opium poppy (*Papaver somniferum* L.). Genetika-Belgrade 2011; 43(1) 113-128.

[58] Kumar B and Patra NK. Inheritance pattern and genetics of yield and components traits in opium poppy (*Papaver somniferum* L.). Industrial Crops and Products 2012; 36(1) 445-448.

[59] Azcan N, Kalender BO and Kara M. Investigation of Turkish poppy seeds and seed oils. Chemistry of Natural Compounds 2004; 40(4) 370-372.

[60] Krist S, Stuebiger G, Unterweger H, Bandion F and Buchbauer G. Analysis of volatile coumpounds and Triglycerides of seed oils extracted from different poppy varieties (*Papaver somniferum* L.). Journal of Agricultural Food Chemistry 2005; 53 8310–8316.

[61] Ozcan MM and Atalay C. Determination of seed and oil properties of some poppy (*Papaver somniferum* L.) varieties. Grasas Y Aceites 2006; 57(2) 169–174.

[62] Hakan E, Aziz T and Mehmet MO. Determination of fatty acid, tocopherol and phytosterol contents of the oils of various poppy (*Papaver somniferum* L.) seeds. Grasas y Aceites 2009; 60(4) 375–381.

[63] Francis TR and Kannerberg LW. Yield stability studies in short season maize. I. A descriptive method for grouping genotypes. Canadian Journal of Plant Sciences 1978; 58 1029-1034.

[64] Plaisted R L and Peterson L C. A technique for evaluating the ability of selections to yield consistently in different locations or seasons. American Journal of Potato Research 1959; 36 381-385.

[65] Wricke G. Über eine Methods zur Erfassung der ökologisches Streubreite in Feldversuchen. Zeitschrift für Pflanzenzüchtung 1962; 47 92–96.

[66] Shukla GK. Some statistical aspects of partitioning genotype-environmental components of variability. Journal of Heredity 1972; 29 237-245.

[67] Finlay KW and Wilkinson GN. The analysis of adaptation in a plant-breeding program. Australian Journal of Agricultural Research 1963; 14 742–754.

[68] Perkins JM and Jinks JL. Environmental and genotype-environmental components of variability. Heredity 1968; 23 339-356.

[69] Eberhart SA and Russel WA. Stability parameters for comparing varieties. Crop Science 1966; 6 36-40.

[70] Yadav HK, Shukla S and Singh SP. Assessment of genotype x environment interactions for yield and morphine content in opium poppy (*Papaver somniferum* L.). Acta Agronomica Hungarica 2007; 55(3) 331–338.

[71] Yadav HK, Shukla S, Rastogi A and Singh SP. Non parametric measure of stability for yield and morphine content in opium poppy (*Papaver somniferum* L.). Indian Journal of Agricultural Sciences 2007; 77(9) 596–599.

[72] Yadav HK, Shukla S and Singh SP. Discriminant function analysis for opium and seed yield in opium poppy (*Papaver somniferum* L.). Genetika 2008; 40(2) 109–120.

[73] Sharma JR, Lal RK, Gupta AP, Misra HO, Pant V, Singh NK and Pandey V. Development of non-narcotic (opiumless and alkaloid-free) opium poppy, *Papaver somniferum*. Plant Breeding 1999; 118 449–452.

[74] Chatterjee A, Shukla S and Singh SP. Genetic variability for different quantitative and qualitative traits in M_2 generations of opium poppy (*Papaver somniferum* L.). Journal of Genetics and Breeding 2004; 58 319–322.

[75] Chatterjee A, Shukla S, Mishra P, Rastogi A and Singh SP. Prospects of in vitro production of thebaine in opium poppy (*Papaver somniferum* L.). Industrial Crops and Product 2010; 32 668-670.

[76] Chatterjee A, Shukla S, Rastogi A, Mishra BK, Ohri D and Singh SP. Impact of mutagenesis on cytological behavior in relation to specific alkaloids in Opium Poppy (*Papaver somniferum* L.). Caryologia 2011; 64(1) 14-24.

[77] Chatterjee A, Shukla S, Mishra BK, Rastogi A and Singh SP. Induction of variability through mutagenesis in opium poppy (*Papaver somniferum* L.). Turkish Journal of Agriculture and Forestry 2012; 35 1-11.

[78] Mishra BK, Pathak S, Sharma A, Trivedi PK and Shukla S. Modulated gene expression in newly synthesized auto-tetraploid of *Papaver somniferum* L. South African Journal of Botany 2010; 76 447–452.

[79] Srivastava HK and Singh D. Honeybees foraging response in genetically diversified opium poppy. Bioresource Technology 2006; 97(13)1578-1581.

[80] Losak T and Richter R. Split nitrogen doses and their efficiency in poppy (*Papaver somniferum* L.) nutrition. Plant Soil and Environment 2004; 50(1) 484-488.

[81] Ziska LH, Panicker S and Wojno HL. Recent and projected increases in atmospheric C dioxide and the potential impacts on growth and alkaloid production in wild poppy (*Papaver setigerum* DC.). Climatic Change 2008; 91 395-403.

[82] Szabo B, Lakatos A, Koszegi T and Botz L. Investigation of abiogenic stress-induced alterations in the level of secondary metabolites in poppy plants (*Papaver somniferum* L.). Acta Biologica Hungarica 2008; 59(4) 425-438.

[83] Skarpa P and Richter R. Foliar nutrition of poppy plants (*Papaver somniferum* L.) with selenium and the effect on its content in seeds. Journal of Elementology 2011; 16(1) 85-92.

[84] Millgate AG, Pogson BJ, Wilson IW, Kutchan TM, Zenk MH, Gerlach WL, Fist AJ and Larkins PJ. Morphine-pathway block in top1 poppies. Nature 2004; 431-413.

Chapter 9

Castor Breeding

Máira Milani and
Márcia Barreto de Medeiros Nóbrega

Additional information is available at the end of the chapter

http://dx.doi.org/10.5772/56216

1. Introduction

Produced from the seeds of *Ricinus communis,* castor oil is an important feedstock for the chemical industry because it is the only commercial source of ricinoleic acid, a hydroxy fatty acid, which comprises about 90% of the oil. In addition to the traditional uses of ricinoleic acid, there is also a demand for vegetable oil to be used as biofuel and for nem products derived from the castor oil. Due to the increasing demand in the global market, there is a short supply of castor oil and this trend seems to get worst every year. Castor is an ideal candidate for production of high value, industrial oil feedstocks because of the very high oil content (48-60%) of the seed, and the extremely high levels of potential oil production [1] Due to the ricinoleic acid, castor oil and its derivatives are of great versatility being used in synthesis routes for a large number of products and are increasing rapidly [2,3]. In some places of the world it is used like an ornamental due to their vibrant leaf and floral coloration [4].

All over the world, cultivation is done by small farmers in countries such as India, China, and Brasil, and FAO statistics report seed yield averages of 1,104.8; 911.8; and 701.1kg/ha respectively for these countries (Figure 1). In Brazil and in India, the production is made in arid or semiarid regions. In these environments, the rainfall, is generally erratic and low, and the availability of water is the major factor affecting yield.

In Brazil, the production of castor oil is concentrated in the semi-arid northeast, mainly in the state of Bahia, which accounts for more than 80% of the production and acreage [6, 7]. The culture system used by small producers in Brazil usually involves intercropping with food crops mainly maize and beans, and low adoption of technologies. The whole system of production, from planting to processing is manual [8]. Mostly the use of local varieties with long cycle and uneven seed maturation, little or no soil tillage and fertilization. Using such technology farmers have low-income, and the national seed yield of castor is low as 600 kg/ha

[7]. These values are too low to make the production profitable. The cultivars developed by Embrapa Cotton for the traditional areas of cultivation of castor, produce an average of 1500 kg/ha of castor in farmers fields [9].

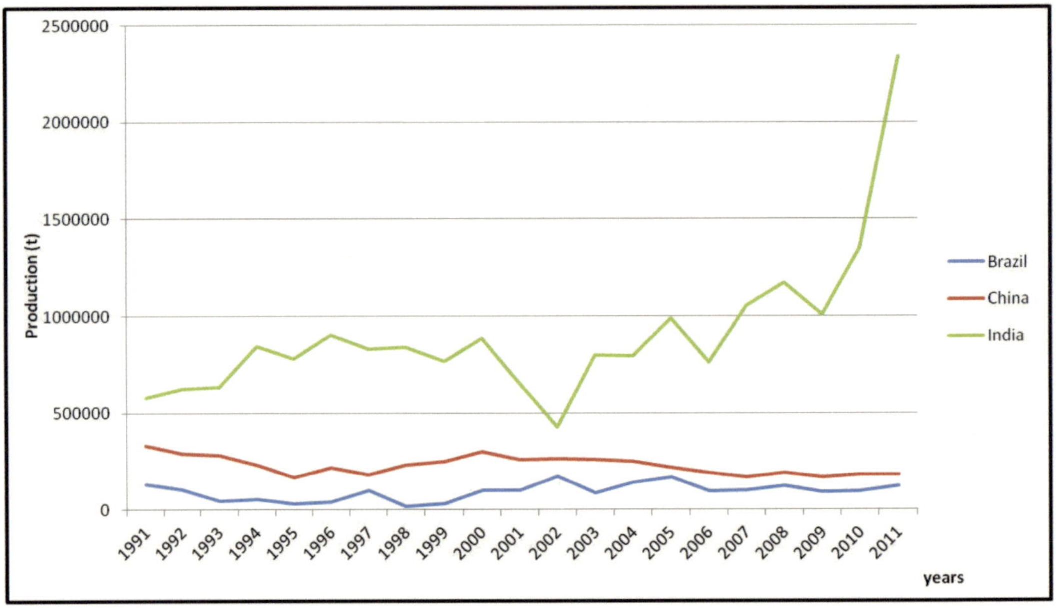

Figure 1. Yield of castor seed in the three main producers countries in twenty years. Data Source: [5]

The populations synthesized by the breeding program of Embrapa Cotton have been evaluated along with public and private partners since 1987. The Research Group mainly evaluates selected genotypes based on the behavior per se of individuals or populations. The main objective is to obtain cultivar that are more productive and adapted to the environment of each growing region, to the production system, and the technological level applied.

The program aims to develop cultivars that are indehiscent, short, and easy to harvest. Earliness of seed maturation is also desired.

2. Genetic resources

The taxonomy and geographic distribution were thoroughly studied and documented earlier in USSR [10], USA [1], Brazil [11] and India [12,13,14]. Castor is reported to have a polyphyletic origin, both India and Africa were considered as the origin of castor based on its widespread cultivation, documents of its medicinal uses and physical evidences. Due to its widespread survival and perennial nature, all possible transitions from an uncultivated plant to a weedy plant and from semi cultivated to a field crop exist and there is no gap between uncultivated and cultivated castor.

The genetic diversity in castor is restricted due to its monotypic existence. Six subspecies viz., persicus, chinensis, zanzibarinus, sanguineus, Africans, Mexicans were identified based on eco-geographical grouping [12, 10, 15]. However, there is no difference in the chromosome number (2n=20) among the sub-species and they all can cross easily with each other [12, 16].

According [17] and [18], the castor can be classified as:

- Superdivision: *Spermatophyta* - Seed plants
- Division: *Magnoliophyta* - Flowering plants
- Class: *Magnoliopsida* - Dicotyledons
- Subclass: *Rosidae*
- Order: *Euphorbiales*
- Family: *Euphorbiaceae* - Spurge family
- Genus: *Ricinus* L. - Ricinus
- Species: *Ricinus communis* L. - Castor

According [19], castor must be classified as Angiospermae, Eudicotyledone, Rosanae and Malpighiales.

Although generally known as "castor bean", this plant is not a legume, and the term "bean" should be discontinued in favor of castor plant and castor seed [15] 2000). Avoiding to use the term bean is really important because these seed and the whole plant are very poisonous and should not be eaten.

A great variation in phenotypic expression is observed due to its cross-pollinated nature. Example of high variability in morphological characters are stem color, epicuticular wax

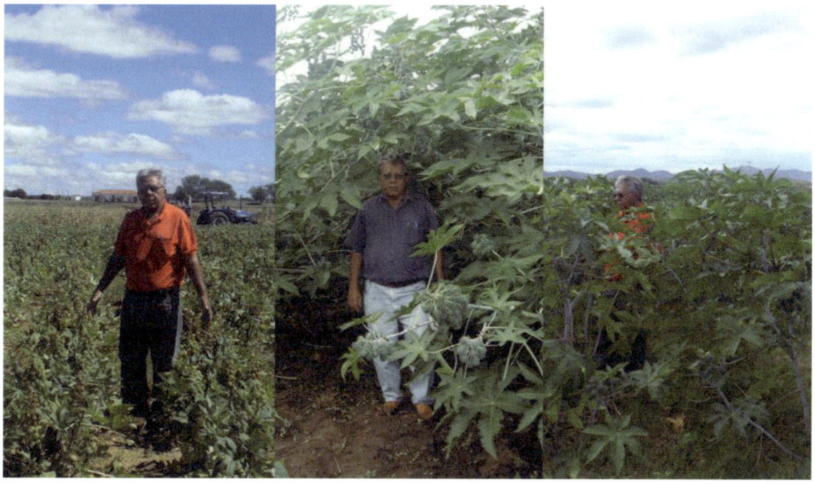

Figure 2. Examples of castor bean plants with different height. Photos: Máira Milani, Embrapa Cotton.

(bloom wax), plant height (Figure 2), presence of spines on capsules (Figure 3), branching pattern, leaf shape, sex expression (Figure 4), seed color, and response to environmental conditions. Wide variation was observed in several morphological traits in the germplasm collections in India, USSR and elsewhere [14, 20, 15]. Also for quantitative traits its genetic polymorphism is exploitable in breeding programs [21, 22, 23, 24].

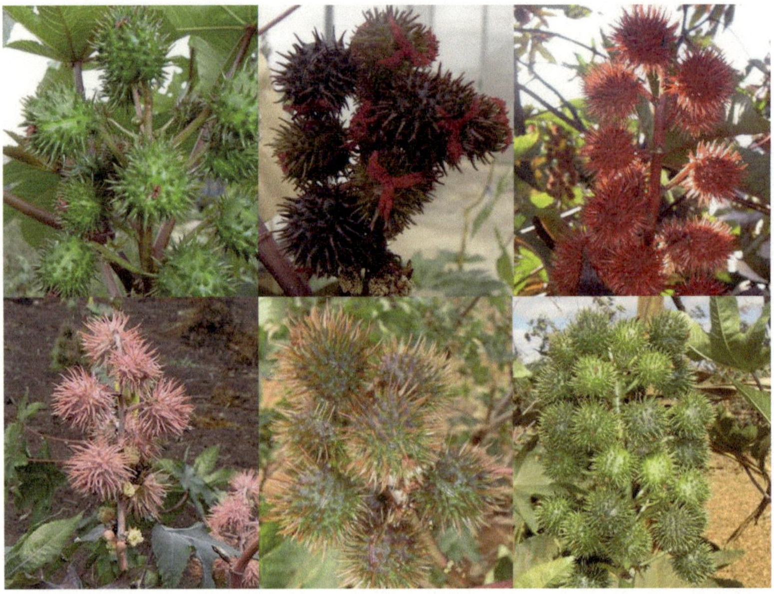

Figure 3. Examples of different colors in the fruits of castor bean. Photos: Máira Milani, Embrapa Cotton.

Germplasm banks are the basic providers of useful genes and genotypes needed to achieve the desirable genetic improvement in breeding programs; however, the resources available in castor germplasm worldwide have been barely tapped for castor genetic improvement and the majority of them have been poorly characterized [25]. The use of genetic resources by the global castor community could be increased if there were characterization of accessions, consolidated reports on available resources, free accession to information on banks, and uniform data collection standards among repositories [25].

These enhancements would allow an estimate of the genetic variability with single collections without the flux of accessions between countries. Germplasm characterization would also be easier if fast, non-destructive, and reliable screening methods were developed. An example is the quick and non-destructive method for estimating ricinoleic fatty acid content by Nuclear Magnetic Resonance in seeds [26].

Normally, castor is monoecious, with pistillate flowers on the upper part of raceme and staminate flowers on the lower part (Fig. 4a). This type is referred to as normal monoecious. Another type, referred as interspersed monoecious, has pistillate and staminate flowers interspersed along the entire raceme axis. The proportion of pistillate and staminate flowers

http://dx.doi.org/10.5772/56216

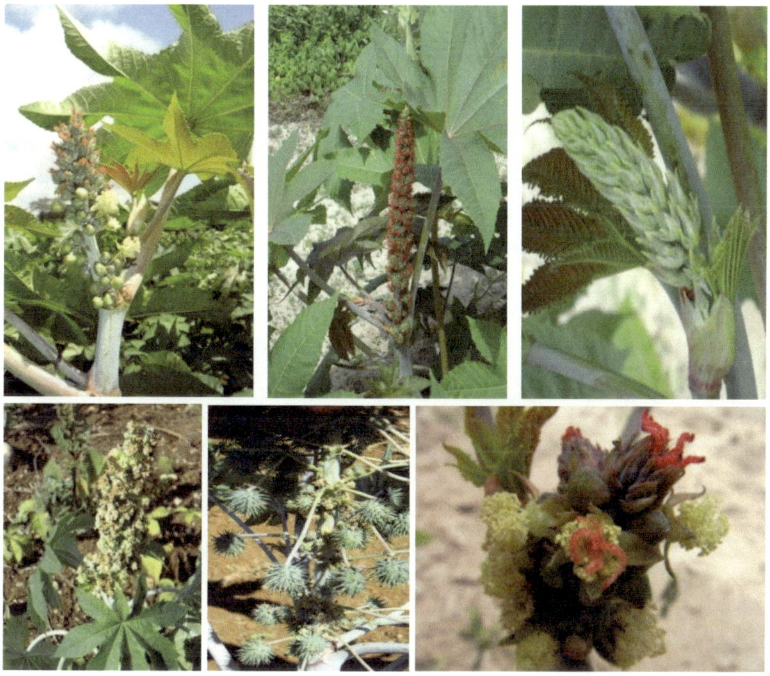

Figure 4. Arrangement of male and female flowers in racemes of castor: a)monoic normal; b and c) gynodioc; d) androdioic; e)interspersed; f) monoic bearing some perfect flowers.

among racemes can vary widely both within and among genotypes. It can also be influenced considerably by environment [27]

In normal monoecious varieties, the percentage of pistillate flowers along the raceme axis is usually the highest on the first raceme, with a decreasing percentage on subsequently developed racemes. With the decrease in pistillate flowers, there is a proportional increase in the number of staminate flowers [27]. This within plant variation is generally associated with the seasons. Female tendency is highest in spring and early summer; male tendency is highest in mid and late summer. Temperature is probably the main environmental component affecting sex. Moderate temperatures promote female flowers while high temperature promote male flowers. However, age of plant and nutrition can also influence sex expression. Femaleness is strongest in young plants with a high level of nutrition. Maleness is strongest in old plants with a low level of nutrition [28].

In addition to monoecism, a subtype of dioecism occurs in plants with only pistillate flowers along the entire raceme axis of all racemes [27]. The counterpart, plants with only staminate flowers, can occur in extreme climatic conditions, with high temperature or water deficit (Fig. 4d).

There are three types of pistillate lines (employed for hybrid production): N, S, and NES. In the N type, the femaleness is controlled by a recessive gene (ff). In the S type, femaleness is controlled by a polygenic complex with dominant and epistatic effects in which the plant starts as female, but a reversion can occur at any time. In the NES type, the plant has the recessive gene (ff) that allows it to start as female, but the presence of environmentally sensitive genes triggers a sexual reversion when temperature is higher than 31 °C [29,30, 31].

The development of pistillate lines has allowed breeders to successfully utilize heterosis (hybrid vigor) in castor. Prior to the development of pistillate lines, inbred lines having many female flowers were used as female lines. Commercial exploitation of heterosis in India was instantly adopted after the development of VP-1, a S type stable pistillate line derived from TSP 10 R (Texas Stable Pistillate 10R) introduced from the USA [31]. Several pistillate lines were developed using VP-1 source of pistillate expression [32,33,34]. Other pistillate lines were developed using NES type of sexual expression but GCH-6 is the only commercial hybrid based on that system. Several other sources of pistillate lines were identified by screening 1 250 accessions from the germplasm bank at DOR, India [25, 34].

The adoption of male-sterile lines could be an alternative to pistillate lines for the production of hybrid seeds. Some studies were performed looking for genotypes with male sterility or inducing it through mutation [35], but we did not find any reference to a genotype expressing male-sterility for adoption into hybrid development programs.

A male flower, after opening, releases viable pollen grains for 1 to 2 days. The best environmental conditions for pollen dispersal are at a temperature between 26 °C to 29 °C and relative humidity of 60%, which may vary according to the cultivar. The pollen contain allergenic substances similar to those found in the seeds, which are of protein nature, such as ricin, robina, crotin, and circina Arbina [15] 2000). High temperatures, plant age, and short day length favor the appearence of male flowers.

Regarding the female flowers, the literature shows that stigmas become receptive before the anthesis of male flowers. However the existence of this short protogynous phase [36] is not accepted by most researchers [37] who claim the male flowers reach maturity first and anthesis usually occurs in a short period of time before the opening of the female flowers [1]. In this way, there is a large source of pollen for the first pistillate flowers that open and become receptive. The stigma is fully receptive a few hours after the flower opens, but it is difficult for pollination to occur shortly after the opening of the flower. The stigma remains receptive after anthesis, , for a period of 5 to 10 days depending on environmental conditions [38].

Castor has a mixed mating system generating both selfed and cross fertilized offspring. Under natural conditions, cross pollination in castor can exceed 80% [11], but the actual level of cross pollination is dependent on both genotype and environmental conditions. Since pollination occurs mostly by wind, genetic purity of individual accessions can be maintained by planting in isolation by time or space (usually 1,000 m from other accessions) or covering the inflorescence with a paper bag [39]. This later option is labor intensive and expensive, but usually more practical if breeders need just a few seeds. Storing pollen is another option for germplasm conservation. [40] observed that castor pollen grains were viable after being stored at temperatures of -196° C, -80° C, and -18° C for up 30 days and there is evidence that pollen viability would be retained for long periods with cryopreservation at -80° C.

3. Goals of castor bean breeding

Presently the main objectives of the breeding programs around the world are: earliness of seed maturation, plants architecture for mechanized harvest and disease resistance (root not and gray mold). These should be combined with superior productivity of cultivars and at least of 48% oil content of seed. Most breeding programs have searched genotypes with short height (less than 1.5m), height of primary raceme between 20 and 40cm, less than 150 days for harvesting, erect plant and non-shattering fruits.

In some regions, castor has have been selected for increased tolerance to abiotic stresses such as drought, high temperature, salinity, and exchangeable aluminium. Considering that the castor is not a food crop, it is often considered to be cultivated in marginal areas.

The reduction of the toxicity of castor seeds has also been the target of improvement programs. Ricin is a protein toxin found in the endosperm of castor seed capable of inhibiting protein synthesis by enzymatically blocking the ribosomes of eukaryotes [41]. Castor oil does not contain ricin because this protein is insoluble in oil, and any residual ricin is eliminated in the refining process. Ricin content varies among genotypes. The ricin content varied from 1.9 a 16 g/kg among 263 accessions from the USDA Germplasm Bank [42] and from 3.5 to 32.2 in varieties and accessions from the Embrapa Germplasm Bank [43].

The development of new cultivars with traits of interest and adapted to specific microclimates is only possible when there is available knowledge about the extent of genetic diversity of the species [44]. Despite the recent publication of the castor bean genome [45], little is known about the actual genetic diversity of this species. Genetic diversity analyses of castor bean germplasm collections worldwide have showed low levels of variability and lack of geographically structured genetic populations, regardless of marker system used (e.g. [4, 46, 47]). Thus, the remarkable phenotypic variation observed in castor does not seem to reflect a high genetic diversity, similar to the one reported for physic nut, in which variations in epigenetic mechanisms may have a more important role in the diversity of the species than genetic variability per se [48]. Castor diversity is still poorly characterized by means of molecular marker systems [49, 50, 51, 52, 53]. In fact, the species has been overlooked until the late 2000s, when analyses regarding genetic diversity of germplasm collections were first published [46]. Thus, obtaining the desired genotypes implies the characterization of the germplasm banks and the proper publication of these results.

4. Breeding methods

In early phases of breeding programs, more attention is given to qualitative characters, but in later stages of improvement greater emphasis is shifted to quantitative traits such as yield, plant height, days to flowering, and traits associated with agronomic and economic factors.

Because castor has both self and crossed pollination and most of pollination is made by wind, contamination of varieties during seed production is a constant risk. To prevent contamination, it is necessary to isolate the area, physically (1000 meters) or temporally, or the use of self-fertilization using paper bags (Fig. 4). Both strategies are expansive. The self-fertilization is a hand labor and normally demands many people and time. is practically impossible to keep the distance recommended in areas multiplication of lines, where they are multiplied dozens of strains simultaneously because it would require a large extension of the area.

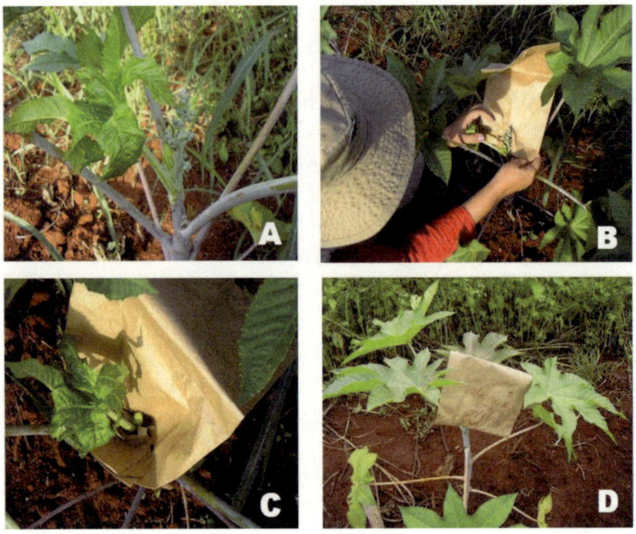

Figure 5. Self fertilization in castor. A) raceme with growing flowers; B) paper bag being placed over the raceme; C) Fixing paper bag; D) Identification. Photos of Marcia B. M. Nobrega, Embrapa Cotton.

Heterosis is a option for the development of hybrid cultivars of castor oil, representing an effective way to increase yield. In castor, this technique is possible due to the occurrence of gynodioecious plants whose genetic control is assigned to a recessive allele. However, the maintenance of female lines in castor increases the costs of production of hybrids. Thus, it is believed that the maintenance and propagation of female lines by micro propagation could be performed in vitro and therefore the purity of the female lines could be easily ensured, and manufacturing costs would be lower. Embrapa Cotton has been testing methods of clonal propagation in vitro and ex vitro in the castor, in order to regenerate and increase germplasm bank accessions, including a few female lines.

The cultivar development is divided into two main phases: pre-breeding and breeding. Both are essential to reaching its ultimate goal,which is to release new productive cultivars with wide adaptation, stability and good acceptance among producers. The pre-breeding, by definition, is the "bridge" between genetic resources and improvement [54]. In addition to the activities of these two steps it is essential to support activities of processes such as evaluation of the rate of outcrossing, asexual multiplication (in vitro and ex vitro), seed multiplication, and others. Each process is very important for the outcome. On average, the development of cultivars takes 10 to 12 years from the selection of germplasm to the legal process of plant variety protection.

Embrapa Cotton with partners developed four castor cultivars using methods applied for inbreed populations: BRS Nordestina, BRS Paraguaçu, BRS Energia e BRS Gabriela. These varieties are recommended for the states of North and Northeast of Brazil.

BRS Nordestina stands out from the average height of 1.90 m, greenish stems with the presence of wax, conical racemes, semi-dehiscent fruits, and black seeds. The period between emergence and first flowering raceme is 50 days, on average, while the average weight of 100 seeds is 68 g, and the oil seed content is 48%. The average yield is 1,500 kg/ha under conditions of normal rainfall in the Northeast semiarid region. The period between the emergencee until the last harvest is 250 days. The BRS Paraguaçu has an average height of 1.60 m, purple wax stem, oval raceme, semi-dehiscent fruits and black seeds. The period from emergence to flowering is 54 days, while the average weight weight of 100 seeds is 71g, and the oil seed content is 47%. The average productivity is 1,500 kg/ha under rainfed conditions of the semiarid region of the Northeast. Earliness is a key feature of BRS Energia, whose average cycle is 120 days between emergence and maturation of the last racemes. The appearance of the first raceme occurs about 30 days after germination. The yield of this cultivar is 1.800kg/ha under the same climatic conditions of the others. The average plant height is 1.40 m, 100 seed weight is around 40 g

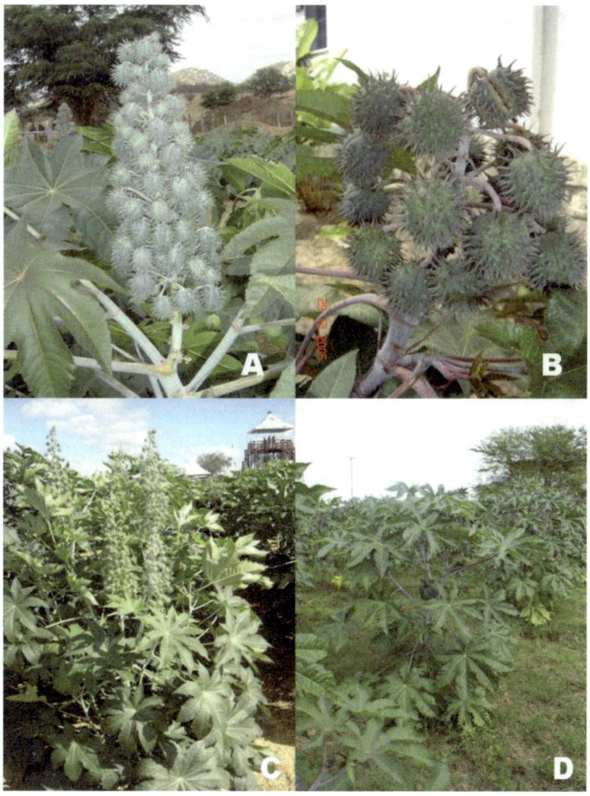

Figure 6. Embrapa´s castor cultivars: (A) BRS Nordestina, (B) BRS Paraguaçu, (C) BRS Energia, and (D) BRS Gabriela. Photos of Máira Milani, Embrapa Algodão.

and the seed oil content is 48%. The BRS Gabriela has the highest seed oil content, 50% on average. It has a mean cycle of 150 days, productivity of 1900 kg/ha. The racemes have a round shape, immature green fruit with wax, an average density of spines, average density of fruit and green pink spines. Under extremes of precipitation (high or low), the density of fruits in racemes can be sparse. The fruits are indehiscent.

4.1. Mass selection

Mass selection consists in the selection of superior types and the discharge of undesirable types within a plant population. It is used for imprioved cultivars or established local types to improve, or standardize traits of economic importance.

Mass selection is the most effective method for characteristics with high heritability in populations with high levels of natural genetic variability. Two procedures are useful in increasing the efficiency of the mass selection in populations of castor: the self-fertilization of the selected plants to prevent cross pollination, and the use of controlled selection techniques to reduce environmental variation [55]. Mass selection was used to develop IAC-38, an important dwarf castor cultivar in Brazil [11]

4.2. Individual plant selection with progeny tests

This method consists in selecting individual plants and the subsequent study of their offspring in progeny trials. It is based on the principle that the breeding value of a plant may be measured by the performance of its progeny. It is a straightforward procedure to achieve greater uniformity and increased production in castor. The method of progeny test is highly effective for the improvement of populations of castor with high levels of natural genetic variability. This method was successfully used in the development of the high yielding cultivar 'Guarany' [56]

4.3. Methods involving sexual hybridization

When populations of castor with sufficient natural genetic variation for agronomic characteristics are not available, it is necessary to generate variability by producing hybrids between different lines or cultivars [55]. The choice of the parents of these populations must be based on their agronomic performance within the targeted production region, and diallel cross can be used if there are several promising parents or cultivars [55].

The pedigree method is adequate for simultaneous selection of several traits. This methods has been used to develop the cultivar IAC-2028, a dwarf and not-shattering genotype in Brazil [57].

The bulk method is the most effective option when the main objective is to improve the adaptation of castor to stress conditions such as drought, acid soils, high levels of salt and resistance to diseases [55]. The backcross method of selection is the most effective when there is a need to improve some simply inherited, qualitative characteristic in a commercial cultivar or promising elite line. The non-recurrent parent must have the characteristic absent from the recurrent parent. The method of backcrossing is especially effective in castor for the improvement of characteristics such as seed shattering, flower height, and disease resistance [55].

Recurrent selection is defined as successive cycles of selection and recombination of selected lines or individual plants [55]. It is not often used for castor selection, but it has been successful on the reduction of height of the cultivar Guarani [58, 59]. In each of five cycles of selection, plant height was reduced by 28 cm, 13 cm, 19.9 cm, 11.7 cm and 3.4 cm [59].

In the last three decades, India has made significant progress in the development of hybrids [60]. The availability of pistilate lines, like the VP-1, was the base for launching hybrids such as GAUCH-1, GCH-2, and GCH-4 during 1990s and ten more high yielding hybrids later on [60].

The first commercial castor hybrid, 'GCH 3', was developed in India and had high seed yield potential (88% superior to the most planted cultivars at that time), drought tolerance, medium maturity time (140-210 days) and high oil content (46%). Since then, a total of 15 hybrids were released in India, some of them with resistance to fusarium wilt and high seed yield potential [34]. The advantages of hybrids over cultivars resulted in a predominance of hybrids (50 to 60%) in the castor production in India. In the State of Gujarat, the use of hybrid seed is up to 95% of the cultivated area. In Gujarat, where castor is cultivated mostly under irrigated conditions, the adoption of hybrid seed has caused an increase in seed yield from 350 to 1 970 kg/ha within a few years [34].

The intensity of heterosis on castor seed yield depends on both the genetic diversity and individual combining ability of the parents [61, 62, 63, 64, 32, 33, 34]. More studies on genetic diversity and combining ability are necessary for supporting the development of hybrids.

An alternative method for selecting castor hybrids was successfully evaluated by Toppa [65]. The method of cryptic hybrids was proposed by Lonqquist [66] for maize, consisting of simultaneous self-pollination and crossing in the same plant, allowing the selection of the best progeny at each cycle. Because castor has a low endogamic depression and produces more than one raceme per plant, the method can be employed. After four cycles of selection, the 12 cryptic hybrids had higher seed yield (1,675 kg/ha) than the 12 conventional hybrids (1,550 kg/ha) evaluated over two years in two locations [65].

5. Challenges

The scarcity of labor that has been observed in rural areas over the past decade, has raised the costs of operation management and cultivation. A research group in Brazil has been focusing on the research for indehiscent cultivars with shorter plants to facilitate mechanical harvesting operations. Also earlier genotypes have been obtained to reduce the residence time of the crop in the field.

In a review of the challenges to reach greater productivity with the castor [67], the authors mention that the main challenge in developing cultivars is the castor plant adaptation to

Combine harvesting. Both cultivars as machines, require further adjusted in order to obtain more efficiency in the process of Combine harvesting.

Nowadays, breeders look for plants that could be adapted for a variety environmental conditions including the increased ambient temperature caused by Global Climate Change.

Author details

Máira Milani and Márcia Barreto de Medeiros Nóbrega

Embrapa Cotton, Campina Grande, Paraíba, Brazil

References

[1] Brigham RD. Castor: Return of an old crop. In Janick J; Simon JE (ed.) Progress in New Crops. New York: Wiley, 1993. 380-383.

[2] Chierice GO; Claro Neto S. Aplicação industrial do óleo. In: Azevedo DMP; Beltrão NEM (Ed.). O Agronegócio da mamona no Brasil. Brasília, DF:Embrapa Informação Tecnológica, Campina Grande: Embrapa Algodão, 2007, 417-447.

[3] CASTOROIL.IN Comprehensive Castor Oil Report: A report on castor oil & castor oil derivatives, in: http://www.castoroil.in/reference/report/report.html. (Accessed 31 january 2013)

[4] Foster JT, Allan GJ, Chan AP, Rabinowicz PD, Ravel J, Jackson PL. Single nucleotide polymorphisms forasses sing genetic diversity in castor bean (Ricinus communis). BMC Plant Biol. , 201010:13-23. doi:10.1186/1471-2229-10-13

[5] FAOSTAT http://faostatfao.org/site/567/DesktopDefault.aspx?PageID=567#ancor 2012 (accessed 12 november 2012)

[6] Carvalho BCL. Manual do cultivo da mamona. Salvador: EBDA. 2005

[7] CONAB. Série histórica: mamona. Brasília, DF: Central de Informações Agropecuárias. http://www.conab.gov.br/conteudos.php?a=1382&t=2. (Accessed 31jan2013)

[8] Savy Filho A. Mamona: tecnologia agrícola. Campinas: Emopi, 2005

[9] Freire EC; Lima EF; Andrade FP; Milani M; Nóbrega MBM. Melhoramento genético. In: Azevedo DMP; Beltrão NEM (Ed.). O Agronegócio da mamona no Brasil. Brasília, DF:mbrapa Informação Tecnológica, Campina Grande: Embrapa Algodão, 2007. 169-194

[10] Moshkin VA. Castor. New Delhi: Amerind; 1986

[11] Savy Filho A. Castor bean breeding. In: Borém A (Ed.) Improvement of Cultivated Species. Viçosa: Federal University of Viçosa, 2005

[12] Kulkarni LG, Ramanamurthy GV. Castor. New Delhi: Indian Council of Agric Res., 1977

[13] DOR. Castor in India. Hyderabad: Directorate of Oilseeds Research. 2003

[14] Anjani K. Extra-early maturing germplasm for utilization in castor improvement. Ind. Crops Products 2010, 31, 139-144

[15] Weiss EA. Oilseed crops. 2nd ed. Oxford: Blackwell Science, 2000

[16] Atsmon D. Castor. In: Röbbelen G, Downey RK, Ashri A (Eds.) Oil Crops of the World. New York: McGraw Hill, 1989; p 348–447,

[17] Vidal WN, Vidal MRR. Fitossistemática: famílias de angiospermas.Viçosa: UFV, 1980. 59.

[18] Popova GM, Moshkin VA. Botanical classification. In: Moshkin VA (Ed.). Castor. New Delhi: Amerind, 1986

[19] Angiosperm Phylogeny Group III. An update of the Angiosperm Phylogeny Group classification for the orders and families of flowering plants: APG III. Botanical Journal of the Linnean Society, London, 2009, 161: 105 – 121

[20] Moshkin VA, Dvoryadkina AG. Cytology and genetics of qualitative characters. In: Moshkin VA Castor. New Delhi: Amerind, 1986. 93-102

[21] Uguru MI, Abuka IN. Hybrid vigour and genetic actions for two qualitative traits in castor plant (Ricinus communis L.). Ghana Journal. Agric. Sci. 1998; 31: 81 – 82

[22] Bahia HF, Silva SA, Fernandez LG, Ledo CAS, Moreira RFC. Divergência genética entre cinco cultivares de mamoneira. Pesquisa Agropecuária Brasileira, 2008. 43, 357-362.

[23] Bezerra Neto FV, Leal NR, Gonçalves LSA, Rêgo Filho LM, Amaral Júnior AT. Descritores quantitativos na estimativa da divergência genética entre genótipos de mamoneira utilizando análises multivariadas Rev. Ciênc. Agron., 2010, 41, 294-299

[24] Nóbrega MBM, Geraldi IO, Carvalho ADF. Avaliação de cultivares de mamona em cruzamentos dialélicos parciais. Bragantia 2010. 69. 281-288

[25] Anjani K. Castor genetic resources: a primary gene pool for exploitation. Ind. Crops. Products 2012.35:1-14 doi: 10.1016/jindcrop.2011.06.011.

[26] Berman P, Nizri S, Parmet Y, Wiesman Z. Large scale-scale screening of intact castor seeds by viscosity using time domain NMR and chemometrics. J. Am. Oil Chem. Soc. 2010. 87:1247-1254.doi:10.1007/s11746-010-1612-z.

[27] Zimmerman LH, Smith JD. Production of F1 seed in castorbean by use of sex genes sensitive to environment. Crop Science, 1966, 6: 406-409

[28] Shifriss O. Sex Instability in Ricinus. Genetics, 1956, 41: 265–280.

[29] Zimmerman, L. H. Castorbeans: a new crop for mechanized production. Adv. Agron. (1958). X:, 257-288.

[30] Shifriss, O. Conventional and unconventional systems controlling sex variations in *Ricinus*. J. Genet. (1960).

[31] Ankineedu G, Rao GP. Development of pistillate castor. Indian J. Genet. Plant Breeding 1973, 33:416-422

[32] Lavanya C, Ramanarao PV, Gopinath VV. Studies on combining ability and heterosis in castor hybrids. Journal of Oilseeds Research 2006, 23:174-177.

[33] Pathak HC. Crop Improvement in Castor. In D.M. Hegde (ed.) Vegetable Oils Scenario: Approaches to Meet the Growing Demands. Hyderabad: Indian Society of Oilseeds Research, 2009. 82-94

[34] Lavanya C, Solanki SS. Crop improvement of castor. The challenges ahead. In Hegde DM (ed.). Research and Development in Castor. Present status and future strategies. Hyderabad: Indian Society of Oilseeds Research, 2010, p 36-55

[35] Chauhan SVS, Singh KP, Kinoshit T. Gamma-ray induced pollen sterility in castor. J. Fac. Agric. Hokkaido Univ. 1990.64, 229-234

[36] Gurgel JT. Estudos sobre a mamoneira (Ricinus communis L.). Thesis for teaching profession. ESALQ/USP; 1945

[37] Tavora FJAF. A cultura da mamona. Fortaleza: Epace, 1982

[38] Moreira JAN, Lima EF, Farias FJC, Azevedo, DMP. Melhoramento da mamoneira (Ricinus communis L.). Campina Grande. Embrapa/CNPA, 1996

[39] Rizzardo RAG. O papel de Apis mellifera L. como polinizador da mamoneira (Ricinus communis L.):avaliação da eficiência de polinização das abelhas e incremento de produtividade da cultura, MS thesis.Universidade Federal do Ceará; 2007

[40] Vargas DP, Souza SAM, Silva SDA, Bobrowski VL. Pollen grain analysis of some cultivars of castor-oil plant (Ricinus communis L., Euphorbiaceae): conservation and viability. Arquivos do Instituto Biologico 2009. 76, 115-120

[41] Khvostova IV. Ricin: the toxic protein of seed. In: Moshkin VA (Ed.) Castor. New Delhi: Amerind Publ., 1986. p 85–92

[42] Pinkerton SD, Rolfe RD, Auld DL, Ghetie V, Lauterbach BF. Selection of castor with divergent concentrations of ricin and Ricinus communis agglutinin. Crop Sci. 1999; 39:353-357

[43] Baldoni AB, Carvalho MH, Sousa NL, Nobrega MBM, Milani M, Aragão FJL. Variability of ricin content in mature seeds of castor bean. Pesquisa Agropecuária Brasileira, 46, , 2011. 776-779

[44] Gepts, P. Crop domestication as a long-term selection experiment. In: Janick J. (Ed.) Plant Breeding Reviews, Habaken: John Wiley & Sons, Inc., (2004). , 24, 1-44.

[45] Chan AP, Crabtree J, Zhao Q, Lorenzi H, Orvis J, Puiu D, Melake-Berhan A, Jones KM, Redman J, Chen G, Cahoon EB, Gedil M, Stanke M, Haas BJ, Wortman JR, Fraser-Liggett CM, Ravel J, Rabinowicz PD. Draft genome sequence of the oilseed species Ricinus communis. Nat. Biotechnol. 2010; 28:951-956. doi:10.1038/nbt.1674.

[46] Allan G, Williams A, Rabinowicz PD, Chan AP, Ravel J, Keim P. Worldwide genotyping of castor bean germplasm (Ricinus communis L.) using AFLPs and SSRs. Genet. Resour. Crop Evol. 2008; 55:365-378.doi:10.1007/s10722-007-9244-3

[47] Qiu LJ, Yang C, Tian B, Yang JB, Liu AZ. Exploiting EST databases for the development and characterization of EST-SSR markers in castor bean (Ricinus communis L.). BMC Plant Biol. 2010; 10:278-287. doi:10.1186/1471-2229-10-278

[48] Yi C, Zhang S, Liu X, Bui H, Hong Y. Does epigenetic polymorphism contribute to phenotypic variances in Jatropha curcas L.? BMC Plant Biology 2010; 10: 1-9

[49] Billotte N, Jourjon M, Marseillac N, Berger A, Flori A, Asmady H, Adon B, Singh R, Nouy B, Potier F, Cheah S, Rohde W, Ritter E, Courtois B, Charrier A, Mangin B. QTL detection by multi-parent linkage mapping in oil palm (Elaeis guineensis Jacq.). Theoretical and Applied Genetics, 2010; 120, 1673-1687

[50] Feng S, Li W, Huang H, Wang J, Wu Y. Development, characterization and cross-species/genera transferability of EST-SSR markers for rubber tree (Hevea brasiliensis). Molecular Breeding, 2009; 23: 85-97

[51] Sayama T, Hwang TY, Komatsu K, Takada Y, Takahashi M, Kato S, Sasama H, Higashi A, Nakamoto Y, Funatsuki H, Ishimoto M. Development and application of a whole-genome simple sequence repeat panel for high-throughput genotyping in soybean. DNA Research, 2011; 18:107-115

[52] Sraphet S, Boonchanawiwat A, Thanyasiriwat T, Boonseng O, Tabata S, Sasamoto S, Shirasawa K, Isobe S, Lightfoot DA, Tangphatsornruang S, Triwitayakorn K. SSR and EST-SSR-based genetic linkage map of cassava (Manihot esculenta Crantz). Theoretical and Applied Genetics, 2011; 122: 1161-1170

[53] Talia P, Nishinakamasu V, Hopp HE, Heinz RA, Paniego N. Genetic mapping of EST-SSRs, SSR and In Dels to improve saturation of genomic regions in a previously developed sunflower map. Electronic Journal of Biotechnology, 2010; 13: 6

[54] Nass LL. Utilização de recursos genéticos no melhoramento. In: Nass LL, Valois ACC, Melo IS, Valadares-Inglis MC. Recursos genéticos e melhoramento de plantas. Rondonópolis: Fundação MT, 2001; 29-56

[55] Auld DL, Zanotto MD, Mckeon T, Morris JB. Castor. In: Vollmann J, Rajcan I. (ed.) Oil Crops - Handbook of Plant Breeding. New York: Springer, 2009, 316-332

[56] Amaral JGC Genetic variability for agronomic characteristics between self pollinated lines of castor (*Ricinus communis* Lcv. AL Guarany. Ph. Dissertation, College of Agronomic Sciences, São Paulo State University; (2003).

[57] Savy Filho A, Amorim EP, Ramos NP, Martins ALM, Cavichioli JC. IAC 2028: nova cultivar de mamona. Pesq. agropec. bras., 2007, 42:449-452

[58] Zanotto MD, Amaral JGC, Poletine JP. Recurrent selection with use of self pollinated lines for reduction of the height of plants of castor (Ricinus communis L.) in a common Guarani population. Proc. Congresso Brasileiro de Mamona, 1st, 2004, 1:1-5. Campina Grande. Embrapa Algodão, Campina Grande, 2004

[59] Oliveira IJ, Zanotto MD. Efficiency of recurrent selection for reduction of the stature of plants in castor (Ricinus communis L.). Cienc. Agrotecnol. 2008, 32:1107–1112. doi: 10.1590/S1413-70542008000400011.

[60] Sujatha M, Reddy TP, Mahasi MJ. Role of biotechnological interventions in the improvement of castor (Ricinus communis L.) and Jatropha curcas L. Biotechnol. Adv. 2008; 26:424–435. doi:10.1016/j.biotechadv.2008.05.004

[61] Costa MN, Pereira WE, Bruno RLA, Freire EC, Nóbrega MBM, Milani M, Oliveira AP. Genetic divergence on castor bean accesses and cultivars through multivariate analysis. Pesquisa Agropecuária Brasileira, 2006; 41:1617-1622. doi: 10.1590/S0100-204X2006001100007

[62] Golakia PR, Madaria RB, Kavani RH, Mehta DR. Gene effects, heterosis and inbreeding depression in castor, Ricinus communis L. Journal of Oilseeds Research, 2004; 21:270-273

[63] Lavanya C, Chandramohan Y. Combining ability and heterosis for seed yield and yield components in castor. Journal of Oilseeds Research, 2003;20:220-224

[64] Ramana PV, Lavanya C, Ratnasree P. Combining ability and heterosis studies under rainfed conditions in castor (Ricinus communis L.,). Indian Journal of Genetics and Plant Breeding, 2005, 65:325-326

[65] Toppa EVB. Análise comparativa da produtividade de híbridos de mamoneira (Ricinus communis L.) obtidos por meio da hibridação convencional e do método dos híbridos crípticos. Ph dissertation, FCA/Unesp. 2011

[66] Lonnquist JH, Williams NE. Development of maize hybrids through among full-sib families. Crop Sci. 1967; 7:369-370

[67] Severino LS, Auld DL, Baldanzi M, Cândido MJD, Chen G, Crosby W, Tan D, et al. A Review on the Challenges for Increased Production of Castor. Agronomy Journal, 2012; 104(4):853–879. doi:10.2134/agronj2011.0210

Participatory Plant Quality Breeding: An Ancient Art Revisited by Knowledge Sharing. The Portuguese Experience

Maria Carlota Vaz Patto,
Pedro Manuel Mendes-Moreira, Mara Lisa Alves,
Elsa Mecha, Carla Brites,
Maria do Rosário Bronze and Silas Pego

Additional information is available at the end of the chapter

http://dx.doi.org/10.5772/52951

1. Introduction

1.1. Participatory plant breeding and on-farm conservation

Since the first domestications of wild plants about 12.000 years ago, farmers have been responsible for the development and conservation of thousands of crop landraces in hundreds of species [1]. Farmers put aside, for the next generation, a part of the harvested seed. Depending on the crop and the farmer, selection is carried out to obtain a crop answering better to the wishes of the growers and communities [2].

Following [3] definition: "a landrace is a dynamic population(s) of a cultivated plant that has historical origin, distinct identity and lacks formal crop improvement, as well as often being genetically diverse, locally adapted and associated with traditional farming systems".

Especially in more favorable environments, landraces are being replaced by modern varieties, which are less resilient to pests, diseases and abiotic stresses and thereby losing a valuable source of germplasm for meeting the future needs of sustainable agriculture in the context of climate change. However, landrace cultivation persists in less favorable environments [4]. This persistence is not due to increased productivity levels but because of their increased stability, accomplished through generations of natural and deliberate selection for favorable genes for resistance to biotic and abiotic stresses and intergenotypic competition and compensation [5]. They may also be kept by their dietary or nutritional value, taste, or for the price premium they attract because of high-quality traditional properties that compensate for lower yields [6]. This seems to be the case of the maize (*Zea mays* L. ssp. *mays*) landraces in Portugal that survived based on their quality traits such as technological capacity and aroma characteristics highly valued for bread production [7]. This bread making ability seems to depend on a range of particular traits not found on the available commercial hybrid varieties, and this is probably why maize landraces have not, in these regions, been totally replaced by hybrid varieties. As long as farmers themselves find it in their best interest to grow traditional varieties, both farmers and society as a whole will benefit at no extra cost to either partner [8].

As reviewed in [9], the food price crisis of 2008, sustained high prices, and more recent peaks observed in 2011 and 2012 have brought agriculture back onto global and national agendas. By 2050, global population is projected to increase by about one third, which will require a 70% increase in food production. To meet this need we should focus again on shifting the crop yield frontier, but also increasing production in more marginal environments through the increase of resistance to stress and improving competitiveness and sustainability. Traditional varieties continue to be fundamental in trying to achieve this global food security [6]. The erosion of these resources results in a severe threat to the world's long-term food security. Although often neglected, the urgent need to conserve and utilize landraces genetic resources as a safeguard against an unpredictable future is evident [10]. Farmers can contribute to this objective. The conservation and use of traditional varieties by farmers might be increased or at least sustained if more information on their good characteristics (adaptive, quality) is gather and disseminated among farmers and consumers and if the materials themselves are enhanced (breed). On-farm participatory breeding may have a significant and positive influence by encouraging farmers to adopt simple population improvement methodologies allowing them to do better with their own landraces [7].

1.2. Addressed problems and advantages

Conventional plant breeding (CPB), emerged in the early part of the 20th century, based on Darwin's theory of evolution through selection and the genetic mechanisms of evolution developed by Mendel and others [11, 12], has become increasingly isolated from the traditional plant breeding performed by farmers. The emphasis of this conventional breeding has typically been on developing modern varieties with high yield and geographically wide adaptation to optimal, relatively uniform growing environments [13, 14]. This contrasts with farmer breeding and farmers' local varieties, which are usually assumed to have narrow geographical adaptation to marginal, relatively variable growing environments, and high yield stability in those environments from year to year [1]. Modern agriculture, conventional breeding and the liberal use of high inputs has resulted in the loss of genetic diversity and the stagnation of yields in cereals in less favorable areas [5].

With the development of modern sustainable low-input agriculture in industrialized countries, for economic and environmental reasons, emphasis has recently been placed on local adaptation, on preservation of genetic diversity and on quality. This has resulted largely from the increasing awareness of the limits to conventional breeding as a consequence of increasing scarcity and decreasing quality of production resources in the low stress environments of modern agriculture [15]. Also the awareness that future increases in productivity may depend on increasing yields in high stress environments and on the maintenance of the available genetic variation, has motivated emphasis on specific or narrow adaptation and on genetic diversity conservation [15]. Conventional plant breeding has been successful in favourable environments, or in those which can be made favourable (e.g. by the use of inputs), but is less successful in traditional low-input or organic farming systems with higher stress growing conditions especially in small-scale farms.

Under this scenario, participatory research approaches have emerged as a relevant and necessary response to the problem of conserving genetic diversity also in industrialized countries [16]. Participatory plant breeding (PPB) programs are arising world-wide to meet the needs of farmers in low-input and organic environments that are normally overlooked by conventional crop breeders.

Several scientists, as reviewed by [17] discriminate among different types or modes of PPB, which are not necessarily mutually exclusive. However we agree with [18] on that the definition of PPB does not imply pre-assigned roles, or a given amount of collaborative work, nor imply that farmers and breeding institutions are the only partners. Experience in practicing PPB tells us that a true PPB program is a dynamic process with permanent collaboration, where both the roles of partners and the extent and the manner in which they collaborate, change with time. As farmers become progressively more empowered the type or mode of participation also evolves.

In PPB programs, farmers are invited to interact with professional breeders in their own farm and intervene at different stages of the breeding program, such as the generation of diversity, selection and seed multiplication. PPB helps farmers and breeders to communicate more efficiently with each other so that breeders can use their knowledge of biological theory, statistical design and analysis, to help the farmers' selection and access to a wide range of genetic diversity. Farmers can use their knowledge of their crops and environments and learn simple population genetics methodologies that will help them to progress more rapidly and efficiently in their seed selection. This collaboration should lead to varieties that better meet farmers' needs and conditions and conserve crop genetic diversity *in situ*, thus contributing to sustainable agriculture [15]. PPB exploits the potential gains of breeding for specific adaptation through decentralized selection, defined as selection in the target environment, and is the ultimate conceptual consequence of a positive interpretation of genotype x environment interactions [19].

Conventional plant breeding has aimed at pure lines and increasingly use of hybrids, resulting in a decrease of genetic diversity in conventional varieties. Also genetic diversity at the regional level is decreasing with few varieties grown over large areas [20]. In PPB, biodiversity is maintained or increased because, besides the use of heterogeneous populations with an inherent high level of diversity, different varieties are selected at different locations. With PPB, decision on which variety to release depend on the initial adoption by farmers; the process is demand-driven. This is expected to increase adoption rates and also reduce production risks, since the farmers gain knowledge of the variety's performance as part of the selection process [19].

The essential advantages of PPB over CPB involve: better targeting of local environmental conditions, better definition of selection criteria important to the end-users, faster and higher adoption of improved cultivars by the farmer and increase/maintenance of genetic variability. PPB also gives voice to farmers and elevates local knowledge to the role of science [19].

Participative approaches to agricultural research and development are now extensively used throughout the world to help define and address the practical research needs of farmers. They have proved useful in solving practical problems in complex and diverse farming systems, characteristics typical of organic farming and low input systems. In the case of maize breeding, very effective PPB projects are reported all over the world. This is the case of the Andean region (Ecuador, Peru and Bolivia) [21], Brazil [22, 23], China [24], Ethiopia [25], Ghana [26], India [27, 28], Kenya [29], Mexico and Honduras [30], Nepal [31] and in Nigeria [32]. In Portugal, a very successful long running PPB project in maize (the VASO project, Vale do Sousa - Sousa Valley) is on going since 1984 [33]. This PPB project was developed to cover the needs of small maize farmers, with scarce land resources, in polycropping systems for human uses (bread production). This project has recently been enlarged and extended to other regions of the country and special attention is now given to quality traits such as nutritional and health beneficial quality aspects besides the already considered technological ability for bread production.

2. Maize participatory breeding in Portugal – VASO project

2.1. Historical prespective

Maize domestication resulted from a single event involving its wild progenitor teosinte (*Z. mays* subspecies *parviglumis*), introgression from other teosinte types and the segregation into two germplasmpools between which much hybridisation occurred (reviewed by [5]. Portugal, by its privileged historical and geographical position as an enter point of new species into Europe, was among the first European nations to adopt maize (*Zea mays* L.) in its agricultural systems, more than five centuries ago [34]. The idea of hybridization among different maize introductions all over the country, rather than a slow northward dispersion accompanied by selection for earliness from one only germplasm introduction is supported in the case of Portugal (and Spain). The Iberian maize germplasm display no close relationship with any American types, but sharing alleles with both Caribbean and North American flints [35, 36].

After its introduction in the 16th century, maize spread rapidly throughout the country leading to an agricultural revolution, enhancing the rural population's standard of living. Numerous landraces (open pollinated varieties, OPV) have been developed during the centuries of cultivation, adapted to specific regional growing conditions as well as farmer's needs.

However, after World War II, Portugal was one of the first European countries to test the American maize hybrids which initially were not well accepted by the Portuguese farmers due to several handicaps such as late maturity or kernel type, not fitted for food or poly-cropping systems. Nevertheless, several breeding stations were established within Portugal at that time, from North to South, in the cities of Braga (NUMI), Porto, Viseu, Elvas and Tavira, releasing adapted hybrid varieties based on inbreds developed from Portuguese and American germplasm. This was the case specially of NUMI and the breeding station at Porto with their famous white flint double-crosses being the preferred seed by the Portuguese farmers, during the 60's and 70's. In fact, during that period of time the commercial yellow dent hybrids from the international seed companies never reached the same level of preference by our farmers, who needed a type of plant with a cycle that could fit their poly-cropping system and with a type of quality kernel for human consumption and not for feed. Accordingly, an enormous decrease in the number of cultivated landraces occurred by replacement with hybrid varieties. Due to this, a growing concern that numerous Portuguese maize landraces may have been lost forever started to be felt since the late 1970's. This awareness of genetic erosion led Silas Pego to initiate collection missions for maize in 1975. In the following years a more in-depth collection supported by FAO/IBPGR covered the entire country in successive missions. These materials gave rise to the first long-term cold storage facilities, the precursors of the present Portuguese Plant Germplasm Bank (BPGV), with one of the best European maize germplasm collections (ca 3000 landraces accessions) [37].

After Portugal and Spain entered the European Community, in 1986, a new political reality took place with a consequent change in our agriculture policy, smashing down the traditional small farming characterized by a poly-cropping, quality oriented and sustainable agriculture. In two decades these small farmers were pushed to bankruptcy. Also later on, during the 1980's, the scientific community became aware of the importance of the genetic resources co-evolution and the need for *in-situ* / on-farm conservation. The main question now was, how to restore this sustainable and quality oriented agricultural system in Portugal, and bring it back to business? Why not to apply some science to those genetic resources that had been selected by our traditional farmers during the last four centuries?

To provide an incentive for *in-situ* conservation of traditional maize landraces Silas Pego had the idea of engaging local farmers and their seeds in a participatory maize breeding program. By doing this, his goals were not only to conserve, but also to improve the social well-being of this rural community by increasing farmers' income through rising yields from some of their own seeds. To bring that idea to practice he led, in 1984, a detailed survey on farmer's maize fields at «Vale do Sousa» Region (Sousa Valley Region) in the North-west of Portugal. The collected materials were the starting point of a PPB project, with simultaneous on-farm breeding and on-farm conservation objectives (VASO- "Vale do Sousa"- project). This project aimed to answer the needs of small farmers (e.g., yield, bread making quality, ability for polycropping systems) with scarce land availability due to a high demographic density, where the American agriculture model did not fit and the multinationals had no adequate market to operate. From our previous knowledge of the small farming reality of the mountainous North of our country we knew that a project oriented to one crop integrated within a system should be oriented under a general developmental framework, understood and accepted by the farmer. This would require a different philosophic approach that we coined as *integrant philosophy* in opposition to the *productivist philosophy*. While in this last model the plant breeder occupies the center of decision, in the *integrant philosophic approach* is the farmer who occupies that position. Furthermore, we needed to link our philosophy with the basic formula of any production system: energy + raw material+ science = final product. This commanded our decisions, preference for renewable energy instead of fossil, local genetic resources instead of exotic germplasm, and an adequate breeding methodology accessible to the farmer's understanding and participation. Besides, a set of parallel decisions came along, as:

1. start with the farmer's genetic resources,
2. move to the farmer's place and develop the project at his own plots,
3. work side-by-side and let the farmer be the decision maker,
4. respect the agricultural system and the farmer's preferences and
5. always be ready to share knowledge and enthusiasm.

If we could get at least some of these achievements, we needed to be sure that they had to be reached at the farmer's speed and under his own constraints. This model also embraced a quality oriented perspective (human food) where the quality factor must be financially valorized in order to sustain the agricultural system.

To implement this project several main decisions had to be made, such as the choice of the location to represent the region, the farmer to work with side-by-side, the germplasm source, and the breeding and management methodologies to apply.

2.2. General procedures

In this section, and taking the VASO project as a model, a generalised description of the most important decisions to be made on a maize PPB project implementation is presented.

As in any collaborative approach all the plans and decisions have to be made between all the involved partners and with that purpose breeders need to meet with local farmers and discuss selection strategies to understand farmer's objectives and constraints. Following this, four main decisions must be taken to implement correctly the participatory breeding approach:

2.2.1. Farmers, breeders and environmental choices

The selected farmer's fields must be located in a traditional production area where the crop to be breed is important and where support from local authorities/farmers associations is guaranteed. Farms should represent the different soil and climatic conditions under which the crop is grown, the different size of farms and farm types.

In the case of the VASO project, the Sousa Valley was chosen after the results of the 1984 survey and taking in account several factors:

a. At that time only 15% of the Portuguese farmers were using hybrid seeds. However, in the fertile Sousa Valley this percent was higher - 25%. This meant that even in this region 75% of the farmers were still using their own regional varieties of maize. This created a perfect situation for developing alternative production systems.

b. That region was known as a source of the best inbred lines which were in the basis of one most successful double cross national hybrids – HP21.

c. A previous sociological survey that had been carried out by a small team of scientists had raised a general and thorough picture of the local rural society and its organized structures. Out of it came the information of a private farmers' association (CGAVS) – Center for Agriculture Management of the Sousa Valley – that was open to collaborate and was offering its headquarter facilities as a basis for the maize breeder.

d. The region was among the national most populated areas, with good soil quality and plenty of water supplies.

e. Both the communities of the closest town Lousada, and the Agriculture Cooperative of another close town Paredes, were willing to follow the project.

f. After a national contest promoted by the Portuguese Ministry of Agriculture, it came out that the national winner, with a long cycle yellow dent single cross hybrid, was located in the Sousa Valley. To run a maize breeding project in a place where our national champion was located, certainly was a natural challenge.

Choosing the right person to work with is also a major decision on participatory approaches, where the work is carried out side-by-side and the power of decision shared. A high farmer initial acceptance of this type of approach and enthusiasm for joining this kind of projects are the best guarantee of success. Nevertheless, a careful respect of the breeder for the local traditional agriculture is also crucial.

The farmer' selection in the VASO project was made having into account both a previous information obtained in the mentioned sociological survey, and from direct contacts within the farmers' organization CGAVS. From this collected information, the most willing and also contradictory people were chosen. In its beginning only 3 farmers were directly involved.

In the process of choosing the right person, it is very important, as highlighted by [18], to clarify

i. what plant breeding can offer and how long it can take;

ii. what sort of commitment in land, time and labor is required from the farmer;

iii. what are the risks for the farmer and how these can be compensated for (in-kind compensation vs. money); and

iv. what overall benefits farmers can expect if everything goes well.

These farmers will need to be trained/updated with practical examples of how selection could be improved. The plant breeder will have to take into account the selection objectives of the farmer and the farmer will learn simple population genetics methodologies that will help him to progress more rapidly and efficiently in their seed selection.

In a PPB program it is very important to maintain contacts with farmers beyond and besides specific scientific activities. These 'courtesy' visits are not only instrumental in building and maintain good human relationships between scientists and farmers by bridging gaps, but are an incredibly valuable reciprocal source of information [18].

In the VASO project the initial enthusiasm of some of the contacted farmers that still today collaborate with the project was fundamental. Also the support of a local elite farmers' association (CGAVS) which agreed to be part of the project was very beneficial to the success of the project.

2.2.2. Starting germplasm and variability generation

According to the VASO philosophy, the project should start by using local landraces as its genetic resources, selected by the breeder as the most representative of the local farming. A survey was made by the breeder in 1984 during the summer time along the maize fields of that region in a close look for particular plant phenotypes and ear size. Further, at harvest time, several sets of store houses ("*sequeiros*") were visited and farmers contacted. From this first survey two regional varieties were selected: "Pigarro", a white flint type FAO 300 cycle with strong fasciation expression, used in the best soils for human consumption, and "Amarelo miúdo" ("Amiúdo"), a yellow flint type FAO 200, adapted to the poorest soils with low ph, water stress and aluminum toxicity, but also with quality for bread production. Afterward, the VASO project was also conserving additional landraces such as "Basto", "Aljezur", "Aljezudo", "Castro Verde", "Verdial de Aperrela" and "Verdial de Cete". In parallel with the landraces approach, a synthetic population, Fandango, was also included [38].

So, as highlighted from the VASO project, one of the prerequisites for the implementation of a PPB project is the existence of local adapted germplasm. In this way the farmer's selection pursued over several centuries (quality preferences) will be respected and the environmental adaptation already achieved either for the soil or climate will be assured [33].

The inclusion of high quality parents is of particular importance when considering the quality objectives of the population. Quality is difficult for farmers to access if they grow a crop for the commercial market, and is not necessarily improved by natural selection [39].

When needed, genetic diversity can be generated by crossing genetically diverse and adapted local cultivars as starting genetic base. Other foreign materials (exotic germplasm) can also be added after this point to overcome any limitation typical from the local cultivars (as disease susceptibility).

2.2.3. Breeding methodologies

Technically the process is similar to conventional breeding, with three main differences. Trials will be grown in farmers' fields rather than on-station, covering a range of target environments and using farmer's agronomic practices and levels of inputs. Selection will be conducted jointly by breeders and farmers (and other end-users when appropriate), so that farmers participate in all key decisions. This process can be independently implemented at a large number of locations [19].

The goal of any plant breeding is to develop a plant population composed of phenotypes that meet farmers' criteria, and that farmers will, therefore, adopt and maintain. So selection criteria must consider farmers objectives like quality traits, such as flavour or nutritional value, pest and disease resistance and enhanced capacity to survive in highly changeable environment typical of low input/organic farming systems (yield stability) through genetic diversity maintenance or enhancement.

The choice of the breeding methods cannot be made without considering whether and how farmers are handling genetic diversity. An issue related to the choice of the breeding method is how much breeding material farmers can handle. The choice of the breeding method also depends on the desired genetic structure of the final product, i.e. pure lines, mixtures, hybrids or open pollinated varieties [18].

Common mass selection, usually performed by all farmers, consists on the identification of superior individuals in the form of plants from a population, and in the case of crops like maize, the bulking of seed to form the seed stock for the next generation [40]. It requires relatively little effort compared with other selection methods and, practiced season after season with the same seed stock, has the potential to maintain or even improve a crop population, depending upon the heritabilities of the selected traits, GxE for the trait, the proportion of the population selected, and gene flow in the form of pollen or seeds into the population [15]. PPB is a cyclic process where the best selections will be used in further cycles of recombination and selection or selection will just give rise to experimental cultivars, to be tested again on the farmers' fields.

Within the VASO project a tacit agreement was made between the breeder and the farmer involved. While the breeder would apply his breeding methodologies, the farmer would continue a parallel program with their own mass selection criteria, starting with the same initial populations. With this agreement the breeder had to accept low-input and intercropping characteristics, as well as to accept and respect the local farmer as the decision maker. On the other hand the farmer was able to compare the effectiveness of the two breeding systems allowing him to base his decisions on solid grounds. Due to the choice of locally adapted germplasm, diversity and quality were considered as selection priorities.

In relation to the selection approach followed by the VASO project the breeder initially opted by the *S2 lines recurrent selection*, due to its potential for favoring a good amount of additive gene action. This methodology worked very promisingly with the "Pigarro" germplasm, but not so good with "Amiúdo". In fact, while we could observe a surprisingly low inbreeding depression when we tested the S2 lines of "Pigarro", a different situation came out from the S2 lines of "Amiúdo". Here, the inbreeding depression was so high that we had to move to the *S1 lines recurrent selection methodology*. On the other hand, farmers were advised to use improved mass selection approaches, such as with a two parental control (*stratified mass selection*), where selection takes place not only after harvesting, at the storage facilities (ear traits), but also during crop development in the field such as in a cross pollinating species before pollen shedding, for the male parent selection by detasselling all undesirable plants, and before harvesting, for the female parent selection (ear size, root and stalk quality and indirectly pest tolerance; [33]). As the time was passing by, the Common Agriculture Policy (CAP) from the EU, which favored the big farming oriented for feed production, pressed the small farming to bankruptcy. As a consequence, our VASO project also suffered a sudden lack of governmental support leaving the breeder without any support to adequately pursue the mentioned methodologies, both requiring a big amount of hand pollinations. Again, the breeding methodology had to be changed, now for *stratified mass selection* to all the other landraces in the project.

The improvement program included yield, lodging performance, pest and disease tolerance, and indirectly, adaptation to climate changes.

During the VASO project, some pre-breeding methodologies were developed such as the HUNTERS (High, Uniformity, aNgle, Tassel, Ear, Root lodging and Stalk lodging) or the Overlapping Index [7, 38]. These are nowadays very useful on our PPB maize landrace selection on-farm.

In all cases in the VASO project, the traditional poly-cropping technology was followed: surrounded by vineyards, the plots were usually planted with three main crops: maize *(Zea mays L.)*, beans *(Phaseolus vulgaris L.)* and a forage crop *(Lolium perene L.)*. The first two simultaneously planted along the same row in May and the forage later on in July between the rows. This organic system has three main sustainable advantages:

1. a probable symbiosis between a *Leguminosae* (beans) and *Rhyzobium sp*, as a natural source of nitrogen for the *graminea* (maize),

2. any possible plant damage or failure along the row could be compensated in favor of the other crop to which was allowed more sunlight and

3. after harvesting the maize crop in September the soil was already covered with a forage layer that not only functions as a protection against erosion but also as a source of 3-4 cuts of forage for animal feeding during the winter.

2.2.4. Seed management and dissemination

Since the beginning of the VASO Project, phenotypic data were collected and seed of each selection cycle, either from phenotypic recurrent selection or from S2 recurrent selection, was kept at 4ºC in our national Plant Germplasm Bank (BPGV) cold storage facilities [38].

Several maize OPVs were selected within this project with the joint collaboration of the breeder Silas Pego and the farmers.

The seed however has not yet been nationally distributed /commercialized due to the lack of appropriate legislation allowing the certification of OPV with a certain level of heterogeneity. These aspects will be further developed under the PPB success evaluation and the seed dissemination and ownership sections.

2.3. PPB Vaso project success evaluation

During more than a quarter of a century of continuous participatory on-farm maize breeding, some *ups* and *downs* came along, mainly influenced by political fluctuations that affected both the governmental support and the market prices of its quality oriented output. In 2001, the mayor of the town of Lousada presented the situation of the VASO project governmental funds cutting to his general assembly that unanimously decided to substitute our Ministry of Agriculture institution (DRAEDM) as the sponsors of this long term PPB project.

In spite of these *ups* and *downs,* our main achievements can be centered in three areas:

1. breeding output,
2. technological improvement and
3. seed diffusion.

2.3.1. Breeding output

All the outputs from this project are improved OPVs. "Pigarro" is the one which received our main investment in breeding, with several cycles of *S2 lines recurrent selection* and repeated cycles of *stratified mass selection.* Its yield level is now between 8 and 9 t/ha, and is the type of seed that better fits the high quality standards of our most famous maize bread – *Broa de Avintes.* "Amiúdo" went to some cycles of *S1 lines recurrent selection* and fits the conditions of tolerance to soil (low ph and Al) and water stress. As a yellow vitreous flint and small kernel size, this quality enables this variety to be used both for maize bread as well as for the specific market of feed for carrier-pigeons and pigeon breeding. "Fandango", an ear size champion (at the Sousa Valley best ear contest), had its original FAO700 cycle reduced to FAO600 and a competing yield over 10 t/ ha. A set of other improved varieties like "Aljezur" FAO 400 yellow flint, "Aljezudo" FAO 300 yellow flint, "Castro Verde" FAO 600 yellow flint, and some others, complete a minor output that can be improved in future attempts.

Yield trials for evaluation at the farmer's place, were the most difficult task to carry out in a way to fit the levels of statistical significance. Nevertheless for "Fandango" and "Pigarro" OPVs these trials were already established, and for some of the other VASO OPVs are now under way. In the already established evaluation trails we should take into account the original specific objectives defined for the farmers' and breeders' selections. For the "Pigarro" *stratified mass selection* the farmer aimed at obtaining bigger size ears while maintaining the flint and white type of kernel. The breeder with its alternative *S2 lines recurrent selection* method aimed at increasing favorable alleles both for yield, ear placement and stalk quality. For the "Fandango" *stratified mass selection* the farmer was looking for big ear size maximization and the breeder for yield maximization. Evaluation field trials for selection gain on these two OPVs were established in several locations in Portugal and in the case of "Fandango", also in the USA [38, 41]. The statistical analysis indicated that *stratified mass selection* in "Pigarro" lead to an increase in days to silk and anthesis, ear diameter, kernel row number and fasciation. On the contrary, ear length decreased significantly [38]. Molecular SSR marker data, from [42], on three selection cycles (C0-1984, C9-1993 and C20-2004), revealed that no effective loss of genetic diversity has occurred during the selective adaptation to the farmer's needs and the regional growing conditions. Variation among selection cycles represented only 7% of the total molecular variation, indicating that a great proportion of the genetic diversity is maintained in each selection cycle. Genetic diversity has not been reduced from the "Pigarro" bred before 1984 to those examples improved after 2004, but the genetic diversity maintained is not exactly the same. Mass selection seems to be an effective way to conserve diversity on-farm, and interesting phenotypic improvements were achieved as the bigger ears farmers' objective [42].

On the other hand, the response to the "Pigarro" *recurrent selection by S2 lines* indicated that after three cycles of selection, days to silk, uniformity and the cob/ear ratio increased significantly, but also without a significant yield increase [38].

The "Fandango" *stratified farmers mass selection* evaluation performed in Portugal revealed that the ear length and the thousand kernel weight decreased significantly and simultaneously plant and ear height increased significantly [41], accomplishing the bigger ears farmers' objective. These traits had no significant changes during the selection cycles performed by the breeder. Additionally, days to silk had a significant increase during selection. For yield no significant changes were observed during selection when all the evaluation locations were considered. Nevertheless, when considering only the trials performed at the location where the PPB took place (Lousada), a significant yield increase was recorded especially during breeders selection cycles (3.09% gain per cycle per year), being less pronounce during farmers selection cycles (only 0.63% gain per cycle per year). The lack of significant progress in yield for both "Pigarro" and "Fandango" can be explained by low selection intensity due to the exclusion of stalk lodged plants in the basic units of selection [38, 41] what must be taken into consideration in future selections for yield increase.

Both selection methods used in "Pigarro" and "Fandango" different phases of selection, suggest that *stratified mass selection* is better than *S2 lines recurrent selection* due to the following reasons: *Stratified mass selection* is a cheaper methodology, technically more accessible to farmers, with one cycle of selection completed each summer, without reducing the conserved genetic diversity [41].

The evidence of genetic diversity maintenance by this PPB project with simultaneous phenotypic improvement, fundaments the preservation of these on-farm selection programs where threatened landraces of great interest for future use in breeding programs and for developing new farming systems are preserved.

2.3.2. Tecnological improvement

A modified planting system was developed in such a way that two rows of beans (20 cm apart) were planted between two consecutive rows of maize (130 cm apart). The difference to the original technology was that one row of maize was eliminated, but the seed density was maintained by doubling the plant density along each row. On one hand, this higher plant density was compensated by the larger space between rows that the plants could take advantage from. On the other hand, the now separated rows of beans, due to its fast growing, rapidly covered the soil avoiding weeds. This new technology, besides being weed control efficient, facilitates harvest of beans in July and the following planting of the forage crop over that empty space between rows of maize. Additionally, it had a final positive effect in September at the harvest of maize, because the soil was already protected against the erosion from the rainy season that was coming in. Moreover, during fall and winter, 3 or 4 cuts of forage could be made for animal feeding.

Another technological improvement was discovered by the farmer. In a certain morning of June, when the maize was in its four to five leaves stage, the farmer was observing an intense flight of birds over the maize field. With a closer look he noticed that birds were catching the larvae of the pest *Agrotis segetum* L. He then realized that the soil was still humid from his irrigation the afternoon before. Our conclusion became obvious: the larvae were superficial because the soil was still cold, but go underground when the sun heats. We realized that a sustainable insect control tool was available and a light superficial irrigation became usual in each afternoon.

2.3.3.Seed difusion

The diffusion of the improved seeds from this VASO project, while limited to the Sousa Valley area, has been very easy, as expected. Farmers are always ready to share seeds and it happens frequently. However, a private initiative from a local farmers' cooperative (Cooperativa Agricola de Paredes), in the early 90's, with a regional contest for maize - *The maize best ear of the Sousa Valley* turned to be the best diffuser of our seeds since they became quickly champions of ear size. Among our improved varieties the long cycle "Fandango" became a real champion beating, year after year, the best commercial hybrids in ear size. One of our collaborative farmers, *Francisco Meireles,* became the most rewarded Portuguese farmer, with more than 50 trophies. This has contributed to the recognition of the farmer by the community, but also attracted new farmers and new germplasm to this PPB project that in this way could be identified and preserved on-farm by the same approach [38].

3. Participatory plant quality breeding in Portugal

Presently, in particular Portuguese regions, known by their high quality maize bread, farmers keep on cultivating their traditional landraces. Traditionally selected landraces are mainly white kernel flint types, demonstrating quality over yield and maintaining genetic diversity to increase adaptability to a large variety of edaphic/climatic conditions, such as drought or aluminium toxicity [37].

Maize is definitely a deep-rooted crop in the Portuguese rural tradition and the available genetic variability of its landraces offers a superb challenge for breeding for special quality traits. Since the on going PPB project at Sousa Valley (VASO) revealed promising breeding results, our objective is to get further support to maintain the actual project and extend it to other maize landraces production areas as a way to increase the use value of this traditional germplasm and by doing so promote *in-situ/on-farm* conservation and halt the serious genetic diversity erosion. The inclusion of organic breeding objectives in the actual PPB project is also being considered to add value to these improved landraces since the low input sustainable farming system typical of the traditional production systems is already very similar to the organic farming directives. In this more recent PPB approach, molecular and detailed quality data will be used in order to increase the effectiveness of selection when appropriate.

3.1. New material and farmers prospection

With the idea of establishing an on-farm conservation project, with farmers' engagement through participatory breeding approaches, to halt the genetic erosion by improving those landraces and increasing their market value, members of our team engaged in a field expedition to the Central region of Portugal to collect enduring landraces [7]. In this region farmers grow maize landraces, known for their good maize bread quality, in association with common bean local varieties, in a traditional intercropping practice. The collected landraces represent important sources of genes and gene combinations not yet available for crop quality breeding programs and due to their intrinsic quality traits (that promoted their maintenance in cultivation) are the best candidates for expanding the already existing participatory breeding program (VASO) to other regions with more emphasis on quality breeding. Around 50 different (yellow and white) maize landraces were collected, characterized using pre-breeding approaches and conserved in cold storage [7]. These landraces, together with other landraces that were subsequently collected from the surrounding regions, represented the basis for the PPB net existing in the country. During this expedition several associated crop (beans, rye and pumpkin) landraces were also collected. The collected bean landraces are also now being characterized at agronomical, genetic diversity and quality level to select the best material to implement also participatory breeding approaches.

During this expedition, the first steps on contacting new farmers to extend the original PPB net were also given and the most enthusiastic farmers meet during those days, are now involved in the participatory research. VASO still continues nowadays and it is the best inspiration for those intending to start their PPB programs. For this reason, VASO initial actors have been invited to give their testimony to the new associated farmers within the actual extended PPB net. This action boosted the program giving new perspectives to the new farmers, and new paths to our program. Some meetings have been prepared to have farmers' perception (e.g. know what are the kernel preferences for maize bread), or where researchers present their achievements to the network, with time for discussion (e.g. soil, agronomic traits, genetic diversity and quality). Along this process an identification of the farmers' profile was made, their motivations and interests (e.g. germplasm development, trials) in order to fully engage them with the project. Even though the majority of farmers has no background on basic statistics (e.g. replication), they do their empirical research. For this reason appreciate the contact with a "practical" academia, where both look in the same direction and where the arena is at their farmers fields. This action demands an intensive networking regarding motivation and science, where future perspectives are discussed, and results depart from farmers' fields.

3.2. Quality breeding objectives

In the national Portuguese panorama we are now more concerned with the landraces still in cultivation and the quality that prevented their replacement by the generalized hybrid use. These materials represent the actual enduring and surviving genotypes and so constitute the best candidates for a quality breeding program. Additionally, these materials should be allowed to pursue a natural evolution under *in situ* conservation and farmers must be rewarded for their contribution to halt the current and continuing loss of plant diversity. The only way to achieve this is to promote a sustainable use of plant diversity, where conservation responsibilities and benefits will be shared with farmers [7]. A participatory approach seems to be the most logical solution. We try to identify ways of supporting farmers in the maintenance of traditional varieties and crop genetic diversity by performing better with their own seeds improved.

Portuguese maize landraces have been preserved on-farm, due to particular quality traits not found on their competing modern hybrid varieties. These landraces are mainly flint type open pollinated varieties (OPV) with technological ability for the production of the traditional maize leavened bread called "broa" that still plays an important economic and social role on Central and Northern rural communities of the country [7].

Due to this, we decided to start studying in more detail the technological ability for bread production of maize landraces as the major quality trait to breed for. However, later on, it has been described that other quality traits, such a flavor or aromas were also contributing to the consumers preferences for bread obtained from traditional maize landraces in detriment of maize hybrid varieties bread [43]. Volatile components responsible for the aroma were then also included into our detailed study. Presently and due to consumers higher concern about the quality of their food and how their diet can influence their well being also antioxidant compounds and their bioactivity are also being analyzed on the flour and bread made from our traditional maize varieties.

Our objective is that our improved varieties will be attractive to consumers, processing industry and farmers, answering health and environmental public concerns and increasing sustainability of farming systems.

3.2.1. Technological ability for bread production

The introduction of maize in the Iberian Peninsula during the fifteenth century produced important changes in agriculture and in the diet of the people. Maize has become highly integrated into Portuguese agriculture and diet, and and appears as the major cereal for bread making in the middle of 19th century. The bread produced at that time was "broa" where maize flour meal was mixed with wheat or rye. Presently, Portuguese rural areas continue to produce "broa", mainly in the northwest parts of the country in a wide variety of recipes, some with protected geographical identification and traditional methods of baking. The quality of "broa" is the result of empirical knowledge that is very closely related to the quality of the maize, kernel processing, blending flours and baking procedures, including fermentation and baking.

There are many traditional recipes to prepare "broa", but the traditional process involves adding maize flour (sieved whole meal flour ranging between 50% and 80%), hot water, wheat and rye flours, yeast and leavened dough from the late "broa" (acting as sourdough). After mixing, resting and proofing, the dough is baked in a wood-fired oven. This empirical process leads to an ethnic product highly accepted for its distinctive sensory characteristics.

The process begins with blanching maize flour in water boiled followed by kneading. Blanching is important to obtain high consistency dough's because in the absence or reduced amount of gluten the dough rheological properties are provided by the starch gelatinization [43]. The addition of sourdough is another important aspect in the preparation of "broa", and its microbial diversity has been characterized [44] with mainly lactic acid bacteria *Lactobacillus* (*brevis, bulgaris plantarum*) being present in addition to yeast (*Saccharomyces cerevisiae*).

In terms of maize physical characteristics, kernel size and shape, weight and density, degree of stress cracks and resistance to milling and compression have all been linked to hardness and this is the primary cause for the large differences in rheological properties of flours which have subsequent effects on processing.

The majority of commercial hybrid maize varieties that are currently grown in Portugal are dent type, but also some flour types can be found, characterized by a soft or floury endosperm respectively. However, in the traditional varieties and landraces predominates the flint type with the hardest kernels, resulting from the presence of a large and continuous volume of horny (vitreous) endosperm. Maize flint type has harder endosperm than dent types, resulting in different viscosity profiles. Flours from maize flint grain have lower peak viscosity and lower retrogradation than dent types [45, 46].

White maize is the preferred choice by northwest rural populations, probably due to cultural and historical reasons that have created food habits. Indeed in the 18th century, when the maize was the main cereal used for bread making, white bread was the most appreciated, symbolizing wealth and prestige [47], in this context white maize flour was the most suitable for blending with wheat flours. However, it is important to understand if there are differences between the rheological behavior of maize flour from white and yellow grains. With this aim, we analyzed a collection of maize OPVs and found no significant correlation between the Colour Chromameter b* - yellow/blue index and viscosity parameters of flours [34]. From the nutritional standpoint, the white grain has the disadvantage that it is devoid of carotenoids, which are important antioxidants for health. Nevertheless, our preliminary results indicate high amounts of other nutritional compounds such as tocopherols.

Kernel processing into milling is an important quality factor for the production of "broa" because it determines the performance of the flour. Dry-milling process is used for the production of maize meal used for bread making and whole grain is processed traditionally in stone wheel mills, moved by water or wind, and nowadays frequently by electricity.

The native starch can be damaged to a greater or lesser extent thereby influencing the flour water absorption capacity and enzymatic attack, especially α-amylase. The type of grinding may also affect ash flour content, which interferes with the evolution of pH during the fermentation step. The grinding mills driven by water occurs at a slower rate, flours obtained with this process have lower ash content, lower proportion of damaged starch, and higher maximum viscosity than obtained in electrical mills [46].

In addition to the "broa" sensory specificities and the need to diversify baking products to fulfill the consumers' appreciation range of traditional breads, there are also reasons related to nutrition disorders that promote the study of maize quality for bread making.

The high indices of chronic diseases, such as obesity and diabetes, increase the demand for the development of breads with starch that is slowly digestible or partially resistant to the digestive process namely resistant starch [48]. "Broa" revealed a greater resistant starch content than the wheat bread [49]. Differences in starch digestibility or type of dietary fiber, the typical fermentation and bread volume also contributes for lower glycemic index of "broa" when compared with wheat bread [49]. Gluten enteropathy (coeliac disease) is another serious chronic disease, caused by an inappropriate immune response to dietary wheat gluten or similar proteins of barley or rye. Maize is a gluten-free cereal, thus suitable to produce foods addressed to celiac patients. The acquired knowledge on "broa" (made from composite maize–rye–wheat flour) is important for facing the challenges of producing gluten-free bread that usually exhibits compact crumb texture and low specific volume [43]. Baking assays were performed and demonstrated that bread making technology could be satisfactorily applied to produce gluten-free "broa" [43].

Strategies to further improve maize kernel quality for "broa" production considering flour rheological properties and nutrients are under intense investigation, mainly focused on viscosity profiles, protein content, carotenoids and tocopherols.

Management of large number of accessions implies adoption of rapid and non destructive tests for efficiently screening quality traits, consequently research on Near Infrared Spectroscopy (NIR) models to estimate maize kernels quality is under progress and it will be of extreme importance as a fast and inexpensive way to support quality PPB.

Moreover, the selection parameters adopted in quality PPB should reflect "broa" consumers' preference and therefore "broa" bread sensory analyzes with consumer panel are being implemented and the data obtained will be used to improve the screening quality maize tests for bread making.

3.2.2.Aroma

Aroma strongly influences food quality and therefore consumer's preferences and acceptability for the products. Sweet, sour, salty, bitter and umami tastes, olfactory responses, oral sensory sensations related with astringency, coolness and pressure, contribute to food aroma [50]. Since olfactory responses involve a huge number of descriptors to distinguish hundreds of different odors, it is not surprising that most of the work developed in aroma research has been related with volatile compounds analysis [51].

Volatile compounds in plants and foods are produced during harvesting and processing, by enzymatic degradation [52]. The type of volatile compounds depends on plant species, genotype, plant part and environmental growing conditions [53]. Alcohols, aldehydes, ketones, hydrocarbons and terpenic compounds are among the main volatile compounds responsible for foods' aroma and most of them are present in trace amounts, which difficult the task of aroma analysis [50]. Drying, handling, milling and storage conditions may affect aroma of foods [50].

Solid Phase Micro Extraction (SPME) combined with Gas Chromatography-Mass Spectrometry (GC-MS) is now the most used technique for the analysis of volatile compounds [52]. Aroma volatile compounds of different maize types and preparations have been studied by SPME-GC-MS. Characteristic odor of dimethyl sulfide has been associated with sweet maize aroma. Other important compounds include 1-hydroxy-2-propanone, 2-hydroxy-3-butanone and 2,3-butanediol. Higher concentrations of such volatile compounds were reported in canned maize, when comparing canned, frozen and fresh maize [50, 54]. In popcorn, 6-acetyltetrahydropyridine, 2-acetyl-1-pyrroline and 2-propionyl-1-pirroline were described as the most important aroma compounds [54]. In maize tortilla and taco shell it was possible to identify an aroma component not previously identified, 2-aminoacetophenone [54].

Information about aroma volatile compounds in Portuguese maize and maize bread, until now, is scarce. In order to characterize these compounds in this national germplasm and respective food products (bread), we studied a collection of 51 Portuguese maize landraces representing the starting material of the present national participatory maize breeding project. Solid Phase Micro Extraction (SPME) combined with gas chromatography and mass spectrometry was used for the analysis. Volatiles were identified based on comparison with mass spectra in reference libraries NIST 21.LIB and Willey 229.LIB and by the Linear Retention Index (LRI). Aldehydes (hexanal, heptanal, nonanal, 2-nonenal (E), and decanal) were identified as main volatile compounds responsible for maize flour aroma being Hexanal the most representative aldehyde compound on the analyzed flour.

The analysis of the aroma volatile compounds released from traditional Portuguese bread ("broa") made from selected maize varieties is under way using the same conditions of analysis.

3.2.2. Phenolic compounds

Phenolic compounds are secondary metabolites produced by plants as protection against fungi, herbivores, UV radiation and oxidative cell injury, revealing also important functions in several aspects of plant life as growth, pigmentation and reproduction [55].

Phenolic compounds can contribute, with other dietary components such as vitamins C, E and carotenoids to the human protection against oxidative stress caused by an excess of reactive oxygen species (ROS) [55, 56]. Their antioxidant activity contributes to the inhibition of oxidative mechanisms underlying several degenerative diseases such as diabetes, cardiovascular diseases, and cancer [57, 58]. Besides their health promoting effect phenolic acids present in maize samples, for example, may contribute indirectly to flavor quality trough inhibition of lipid oxidation [50].

Phenolic compounds can be classified into two major classes, flavonoids and non-flavonoids. Phenolic acids (hydroxybenzoic acids, hydroxycinnamic acids) and flavonoids correspond to soluble compounds (easily extracted with polar solvents such as ethanol, methanol and mixtures with water) which can be separated and identified by High Performance Liquid Chromatography (HPLC) and detected in the UV-Vis and by Mass Spectrometry (MS) [59].

Some studies have been conducted in order to characterize maize polyphenolic content, and vanillic, *p*-coumaric, ferulic, protocatechuic acids, derivatives of hesperitin, quercetin and anthocyanins like cyanidin-3-glucoside and pelargonidin-3-glucoside [60] were identified as the most important ones. The actual knowledge about phenolic compounds bioaccessibility and bioavailability [61], contributing to the protective effect in biological systems, is still scarce.

In common beans (*Phaseolus vulgaris* L.) phenolic compounds (phenolic acids and flavonoids) were mostly described in the seed coat and at lower amounts in cotyledons [58, 62, 63]. Compounds, such as *p*-hydroxybenzoic, vanillic, caffeic, syringic, coumaric, ferulic and synapic acids as well as flavonoids such as quercetin, kaempferol, daidzein, genistein, *p*-coumestrol and anthocyanins like delphinidin and cyaniding were already identified in common beans [63]. It is widely accepted that thermal processing (boiling or steaming treatment) affects phenolic compounds content and antioxidant activity values [64, 65].

In relation to the Portuguese maize and beans germplasm, and to our knowledge, no information on the phenolic compounds as ever been published. So our initial goal was to characterize the flour composition of 51 Portuguese maize landraces and of 32 different varieties of Portuguese beans.

Spectrophotometric assays were performed to determine total phenolic and total flavonoids content in the samples. For maize, total phenolic content ranged from 100.30 ± 4.81 to 206.83 ± 9.55 mg of gallic acid equivalents/ 100g DW (dry weight) and total flavonoids content ranged between 0.69 ± 0.07 and 17.01 ± 0.52 mg of catechin equivalents/ 100g DW. For beans, the total phenolic content ranged between 1.00 ± 0.02 and 6.83 ± 0.31 mg of gallic acid equivalents/g and total flavonoids content ranged between 0.09 ± 0.00 and 2.50 ± 0.01 mg of catechin equivalents/g.

With the main objective of identifying soluble free, soluble conjugated and insoluble phenolic compounds in maize flour by HPLC, acidic and alkaline hydrolysis were performed. The phenolic fraction which presented higher amount of compounds corresponded to the insoluble. Using HPLC with diode array detector (DAD) it was possible to identify *p*-coumaric and ferulic acids as well as aldehydes such as vanillin and syringaldehyde. In bean's extracts, phenolic acids such as caffeic acid and flavonoids such as catechin, quercetin-3-O-rutinosideand kaempferol-3-O-glucoside were identified.

Studies of the antioxidant activity by Oxygen Radical Absorbance Capacity (ORAC) have also started and were already performed for some maize flour extracts. Values obtained range from 364.30-1223.55 μmol Trolox Equivalents Antioxidant Capacity (TEAC)/100g. In bean extracts, values obtained were between 28.99 ± 2.09 and 189.12 ± 10.20 μmol TEAC/g. These ORAC values showed a strong positive correlation with total phenolic content (R=0.9087) and total flavonoids content (R=0.9171), evaluated by colorimetric methods. The results obtained, until now, revealed a great variability of polyphenolic content and antioxidant activity in the samples analyzed anticipating a high potential for quality breeding within these materials.

Future studies for phenolic compounds' identification and quantification by HPLC-DAD and LC-MS/MS will be performed in raw and processed maize, whole beans seeds and beans fractions (seed coat and cotyledons obtained after beans soaking) submitted to acidic, enzymatic and alkaline hydrolysis. Those studies will allow recognition of the digestion impact on maize and beans' phenolic composition and represent very interesting information to provide to the consumer. This information may increase the crops market value and should be taken into consideration on future participatory breeding selection.

3.3. Development of molecular tools for assisting quality selection

Genetics, particularly molecular genetics, provides further information on patterns of diversity distribution and allows the investigation of the relation of observed diversity with environment, social and cultural factors, providing means to reconcile farmer's classification schemes with genetic distinctiveness. It also helps determine whether there is a wide enough genetic base for future improvement of the *in-situ* materials, or whether there is sufficient diversity to provide system resilience [6]. It can also underpin the identification of ways of supporting the maintenance of traditional varieties, such as in supporting protected geographical identification of certain plant or crop product.

Presently, in our extended PPB project we are conjugating the identification of agronomic and specific quality traits with molecular characterization so as to exploit efficiently the local diversity and produce varieties that are superior in marginal environments, but have a broad genetic base and a high quality level. Nevertheless, in Portugal, molecular breeding is still given its first steps.

In this section we will summarize the development of molecular tools to assist the implementation of participatory breeding program focusing on maize improvement for producing high quality bread. One of the key elements for the implementation of a successful breeding program is the existence of decision supporting tools. Different molecular markers are being tested in order to create new decision supporting tools. Among the different classes of molecular markers, we started initially to use simple sequence repeat (SSR or microsatellite) markers that have proven to be the marker of choice for a variety of applications, particularly in breeding [66]. We are now starting to use also single nucleotide polymorphisms (SNPs) molecular markers that are more abundant in the genome and amenable to automation for high-throughput genotyping [67].

Molecular markers are being used to achieve two main research objectives. First we are using molecular markers to evaluate the progress obtained in conserving or increasing diversity through participatory breeding, as already described in the section 2.3 of PPB success evaluation [42]. The genetic diversity of the newly introduced maize and beans landraces into the participatory plant breeding net is now also routinely characterized, with 20 to 22 SSR uniformly distributed throughout the maize and bean genomes respectively. This method enables us to check if sufficient diversity is present to allow selection and to select the most promising landraces in order to increase the genetic diversity by crossing genetically distant landraces. These studies have also allowed us to compare the genetic diversity with quality clustering of landraces [34]. In detail, 46 traditional maize landraces collected from known

http://dx.doi.org/10.5772/52951

high quality maize bread Portuguese regions, plus six participatory improved maize OPVs from the VASO project, were analyzed for eight different parameters related with their technological ability for bread production, and 13 SSR markers. It was possible to classify these OPVs into three distinct clusters based on the quality traits. Nevertheless, no clear clustering based on genetic distances was observed despite the high levels of genetic diversity presented by these Portuguese landraces [34]. Based on the existence of diversity at molecular level and high quality, the Portuguese maize landraces conserved on-farm represent valuable germplasm with high potential for bread quality improvement [34]. This study also provided important information for the selection of landraces to keep under the extended PPB project.

Second, we are developing genetic studies to identify the genes responsible for our quality traits of interest and subsequently develop molecular markers that target those genes and that can be useful for marker assisted selection (MAS). Quality parameters for bread making, such as technological, nutritional and organoleptic traits, are generally characterized by a continuous variation. This continuous variation suggests the influence of several genes, and because of that, it is difficult to grasp by breeders and farmers. It is expected that several of the maize bread quality parameters show quantitative inheritance. The identification of molecular markers that are linked to the controlling genes will be very helpful for the indirect selection through MAS of these complex quality traits. Marker-assisted selection is a powerful tool for the indirect selection of difficult traits at an early stage, before production of the next generation, thus speeding up the process of conventional plant breeding and facilitating the improvement of traits that cannot be improved easily by conventional methods (reviewed by [67]). The identification and location of genes controlling quantitative traits through Quantitative Trait Loci (QTL) analysis has already been successful undertaken on maize nutritional quality [68, 69, 70].

In our genetic studies we started to use a marker-trait association analysis based on biparental populations, where only a few target traits can be mapped within each population. It was possible by using this approach to identify several genomic regions responsible for ear fasciation related traits, widely present in the Portuguese maize landraces (on going research). Nevertheless, to be able to use this information for indirect selection of fasciated phenotypes, several runs of MAS and population development would be needed to narrow down the genomic regions. This method is time-consuming, but very powerful for the genes with large effect and the alleles with low frequency [71].

Another approach to identify molecular markers for using in MAS is association mapping based on linkage disequilibrium (LD). The availability of high-throughput genotyping technology, together with advances in DNA sequencing and the development of statistical methodology appropriate for genome wide mapping analysis in the presence of considerable population structure, in species such as maize, contributed to an increased interest in LD association mapping [72]. This is the approach that we are now following for the quality genetic studies.

Unlike conventional biparental mapping populations, the natural populations used on this type of linkage analysis, are the products of many cycles of recombination and have the potential to show enhanced resolution of QTLs. Success depends on population size, control of population structure and the degree of LD in the population. LD levels vary both within and between species [73]. With this approach, marker–trait association is only expected when a QTL is tightly linked to the marker, because the accumulated recombination events occurring during the development of the lines will prevent the detection of any marker–trait loose association. In maize, the application of this approach has demonstrated the association between several candidate genes and kernel composition traits, starch pasting properties and amylose levels [74].

Using SSR markers, the genetic diversity among inbred lines derived from the Portuguese germplasm collection was evaluated and compared with worldwide maize inbreds representatives [36]. The Portuguese inbred lines have maintained a level of genetic diversity similar to the foreign lines. Moreover, it was concluded that they are derivatives of miscellaneous populations, showing high genetic diversity and consequently representing a potential valuable source of interesting genes to introduce into modern cultivars [36], and a valuable germplasm for association studies.

Until now, no LD analysis or association studies were undertaken on the group of inbred lines of Portuguese origin, neither the identification of genes/QTLs controlling bread making ability. Presently, in order to address this gap, the collection of Portuguese maize inbred lines, derived mainly from Portuguese landraces, is being genotyped using microsatellites to detect population structure and to study LD.

Currently, the national efforts are focused on the study of the genetic control and the environmental effect on the antioxidant and aroma compounds as well as the bread making ability. This study applies an association mapping approach using the previously characterized inbred lines that differ for endosperm types and colors. QTL associated candidate genes will be identify on the basis of positional information of the recently maize cloned genes (reviewed by [75]). Candidate genes will be validated on the enduring landraces [7] and modern improved OPVs (VASO project) that are also being characterized at genetic, nutritional, organoleptic (aroma volatiles) composition and antioxidants bioactivity. Specific molecular markers tightly linked to the identified QTLs will be identified or developed to provide breeders and farmers user-friendly markers to select for superior genotypes for quality maize bread. Additionally, it will allow the exploration of maize local resources and natural quality diversity in the reinvention of traditional maize to produce modern high quality bread with potential health benefits.

3.4. Testing of higher quality experimental cultivars

Nowadays, the most promising maize populations at agronomic, molecular and quality level, collected during the 2005 expedition, are being evaluated and selected under a participatory approach in 13 different locations. This field research has been done in articulation with the original VASO project locations and improved populations, and now is under the supervision of the ESAC researchers. The association of the farmers' perception with the newly available molecular and quality data can be extremely valuable to aggregate or separate populations, creating possible pools with heterosis that will be very useful to generate new populations or inbred lines. All the molecular and quality evaluations performed on these materials are being developed by researchers at ITQB/UNL and INIAV.

After a detailed characterization of the agronomic, genetic, nutritional, organoleptic and technological quality traits of 41 initial maize OPV (from the collecting expeditions plus VASO project), the most interesting materials were selected for the development of hybrid populations with specific quality traits and maintaining genetic diversity. Hybrid populations can contribute to yield improvement and to avoid the collapse of some interesting germplasm. Dialel tests of the best materials are providing indications regarding heterosis among the chosen germplasm. These new populations are now under field evaluations. New synthetic populations with increased precocity are also being developed and are based upon the most superior Portuguese maize OPVs at agronomic level plus some American populations. These synthetic populations are also under field trial evaluation/selection at different farmers fields. Molecular and quality evaluations will follow on all these new developed materials to sustain their improvement.

4. Seed dessimination and ownership

The potential advantages of PPB, such as the faster dissemination of new varieties, higher adoption and increased biodiversity within the crop, can only be achieved if the seed of the new varieties is available in sufficient amounts to all the farmers' community [19]. Although the varieties developed through PPB will have specific adaptation to certain environmental conditions, it is likely that they will also perform well on farms that share similar climates and soil types. It is unlikely that they will spread as far as varieties specifically targeted to have wide adaptation in higher input systems [76], but it is possible that they will benefit many farmers in neighboring areas. Genetically variable materials, such as OPV and synthetics, make more likely their usefulness to farmers in environments that differ from the original selection environment [77].

The global community, through the Convention on Biological Diversity and the International Treaty on Plant Genetic Resources for Food and Agriculture, has recognized the contribution of farmers to the maintenance of genetic resources. Given the actual and potential future impact of PPB, this contribution will increasingly include new PPB' varieties. [78]. Such varieties need recognition and protection.

According to European Union regulations, farmers are allowed to reproduce non-certified seeds for themselves, but they are not able to sell them. Generally, only varieties that are officially registered and listed, after meeting DUS and VCU requirements, can be multiplied by the formal seed system [79]. Formal seed systems were put in place in Europe, in the mid-19th century, as a result of the development of specialized plant breeding products and to create transparency in a seed market where variety names were rapidly proliferating [80]. Current variety registration for commercial purposes requires that the new variety be distinct from all the varieties of common knowledge, uniform in its essential characteristics and highly stable after repeated multiplication (DUS= Distinctness, Uniformity and Stability,

[80]). In addition, testing for cultivation and use values (VCU) was introduced as a requirement for commercial release, in order for farmers to have an independent assessment of the yield, quality and value of the grain [6]. These last ones are the real concerns for farmers, but in practice this evaluation is based mostly on quantitative Weld criteria such as grain yield, maturity time, standing ability and disease resistance, which are easy to measure. Less attention is given to aspects such as storability, cooking quality and by-product use, which may determine the overall value of the variety, especially for small farmers. To this extent, standard VCU tests do not easily reflect the more complex requirements of small-scale farmers and this has been one of the problems of official variety release in meeting the needs of such farmers [79].

This formal system is unfriendly for farmers' varieties such as landraces and new varieties developed through PPB, leaving these varieties outside the legal market of seeds [81]. These varieties are less likely to meet the stringent DUS and VCU criteria because they lack uniformity and rarely perform well across the majority of test sites. Nevertheless, the European Union has recently approved a special treatment for the so called "Conservation Varieties" by which landraces and varieties adapted to local and regional conditions and threatened by genetic erosion can be registered for commercialization under certain conditions (Directive 2008/62/EC from 20 June 2008). The special treatment consists, of

1. a certain degree of flexibility in the level of uniformity that is required, and
2. an exemption from official examination if the applicant can provide sufficient information about the variety through other means such as unofficial tests and knowledge from practical experiences [6].

The varieties obtained in our project can be registered as conservation varieties. In the registration process, the varieties have to be characterized for a minimum number of morphological traits and only less than 10% of the plants can be out of type. Attention is given to the region where the variety is traditionally used as a crop and to where it is naturally adapted. The registration is obtained if description of the varieties, denomination, results from non-official trials, knowledge associated with sow, multiplications and use, and other information is provided to the genetic resources authorities. This information is then evaluated by the national entity (DGADR in the Portuguese case). In the national catalogue of varieties (CNV) the respective location of origin is indicated, and the regions of seed production can be identified besides the seed origin. Seeds are submitted to sampling and quality standards. Storage must be done in close packages and producer labels are required. The conservation varieties may be marketed only in their regions of origin or in additional regions, as long as these regions are comparable, regarding semi-natural and natural habitats, to the region of origin of this variety. The maximum quantity of seed per specie, allowed for commercialization purposes, is 10% of the seeds used annually in the country, if this condition does not exceed the total amount of seed needed to sow 100 ha. In the case of the Portuguese maize varieties, the maximum allowed is 0.3% of the seeds used in the country during a growing season, but limited to 100 ha. This means that conservation varieties, if we consider the maximum of 100 ha, represent 0,073% of the Portuguese maize area (100 ha/137 413 ha) and can represent 10 000€ (20 kg of seed/ha x 5 €/Kg of seed x 100 ha) in Portugal. This data indicate that this germplasm should be used preferably in marginal areas under PPB project. It also indicates that maize PPB projects should be integrated in the food market preferably in those where the direct output is not the seed itself, but for example, the bread that has a higher market value. Nevertheless, in the process of registration of conservation varieties, the PPB farmer alone will not be able to provide all types of unofficial tests and information needed. So supportive associations should step forward and help on this registration process.

In Portugal, such an association has been created in 2010, the ZEA+ association, where a cluster of maize researchers and participatory breeding farmers are joined together. This association was the logical step to fill in the gap at the logistical level to deal with all the information that had been collected at etnobotanical, agronomical, genetic, and molecular and food quality by the national maize cluster of research. This association main objective is the study and promotion of the conservation and valuation of agricultural genetic resources in a perspective of rural development, emphasizing the link with the urban communities. In this way, this association is dedicated to traditional landraces, including conservation and autochthones varieties. It can provide logistical or managing support to germplasm improvement through participatory plant breeding where its associates collaborate. The Zea+ association could contribute to successfully market conservation varieties and to help establish some kind of small seed enterprise for farmers, in order to have a clean source of seed from those varieties. It should also support the registration of improved varieties already validated with field and molecular marker data. This would allow the reinvestment of the potential royalties in science, to provide more information to farmers and researchers.

Besides seed dissemination, it is also necessary to consider the maintenance of the genetic gains achieved. If the improved material is not managed in a systematic way, it may be diluted by physical contamination or out-crossing and thus dissolve back into the local population. The benefits achieved by PPB may then be lost, leaving no secure point of reference to return to in the future [79]. Consequently, this responsibility should be vested by a farmers/researchers association established to produce and market the seed.

This registration possibility does not mean that the process of selection cannot continue, rather than at certain intervals a reasonably defined 'milestone' is set up along the road of improvement [79]. Further enhancement of productivity and stability is achieved through practicing "non-stop selection" within landraces across the marginal production environments, to exploit the useful adaptive variation constantly released by the genome.

5. Future prospectives and market development

At a time when a team of young scientists is taking care of this PPB project, which is reaching it maturation, we can foresee a new future for the Portuguese small farming. Its quality oriented purpose for food, its sustainability and environment friend signature, will be an important piece to bring our sustainable small farming system back to its feet.

In the medium/long term, we expect that the abandoned northern agricultural systems will survive due to the local abundance of water. In these environments maize will play an important role in the production of quality food. In this case, the national germplasm will play an important role in the recovery of our small farming system. Participatory plant breeding is the tool necessary to take advantage of our rich maize germplasm collected in the 70's and preserved in our Portuguese Plant Gene Bank (BPGV), or in same cases still present at our farmers fields. Without such an investment in breeding, to raise their yielding capability to reasonable levels, our genetic resources will remain in a useless tomb or vanish definitely from our farm land.

In scientific terms, we foresee that with this new multidisciplinary team of young scientists new findings will came along, especially at understanding the genetics of important agronomical and quality traits that will translate into improved high quality varieties. The role of this quality oriented varieties, either under open pollination or hybrid form, will fit in a new agricultural system oriented to quality tourism, where maize will represent only a piece, as important as it may be, within this system. Entertainment, like the traditional "desfolhadas" (harvest festivities), historical, architecture, archeological and cultural attractions, together with the combined restoration of old water mills and cob stores, all of this complemented with folkloric music will complete the system.

The potential fixation of our farmers, consequence of the economic recovery, will benefit the most the environment (water management, soil conservation, genetic resources preservation, and the control of forest fires). Farmers will always be the breeder's best allies and the best curators of our genetic resources. New genetic and analytical tools are now available that can help the traditional plant breeding methodologies. Sustainable, quality oriented, and environmental friendly agriculture still has a role to play in countries like Portugal and beyond.

Nevertheless this extended PPB project was only possible due to funding obtained through several national (from Fundação para a Ciência e a Tecnologia, Portugal, POCI/AGR/57994/2004, PTDC/AGR-AAM/70845/2006, PTDC/AGR-ALI/099285/2008) and international (FP7 program, SOLIBAM project) research projects of limited duration. Its survival depends on finding sustainable ways of self-support that may be obtained by higher marketing of improve quality varieties, maintaining genetic diversity, with increased market value, more attractive to the final consumer.

So, further supportive actions to market creation and market promotion should be taken. As adapted from [6] to our national reality, partnerships should be built or strengthen through the organization of meetings involving market-chain stakeholders to discuss how to change market potential. Niche markets for traditional landraces raw materials or traditional landraces food products (maize bread) should be further exploit. This is the case of the gluten intolerant market, to which the 100% maize bread can be an attractive alternative. Also, the general market should be aimed with media advertisement campaigns to improve consumer awareness of important nutritional or ecological-friendly traits from traditional landraces, for example, using the summary of the research project activities. On the same level, an eco-labeling of products (such as the maize bread) obtained from traditional landraces as a commitment to the preservation of biodiversity, could call the attention of consumers. As already highlighted above, the ecological practices of traditional production systems, where

http://dx.doi.org/10.5772/52951

traditional landraces are maintained, should be promoted. Agrobiodiversity ecotourism could be one way of doing so, because it publicizes the diversity of cultivated plants and the associated cultural practices by involving activities as farm and market visits, participation in agricultural activities and food (bread) preparation, food tasting and attending feasts or celebrations associated with agricultural practices. Finally and as a last resource, farmers who provide environmental services, such as conservation functions should be compensated. A governmental direct support could be provided to farmers who cultivated traditional varieties targeted for protection.

Acknowledgements

This research was financially supported by Fundação para a Ciência e a Tecnologia, Portugal (presently by PTDC/AGR-ALI/099285/2008 and Pest-OE/EQB/LA0004/2011) and by the European Commission FP7 SOLIBAM project.

Author details

Maria Carlota Vaz Patto[1,4*], Pedro Manuel Mendes-Moreira[1,2,4], Mara Lisa Alves[1], Elsa Mecha[1], Carla Brites[3,4], Maria do Rosário Bronze[1] and Silas Pego[4,5]

*Address all correspondence to: cpatto@itqb.unl.pt

1 Instituto de Tecnologia Química e Biológica (ITQB)/Universidade Nova de Lisboa, Oeiras, Portugal

2 Escola Superior Agrária de Coimbra (ESAC), Instituto Politécnico de Coimbra, Coimbra, Portugal

3 Instituto Nacional de Investigação Agrária e Veterinária (INIAV), Portugal

4 Associação ZEA +, Penela, Portugal

5 Fundação Bomfim, Braga, Portugal

References

[1] Harlan, J. R. (1992). Crops and man. *(Second ed.). Madison, Wisconsin: American Society of Agronomy Inc. and Crop Science Society of America Inc.*

[2] Zeven, A. C. (2000). Traditional maintenance breeding of landraces: 1. Data by crop. *Euphytica*, 116, 65-85.

[3] Camacho Villa, T. C., Maxted, N., Scholten-Lloyd, M. A., & Ford., B. V. (2005). Defining and identifying crop landraces. *Plant Genetical Resources*, 3, 373-384.

[4] Zeven, A. C. (1998). Landraces: a review of definitions and classifications. *Euphytica*, 104, 127-139.

[5] Newton, A. C., Baresel, J. P., Babeli, P., Bettencourt, E., Bladenopoulos, K. V., Czembor, J. H., Fasoula, D. A., Katsiotis, A., Koutis, K., Koutsika-Sotiriou, M., Kovacs, G., Larsson, H., Pinheiro de Carvalho, M. A. A., Rubiales, D., Russell, J., Santos, T. M. M., & Vaz Patto, M. C. (2010). Cereal landraces for sustainable agriculture: a review. *Agronomy for Sustainable Development*, 30(2), 237-269.

[6] Jarvis, D. I., Hodgkin, T., Sthapit, B. R., Fadda, C., & Lopez-Noriega, I. (2011). An heuristic framework for identifying multiple ways of supporting the conservation and use of traditional crop varieties within the agricultural production system. *Critical Reviews in Plant Sciences*, 30(1-2), 125-176.

[7] Vaz, Patto. M. C., Moreira, P., Carvalho, V., & Pego, S. (2007). Collecting maize (*Zea mays L. convar. mays*) with potential technological ability for bread making in Portugal. *Genetic Resources and Crop Evolution*, 54(7), 1555-1563.

[8] Smale, M., Bellon, M. R., & Aguirre, A. (2001). Maize diversity, variety attributes and farmers' choices in southeastern Guanajuato, Mexico. *Economical Development and Cultural Change*, 50(1), 201-225.

[9] Pingali, P. L. (2012). Green Revolution: Impacts, limits, and the path ahead. *Proceedings of the National Academy of Sciences*, 109(31), 12302-12308.

[10] Hammer, K., Diederichsen, A., & Spahillar, M. (1999). Basic studies toward strategies for conservation of plant genetic resources. *In: Serwinski J, Faberova I. (eds.) Proceedings of the Technical Meeting on the Methodology of the FAO World Information and Early Warning System on Plant Genetic Resources, 21,23 June 1999, Prague, Czech Republic: FAO*, 29-33.

[11] Allard, R. W. (1999). Principles of Plant Breeding. *New York: John Wiley & Sons.*

[12] Simmonds, N. W. (1979). Principles of crop improvement. *London, UK: Longman Group Ltd.*

[13] Evans, L. T. (1993). Crop evolution, adaptation and yield. *Cambridge, UK: University Press.*

[14] Fischer, K. S. (1996). Research approaches for variable rainfed systems-Thinking globally, acting locally. *In: Cooper M, Hamme GL. (eds.) Plant adaptation and crop improvement. Wallingford, Oxford, UK: CAB International in association with IRRI and ICRISAT*, 25-35.

[15] Cleveland, D. A., Soleri, D., & Smith, S. E. (1999). Farmer plant breeding from biological perspective: Implications for collaborative plant breeding. *CIMMYT Economics Working Paper CIMMYT, Mexico DF: CIMMYT*, 99-10.

[16] Enjalbert, J., Dawson, J. C., Paillard, S., Rhoné, B., Rousselle, Y., Thomas, M., & Goldringer, I. (2011). Dynamic management of crop diversity: From an experimental approach to on-farm conservation. *Comptes Rendus Biologies*, 334(5-6), 458-468.

[17] Desclaux, D. (2005). Participatory plant breeding methods for organic cereals: review and perspectives. *In: Lammerts van Bueren ET, Goldringer I, Ostergard H. (ed.) Proceedings for the Eco-Pb Congress, 17-19 January 2005. Driebergen, The Netherlands: Louis Bolk Institute*, 1-6.

[18] Ceccarelli, S. (2012). Plant breeding with farmers- a technical manual. *Aleppo, Syria: ICARDA*.

[19] Ceccarelli, S., & Grando, S. (2007). Decentralized-participatory plant breeding: an example of demand driven research. *Euphytica*, 155(3), 349-360.

[20] Lammerts van Bueren, E. T., Wilbois, K. P., & Ostergard, H. (2007). European prespectives of organic plant breeding and seed production in a genomics era. *University of Kassel at Witzenhausen JARTS*, 89, 101-120.

[21] Danial, D., Parlevliet, J., Almekinders, C., & Thiele, G. (2007). Farmers' participation and breeding for durable disease resistance in the Andean region. *Euphytica*, 153, 385-396.

[22] Teixeira, F. F., de Vasconcellos, J. H., de Andrade, R. V., dos Santos, M. X., Leite, C. E. P., Guimaraes, P. E. O., Parentoni, S. N., Meirelles, W. F., Pacheco, C. A. P., & Ceccon, G. (2011). BRS Cipotanea and BRS Diamantina: maize varieties. *Crop Breeding and Applied Biotechnology*, 11(2), 189-192.

[23] Machado, A. T., & Fernandes, M. S. (2001). Participatory maize breeding for low nitrogen tolerance. *Euphytica*, 122, 567-573.

[24] Song, Y., & Vernooy, R. (2010). Seeds and Synergies: Innovating Rural Development in China. *Bourton Hall, Bourton-on-Dunsmore, Rugby, Warwickshire: Practical Action Publishing*.

[25] Mulatu, E., & Zelleke, H. (2002). Farmers' highland maize (*Zea mays L.*) selection criteria: Implication for maize breeding for the Hararghe highlands of eastern Ethiopia. *Euphytica*, 127(1), 11-30.

[26] Morris, M. L., Tripp, R., & Dankyi, A. A. (1999). Adoption and impacts of improved maize production technology: a case study of the Ghana grains development project. *CIMMYT Economics Program Paper Mexico DF: CIMMYT*, 99-01.

[27] Witcombe, J. R., Joshi, A., & Goynal, S. N. (2003). Participatory plant breeding in maize: a case study from Gujarat, India. *Euphytica*, 130, 413-422.

[28] Virk, D. S., Chakraborty, M., Ghosh, J., Prasad, S. C., & Witcombe, J. R. (2005). Increasing the client orientation of maize breeding using farmer participation in eastern India. *Experimental Agriculture*, 41, 413-426.

[29] Ouma, J. O., Odendo, M., Bett, C., De Groote, H., Mugo, S., Mutinda, C., Gethi, J., Njoka, S., Ajanga, S., & Shuma, J. (2011). Participatory farmer evaluation of stem borer tolerant maize varieties in three maize growing ecologies of Kenya. *African Journal of Agricultural Research*, 6(13), 3021-3028.

[30] Smith, M. E., Castillo, G. F., & Gomez, F. (2001). Participatory plant breeding with maize in Mexico and Honduras. *Euphytica*, 122, 551-565.

[31] Tiwari, T. P., Virk, D. S., & Sinclair, F. L. (2009). Rapid gains in yield and adoption of new maize varieties for complex hillside environments through farmer participation I. Improving options through participatory varietal selection (PVS). *Field Crop Research*, 111(1-2), 137-143.

[32] Olaoye, G., Ajala, S. O., & Adedeji, S. A. (2009). Participatory selection of a maize (*Zea mays L.*) variety for the control of stem borers in a southeastern Nigeria location. *Journal of Food Agriculture and Environment*, 7(3-4), 508-512.

[33] Moreira, P. M. (2006). Participatory maize breeding in Portugal. *A case study. Acta Agronomica Hungarica*, 54(4), 431-439.

[34] Vaz, Patto. M. C., Alves, M. L., Almeida, N. F., Santos, C., Mendes-Moreira, P., Satovic, Z., & Brites, C. (2009). Is the bread making technological ability of Portuguese traditional maize landraces associated with their genetic diversity? *Maydica*, 54, 297-311.

[35] Rebourg, C., Chastanet, M., Gouesnard, B., Welcker, C., Dubreuil, P., & Charcosset, A. (2003). Maize introduction into Europe: the history reviewed in the light of molecular data. *Theoretical and Applied Genetics*, 106, 895-903.

[36] Vaz Patto, M. C., Satovic, Z., Pego, S., & Fevereiro, P. (2004). Assessing the genetic diversity of Portuguese maize germplasm using microsatellite markers. *Euphytica*, 137, 63-72.

[37] Pego, S., & Antunes, M. P. (1997). Resistance or tolerance? Philosophy may be the answer. *In: Pego S, Martins R. (eds.) Proceedings of the XIX Conference of the International Working Group on Ostrinia nubilabis and other maize pests, 30 August-5 September 1997, Guimarães, Portugal. IWGO*, 303-341.

[38] Mendes-Moreira, P., Pego, S., Vaz Patto, M. C., & Hallauer, A. (2008). Comparison of selection methods on 'Pigarro', a Portuguese improved maize population with fasciation expression. *Euphytica*, 163(3), 481-499.

[39] Murphy, K., Lammer, D., Lyon, S., Carter, B., & Jones, S. S. (2005). Breeding for organic and low-input farming systems: An evolutionary-participatory breeding method for inbred cereal grains. *Renewable Agriculture and Food Systems*, 20, 48-55.

[40] Welsh, J. R. (1981). Fundamentals of plant genetics and breeding. *New York: Wiley*.

[41] Mendes-Moreira, P., Vaz Patto, M. C., Mota, M. M., Mendes-Moreira, J. J., Santos, J. P. N., Santos, J. P. P., Andrade, E., Hallauer, A. R., & Pego, S. E. (2009). Fandango':

long term adaptation of exotic germplasm to a Portuguese on-farm-conservation and breeding project. *Maydica*, 54, 269-285.

[42] Vaz Patto, M. C., Moreira, P., Almeida, N., Satovic, Z., & Pego, S. (2008). Genetic diversity evolution through participatory maize breeding in Portugal. *Euphytica*, 161(1-2), 283-291.

[43] Brites, C., Trigo, M. J., Santos, C., Collar, C., & Rosell, C. M. (2010). Maize based gluten free bread: influence of processing parameters on sensory and instrumental quality. *Food and Bioprocess Technology*, 3(5), 707-715.

[44] Rocha, J. M., & Malcata, F. X. (1999). On the microbiological profile of traditional Portuguese sourdough. *Journal of Food Protection*, 62, 1416-1429.

[45] Almeida-Dominguez, H. D., Suhendro, E. L., & Rooney, L. W. (1997). Factors affecting rapid visco analyser curves for the determination of maize kernel hardness. *Journal of Cereal Science*, 25, 93-102.

[46] Brites, C., Haros, M., Trigo, MJ, & Islas, R. P. (2007). Maíz. *In: León A & Rosell C. (eds.) De tales harinas, tales panes: granos, harinas y productos de panificación en Iberoamérica. Córdoba, Argentina: Hugo Báez*, 75-121.

[47] Brites, C., & Guerreiro, M. (2008). O pão através dos tempos. *Lisboa: Apenas Livros, Lda*.

[48] Englyst, H., Kingman, S., & Cummings, J. (1992). Classification and measurement of nutritionally important starch fractions. *European Journal Clinical Nutrition*, 46(2), 33-50.

[49] Brites, C. M., Trigo, M. J., Carrapiço, B., Alviña, M., & Bessa, R. J. (2011). Maize and resistant starch enriched breads reduce postprandial glycemic responses in rats. *Nutrition research*, 31(4), 302-308.

[50] Zhou, M., Robards, K., Glennie-Holmes, M., & Helliwell, S. (1999). Analysis of volatile compounds and their contribution to flavor in cereals. *Journal of Agricultural and Food Chemistry*, 47(10), 3941-3953.

[51] Ruth, S. M., Roozen, J. P., Hollmann, M. E., & Posthumus, M. A. (1996). Instrumental and sensory analysis of the flavor of French beans (*Phaseolus vulgaris*) after different rehydration conditions. *Zeitschrift für Lebensmittel-Untersuchung und-Forschung*, 203, 7-13.

[52] Barra, A., Baldovini, N., Loiseau-M, A., Albino, L., Lesecq, C., & Cuvelier, L. L. (2007). Chemical analysis of french beans (*Phaseolus vulgaris L.*) by headspace solid phase microextraction (HS-SPME) and simultaneous distillation/extraction (SDE). *Food Chemistry*, 101, 1279-1284.

[53] Wei-N, J., Zhu, J., & Kang, L. (2006). Volatiles released from bean plants in response to agromyzid flies. *Planta*, 1-9.

[54] Grosh, W., & Schieberle, P. (1997). Flavor of cereal products- a review. *Cereal Chemistry*, 74(2), 91-97.

[55] Bronze, M. R., Figueira, M. E., & Mecha, E. (2012). Flavonoids and its contribution to a healthier life. *In: Kazuya Yamane, Yuudai Kato (eds.) Handbook on Flavonoids: Dietary sources, properties and health benefits, Nova Publisher.*

[56] Pandey, K. B., & Rizvi, S. I. (2009). Plant polyphenols as dietary antioxidants in human health and disease. *Oxidative Medicine and Cellular Longevity*, 2(5), 270-278.

[57] Heimler, D., Vignolini, P., Dini, M. G., & Romani, A. (2005). Rapid tests to assess antioxidant activity of *Phaseolus vulgaris L.* dry beans. *Journal of Agriculture and Food Chemistry*, 53, 3053-3056.

[58] Cardador-Martinez, A., Loarca-Piña, G., & Oomah, B. D. (2002). Antioxidant activity in common beans (*Phaseolus vulgaris L.*). *Journal of Agriculture and Food Chemistry*, 50, 6975-6980.

[59] Rispail, N., Morris, P., & Webb, J. (2005). Phenolic compounds: Extraction and analysis. *In: Márquez AJ. (ed.) Lotus japonicus Handbook, Springer.*

[60] Pedreschi, R., & Cisneros-Zevallos, L. (2007). Phenolic profiles of Andean purple corn (*Zea mays L.*). *Food Chemistry*, 100, 956-963.

[61] Wotton-Beard, P. C., Moran, A., & Ryan, L. (2011). Stability of the total antioxidant capacity and total polyphenol content of 23 commercially available vegetable juices before and after in vitro digestion measured by FRAP, DPPH, ABTS and Folin-Ciocalteu methods. *Food Research International*, 44, 217-224.

[62] Rocha-Guzmán, E. N., Herzog, A., González-Laredo, R. F., Ibarra-Pérez, F. J., Zambrano-Gálvan, G., & Gallegos-Infante, J. A. (2007). Antioxidant and antimutagenic activity of phenolic compounds in three different colour groups of common bean cultivars (*Phaseolus vulgaris L.*). *Food Chemistry*, 103, 521-527.

[63] Lin, Z. L., Harnly, J. M., Pastor-Corrales, M. S., & Luthria, D. L. (2008). The polyphenolic profiles of common bean (*Phaseolus vulgaris L.*). *Food Chemistry*, 399-410.

[64] Xu, B., & Chang, S. K. C. (2009). Total Phenolic, phenolic Acid, anthocyanin, flavan-3-ol and flavonol profiles and antioxidant properties of Pinto and Black beans (*Phaseolus Vulgaris L.*) as affected by thermal processing. *Journal of Agriculture and Food Chemistry*, 57, 4757-4764.

[65] Aguilera, Y., Estrella, I., Benitez, V., Esteban, R. M., & Martín-Cabrejas, M. (2011). Bioactive phenolic compounds and functional properties of dehydrated bean flours. *Food Research International*, 44, 774-780.

[66] Gupta, P. K., & Varshney, R. K. (2000). The development and use of microsatellite markers for genetic analysis and plant breeding with emphasis on bread wheat. *Euphytica*, 113(3), 163-185.

[67] Varshney, R. K., Hoisington, D. A., & Tyagi, A. K. (2006). Advances in cereal genomics and applications in crop breeding. *Trends in biotechnology*, 24(11), 490-499.

[68] Harjes, C. E., Rocheford, T. R., Bai, L., Brutnell, T. P., Kandianis, C. B., Sowinski, S. G., Stapleton, A. E., Vallabhaneni, R., Williams, M., Wurtzel, E. T., Yan, J., & Buckler, E. S. (2008). Natural Genetic Variation in Lycopene Epsilon Cyclase Tapped for Maize Biofortification. *Science*, 319(5861), 330-333.

[69] Li, Y., Wang, Y., Wei, M., Li, X., & Fu, J. (2009). QTL identification of grain protein concentration and its genetic correlation with starch concentration and grain weight using two populations in maize (*Zea mays L.*). *Journal of Genetics*, 88(1), 61-67.

[70] Simić, D., Mladenović Drinić, S., Zdunić, Z., Jambrović, A., Ledencan, T., Brkić, J., Brkić, A., & Brkić, I. (2012). Quantitative trait loci for biofortification traits in maize grain. *Journal of Heredity*, 103(1), 47-54.

[71] Xu, Y., Lu, Y., Xie, C., Gao, S., Wan, J., & Prasanna, B. M. (2012). Whole-genome strategies for marker-assisted plant breeding. *Molecular Breeding*, 29(4), 833-854.

[72] Rafalski, J. A. (2010). Association genetics in crop improvement. *Current Opinion in Plant Biology*, 13, 1-7.

[73] Flint-Garcia, S. A., Thuillet, A. C., Yu, J., Pressoir, G., Romero, S. M., Mitchell, S. E., Doebley, J., Kresovich, S., Goodman, M. M., & Buckler, E. S. (2005). Maize association population: a high-resolution platform for quantitative trait locus dissection. *Plant Journal*, 44(6), 1054-1064.

[74] Wilson, L. M., Whitt, S. R., Ibáñez, A. M., Rocheford, T. R., Goodman, M. M., & Buckler, E. S. (2004). Dissection of Maize Kernel Composition and Starch Production by Candidate Gene Association. *The Plant Cell*, 16, 719-2733.

[75] Hartings, H., Fracassetti, M., & Motto, M. (2012). Genetic Enhancement of Grain Quality-Related Traits in Maize. *In: Yelda Özden Çiftçi (ed.). Transgenic Plants- Advances and Limitations. Rijeka: InTech,* Available from, http://www.intechopen.com/books/transgenic-plants-advances-and-limitations/genetic-enhancement-of-grain-quality-related-traits-in-maize, accessed 7 August 2012).

[76] Morris, M. L., & Bellon, M. R. (2004). Participatory plant breeding research: Opportunities and challenges for the international crop improvement system. *Euphytica*, 136, 21-35.

[77] Smith, M. E., Castillo, G. F., & Gomez, F. (2001). Participatory plant breeding with maize in Mexico and Honduras. *Euphytica*, 122, 551-565.

[78] Salazar, R., Louwaars, N. P., & Visser, B. (2011). Protecting farmers' new varieties: New approaches to rights on collective innovations in plant genetic resources. *World Development*, 35(9), 1515-1528.

[79] Bishaw, Z., & Turner, M. (2008). Linking participatory plant breeding to the seed supply system *Euphytica*. 163, 31-44.

[80] Bishaw, Z., & van Gastel, A. J. G. (2009). Variety release and policy options. *In: Ceccarelli S, Guimareaes EP, Weltzien E. (eds.). Plant breeding and farmer participation. Rome, Italy: FAO*, 565-587.

[81] Farm Seed Opportunities. (2009). http//www.farmseed.net/home/, accessed).